VIROLOGY RESEARCH PROGRESS

RESPIRATORY SYNCYTIAL VIRUS

PREVENTION, DIAGNOSIS AND TREATMENT

VIROLOGY RESEARCH PROGRESS

Additional books in this series can be found on Nova's website under the Series tab.

Additional E-books in this series can be found on Nova's website under the E-book tab.

VIROLOGY RESEARCH PROGRESS

RESPIRATORY SYNCYTIAL VIRUS

PREVENTION, DIAGNOSIS AND TREATMENT

HANEUL NAM
AND
GIPPEUM KUN
EDITORS

Nova Science Publishers, Inc.
New York

For permission to use material from this book please contact us:
Telephone 631-231-7269; Fax 631-231-8175
Web Site: http://www.novapublishers.com

Library of Congress Cataloging-in-Publication Data

Respiratory syncytial virus : prevention, diagnosis and treatment / editors, Haneul Nam and Gippeum Kun.
p. ; cm.
Includes bibliographical references and index.
ISBN 978-1-62100-835-4 (hardcover)
I. Nam, Haneul. II. Kun, Gippeum.
[DNLM: 1. Respiratory Syncytial Virus Infections. WC 518]

616.2'4--dc23

2011039366

Published by Nova Science Publishers, Inc. † New York

CONTENTS

Preface vii

Chapter 1 Respiratory Syncytial Virus Infection: Diagnostic Investigation, management and preventive strategies 1
Jonathan Gilleland, James Mahony and Bosco Paes

Chapter 2 Respiratory Syncytial Virus: Prevention, Diagnosis and Treatment 79
Young Yoo

Chapter 3 Respiratory Syncytial Virus Infection: Prevention, Diagnosis, and Treatment 123
Beatriz Gómez

Chapter 4 Cellular Immunity and Immunoproteomics of HLA Class I Ligands in HRSV Infection 149
Daniel López

Chapter 5 Respiratory Syncytial Virus Disease and Severity of Illness 165
Parthak Prodhan M. D. and Natan Noviski, M. D.

Index 179

PREFACE

Respiratory syncytial virus (RSV) is an important respiratory pathogen of infants and young children and is the most common cause of lower respiratory tract infection-related hospitalization of children under the age of one. In this book, the authors present current research in the study of the prevention, diagnosis and treatment of RSV. Topics discussed include the genetic variables that play a role in the presentation and the outcome of severe RSV disease; cellular immunity and immunoproteomics of HLA class I ligands in HSRV infection and recurrent infections, chronic sequelae, and risk factors for RSV.

Chapter 1 - In the current era, Respiratory Syncytial Virus (RSV) prevails as the dominant viral pathogen causing bronchiolitis in infants <2 years of age seen either in the emergency room or hospitalized with lower respiratory tract infections (LRI). The burden of illness with RSV infection is substantial, amounting to approximately 33 million cases worldwide in 2005, with accompanying morbidity and significant mortality especially in infants with underlying medical disorders and those living in developing countries. Of equal importance are high complication rates following RSV-related hospitalization inclusive of the consumption of considerable healthcare resources both within institutions and subsequently in the community. In the early phase of illness, RSV presents as an upper respiratory tract infection which is indistinguishable from the common cold. The progression to bronchiolitis and pneumonia occurs abruptly with marked respiratory distress with or without cyanosis. Pathologically, severe inflammatory changes in the lungs with mucus plugging, edema and epithelial sloughing of the airways results in clinical deterioration which merits hospitalization and intensive care in critically ill infants. Diagnosis is established by nasopharyngeal swabs or aspirates using a combination of techniques including enzyme immunoassay, direct fluorescent antibody staining, cell culture, and nucleic acid amplification tests (NAT). Nucleic acid amplification technology, particularly multiplex PCR coupled with fluidic or fixed microarrays, provides a rapid, accurate and comprehensive approach for the detection of multiple respiratory viruses that cause bronchiolitis including RSV, in a single test. Several commercial NATs are now available. More recently, the addition of allelic discrimination and detection of single nucleotide polymorphisms associated with antiviral resistance to multiplex assays coupled with new viral load tests will facilitate optimal treatment of patients during epidemics and nosocomial spread in hospitals.

Numerous, well-conducted clinical trials have systematically failed to identify a sole therapeutic intervention for the treatment of RSV infection. Evaluated strategies include the use of ribavarin, steroids, bronchodilators, epinephrine, leukotrienes, DNase, antibiotics,

Vitamin A and chest physiotherapy. Inhaled hypertonic saline appears safe and promising but further evidence of efficacy either alone or as part of combination therapy is awaited. Treatment of patients with respiratory failure is case dependent due to the heterogeneity of disease presentation and dynamic physiology which clouds clinical endpoints derived from small randomized controlled studies. Guidelines on the timing and optimal mode of positive pressure and mechanical ventilation do not exist. As a result, management of infants requiring respiratory support and critical care tends to represent a fusion of clinical experience, expert opinion, extrapolation of evidence from other respiratory illnesses and a logical approach to trial and error. Studies are in progress to determine if the use of monoclonal antibodies administered in the acute phase of RSV infection, consistently reduces viral load and perhaps severity of illness. Fusion protein inhibitors and drugs that inhibit viral replication and small interfering RNAs that target mRNA in a sequence-specific manner are under investigation.

Primary prevention should focus on thorough hand washing, avoidance of potential risk factors such as smoking, crowded environments, individuals with respiratory illness and strongly encouraging breast feeding. While awaiting the genesis of an effective pediatric vaccine, genetically engineered, humanized monoclonal antibodies comprise the mainstay of RSV prevention. The efficacy and safety of palivizumab has been proven through two large scale multicenter, randomized controlled trials in premature infants ≤35 weeks gestational age, those with bronchopulmonary dysplasia (BPD) and hemodynamically significant congenital heart disease (CHD). The active use of palivizumab internationally has resulted in reduction in RSV related hospitalizations and complication rates in premature infants and those with BPD and CHD. Concomitantly, prophylaxis in infants with underlying medical disorders is steadily increasing and will further impact the burden of disease.

More recently, motavizumab which is 18 times more potent than palivizumab in neutralizing RSV in tissue culture and has a 70-fold greater binding affinity has been demonstrated to be non-inferior to palivizumab in reducing the rate of RSV hospitalization with a 50% relative reduction in RSV-specific outpatient medically attended LRI. Equal efficacy has also been demonstrated through a RCT in infants with significant cardiac disease. What's in the pipeline? In adults an RSV-A vaccine generated adequate neutralizing antibodies to protect against seasonal RSV-A or B illness but further efficacy studies are required. Phase 1 trials to determine the safety, tolerability, immunogenicity and viral shedding of a pediatric, intranasally administered RSV vaccine are evolving.

Chapter 2 - RSV is a leading cause of viral respiratory tract infections (LRI) during infancy and early childhood. By age 2, nearly all children will have had exposure to RSV manifesting as an upper or lower airway infection. RSV is identified as the etiologic agent in approximately 40-90% of patients with bronchiolitis and in 30-50% of those with pneumonia. [1, 2] From a prospective study conducted on children, admitted with an acute wheezing episode, viruses were detected in nasopharyngeal aspirates.

Chapter 3 - Estimates from the World Health Organization indicate that, worldwide, respiratory syncytial virus (RSV) is responsible for 64 million infections and 160,000 deaths per annum. Both short- and long-term morbidity and mortality are particularly significant for infants. RSV accounts for more than 60% of acute lung respiratory tract infection in children and more than 80%, in infants less than a year of age. RSV is recognized as a significant cause of disease in the elderly population, with an average incidence of 5.5%, about twice that of influenza. Outbreaks occur yearly during the winter season and the infection recurs naturally throughout life.

One diagnostic challenge is that respiratory infections, which can be caused by several viral pathogens in addition to RSV, usually present with signs and symptoms that are nearly indistinguishable by clinical diagnosis. The rapid and accurate detection of RSV provides pathogen-specific diagnosis, allows implementation of appropriate measures to control infection, and improves the management of patients.

Current treatment strategies (*e.g.*, ribavirin) for these patients are limited, but several new drug interventions (*e.g.*, MBX300, RSV604, ALN-RSV01) are under investigation. Several other preventive agents and strategies have been developed (*e.g.*, RSV-IGIV, palivizumab) others are in the pipeline (*e.g.*, motavizumab) or are under development. Although RSV was discovered 40 years ago and despite the importance of RSV as a pathogen, there are as yet no safe and effective vaccines. This is due to a number of factors that complicate the development of such a vaccine, with the basic difficulty being that natural infection imparts only transient and partial immunity to re-infection. At present, prophylaxis with passive antibody therapy is the only specific treatment; thus, patient care remains largely supportive.

However, there are good reasons to think that the scene may soon change. As the pace of development of antiviral drugs and vaccines accelerates, novel therapies are set to make a major impact in the management of this very common infection. Although their use and effect are difficult to anticipate, such interventions could ultimately lead to the interruption of transmission of RSV, thereby resulting in profound changes in the impact of RSV on human health. Thus, it is possible that, in the foreseeable future, such therapeutic tools may have a major impact not only on the management of this infection, but also on prevention of the disease.

In this chapter, the authors review the clinical condition of individuals infected with RSV, with a focus on the populations at highest risk and the squeal to the infection. In addition, they review the prevention and treatment strategies that were used in the past and those currently in use for these high-risk patients, as well as possible future strategies for the development of vaccines and antiviral drugs. This review should provide a single, valuable source of information to clinicians and to investigators.

Chapter 4 - Human respiratory syncytial virus (HRSV) is the single most important cause of serious airway illnesses such as bronchiolitis and pneumonia in infants and young children that require hospitalization with an attendant economic burden. Slight infections of this virus are reported in healthy adults while HRSV poses a severe health risk in immunocompromised individuals and in the elderly. Although multiple immune mechanisms are involved in HRSV disease and protection, the $CD8^+$ T lymphocytes are required to clear virus-infected cells. In last decades, several HRSV epitopes restricted by different major histocompatibility complex class I molecules of the mouse (H-2) or human (HLA) have been identified using murine models or cytolytic T lymphocytes of seropositive individuals respectively. In recent years, using high resolution mass spectrometry analysis of complex HLA-bound peptide pools, physiologically processed HLA ligands from HRSV have been identified. This knowledge could be used in the polyepitope vaccine development.

Chapter 5 - RSV is an important respiratory pathogen of infants and young children and is the most common cause of lower respiratory tract infection-related hospitalization of children under one year of age.

RSV infects over 2/3 of the birth cohort within the first year of life. It has been estimated that more than 120,000 infants in the United States are hospitalized annually with RSV infection. Clinical symptoms are the result of increased mucous production, edema and significant air-trapping. Depending on the types and sizes of airways infected, RSV causes bronchiolitis and/or bronchopneumonia.

Severe RSV disease may also lead to hospitalization and/or PICU admission, requiring, occasionally, mechanical ventilation and even ECMO. Due to the magnitude of the RSV disease impact, and the large variation of the clinical picture, the ability to predict severe RSV illnesses has become important in order to provide appropriate resources for the management of severe RSV disease. Many investigators have described the risks factors that increase the likelihood of hospitalization and of severe RSV disease. This review describes the clinical variables associated with severe RSV illness. In addition, there are predictive models, as in the case of the Michigan and the Rotterdam models, which are based on clinical and epidemiological parameters, which address the ability to predict severe RSV disease in previously healthy infants.

The role of co- infection, viral and bacterial, and nosocomial RSV infection is reviewed as well. Additionally, the current status of genetic polymorphism in RSV disease is briefly highlighted.

In: Respiratory Syncytial Virus
Editors: Haneul Nam and Gippeum Kun, pp. 1-78
ISBN 978-1-62100-835-4

Chapter 1

RESPIRATORY SYNCYTIAL VIRUS INFECTION: DIAGNOSTIC INVESTIGATION, MANAGEMENT AND PREVENTIVE STRATEGIES

***Jonathan Gilleland*[1], *James Mahony*[2] *and Bosco Paes*[3]**

[1]Department of Pediatrics (Division of Critical Care),
McMaster Children's Hospital and McMaster University,
Hamilton, Ontario, Canada
[2]McMaster University (Department of Pathology and Molecular Medicine);
Regional Virology and Chlamydiology Laboratory;
Medical Sciences Graduate Program, Hamilton, Ontario, Canada
[3]Department of Pediatrics (Neonatal Division)
McMaster Children's Hospital and McMaster University,
Hamilton, Ontario, Canada

ABSTRACT

In the current era, Respiratory Syncytial Virus (RSV) prevails as the dominant viral pathogen causing bronchiolitis in infants <2 years of age seen either in the emergency room or hospitalized with lower respiratory tract infections (LRI). The burden of illness with RSV infection is substantial, amounting to approximately 33 million cases worldwide in 2005, with accompanying morbidity and significant mortality especially in infants with underlying medical disorders and those living in developing countries. Of equal importance are high complication rates following RSV-related hospitalization inclusive of the consumption of considerable healthcare resources both within institutions and subsequently in the community. In the early phase of illness, RSV presents as an upper respiratory tract infection which is indistinguishable from the common cold. The progression to bronchiolitis and pneumonia occurs abruptly with marked respiratory distress with or without cyanosis. Pathologically, severe inflammatory changes in the lungs with mucus plugging, edema and epithelial sloughing of the airways results in clinical deterioration which merits hospitalization and intensive care in critically ill infants. Diagnosis is established by nasopharyngeal swabs or aspirates using a combination of techniques including enzyme immunoassay, direct fluorescent antibody staining, cell culture, and nucleic acid amplification tests (NAT). Nucleic acid amplification technology, particularly multiplex PCR coupled with fluidic or fixed microarrays, provides a rapid, accurate and comprehensive approach for the detection of multiple respiratory viruses that cause bronchiolitis including RSV, in a single test. Several commercial NATs are now available. More recently, the addition of allelic discrimination and detection of single nucleotide polymorphisms associated with antiviral resistance to multiplex assays coupled with new viral load tests will facilitate optimal treatment of patients during epidemics and nosocomial spread in hospitals.

Numerous, well-conducted clinical trials have systematically failed to identify a sole therapeutic intervention for the treatment of RSV infection. Evaluated strategies include the use of ribavarin, steroids, bronchodilators, epinephrine, leukotrienes, DNase, antibiotics, Vitamin A and chest physiotherapy. Inhaled hypertonic saline appears safe and promising but further evidence of efficacy either alone or as part of combination therapy is awaited. Treatment of patients with respiratory failure is case dependent due to the heterogeneity of disease presentation and dynamic physiology which clouds clinical endpoints derived from small randomized controlled studies. Guidelines on the timing and optimal mode of positive pressure and mechanical ventilation do not exist. As a result, management of infants requiring respiratory support and critical care tends to represent a fusion of clinical experience, expert opinion, extrapolation of evidence from other respiratory illnesses and a logical approach to trial and error. Studies are in progress to determine if the use of monoclonal antibodies administered in the acute phase of RSV infection, consistently reduces viral load and perhaps severity of illness. Fusion protein inhibitors and drugs that inhibit viral replication and small interfering RNAs that target mRNA in a sequence-specific manner are under investigation.

Primary prevention should focus on thorough hand washing, avoidance of potential risk factors such as smoking, crowded environments, individuals with respiratory illness and strongly encouraging breast feeding. While awaiting the genesis of an effective pediatric vaccine, genetically engineered, humanized monoclonal antibodies comprise the mainstay of RSV prevention. The efficacy and safety of palivizumab has been proven through two large scale multicenter, randomized controlled trials in premature infants ≤35 weeks gestational age, those with bronchopulmonary dysplasia (BPD) and hemodynamically significant congenital heart disease (CHD). The active use of palivizumab internationally has resulted in reduction in RSV related hospitalizations and complication rates in premature infants and those with BPD and CHD. Concomitantly, prophylaxis in infants with underlying medical disorders is steadily increasing and will further impact the burden of disease.

More recently, motavizumab which is 18 times more potent than palivizumab in neutralizing RSV in tissue culture and has a 70-fold greater binding affinity has been demonstrated to be non-inferior to palivizumab in reducing the rate of RSV hospitalization with a 50% relative reduction in RSV-specific outpatient medically attended LRI. Equal efficacy has also been demonstrated through a RCT in infants with significant cardiac disease. What's in the pipeline? In adults an RSV-A vaccine generated adequate neutralizing antibodies to protect against seasonal RSV-A or B illness but further efficacy studies are required. Phase 1 trials to determine the safety, tolerability, immunogenicity and viral shedding of a pediatric, intranasally administered RSV vaccine are evolving.

INTRODUCTION

Acute respiratory disease accounts for an estimated 75% of all acute morbidities in developed countries and most of these infections (approximately 80%) have a viral etiology.

Upper respiratory tract infections (URTIs) such as rhinitis, pharyngitis, and laryngitis, are among the most common infections in children, occurring 3-8 times per year in infants and young children with the incidence varying inversely with age. Acute viral respiratory tract infection is the leading cause of hospitalization for infants and young children in developed countries and is a major cause of death in developing countries. [1,2] The Centers for Disease Control and Prevention's National Vital Statistics Report indicates that there are between 12 and 32 million episodes of URTI each year in children aged 1-2 years and over 300,000 children are hospitalized each year in the United States at an annual cost of about $1billion. [3-5] URTI can lead to acute asthma exacerbations, acute otitis media and lower respiratory tract infection (LRTI) such as bronchitis, bronchiolitis, and pneumonia. In 2002, LRTI accounted for approximately 4 million deaths world-wide, and 7% of all deaths. [6] In clinical practice a specific virus is often not identified, due to the lack of available sensitive tests and/or the presence of as-yet unknown pathogens.

Viral Pathogens

The eight new emerging respiratory viruses discovered since 2000 brings the number of known respiratory virus pathogens to at least eighteen. Although the major causes of acute respiratory distress (ARD) in children and adults are influenza A and B, parainfluenza (PIV) 1, 2, and 3, respiratory syncytial virus (RSV), adenovirus, and rhinovirus, a number of other viruses including coronavirus, bocavirus, enterovirus, PIV type 4, Polyomaviruses WU/K1, Parvovirus 4 and 5, and Mimivirus also infect the respiratory tract albeit at a much lower frequency. The clinical importance of some of the newly discovered viruses is currently under investigation. It is now clear that rhinoviruses and coronaviruses, once thought to only cause a common cold presenting as rhinitis or rhinorrhoea, can also cause LRTI and in some cases can be fatal. Of importance is the fact that all of the viruses mentioned above have overlapping clinical presentations, with all of them having the ability to infect both the upper and lower respiratory tract. Attending physicians therefore are not able to identify the causative agent without a laboratory diagnosis. As mentioned above several new respiratory viruses including avian influenza viruses (H5N1, H7N7, H7N3), human metapneumovirus (hMPV), severe acute respiratory syndrome (SARS) Coronavirus (CoV), and human Coronaviruses (HCoV) NL63 and HKU1 have emerged since 2000. The initial diagnosis of these new viruses and indeed the initial understanding of the epidemiology of the outbreaks they caused was only possible through the development of nucleic amplification tests (NATs).

Since the mid 1990s, NATs have played an important role in diagnosing respiratory virus infections but it wasn't until the emergence of SARS-CoV in 2003 that the importance of nucleic acid detection for diagnosing respiratory virus infection was fully appreciated.

NATs have now been developed for all respiratory viruses including the conventional viruses and the latest emerging viruses such as the 2009 pandemic influenza virus. Figure 1 [7] summarizes the infection prevalence for most of the respiratory viruses obtained from several studies conducted in many countries around the world. The range of prevalence for individual viruses reflects both the different seasons that the studies were conducted and also the sensitivity of molecular tests used.

Virus	Prevalence (%)	Number of Studies	Number of Countries
Influenza	6-40	7	5
Parainfluenza virus types 1-4	15-30	4	4
RSV	10-30	4	4
Adenovirus	2-4	4	4
hMPV	1-30	18	10
HCoV OC43	5-30	5	4
HCoV 229E	1-5	3	3
HCoV NL63	1-9	12	9
HCoV HKU1	1-11	9	8
Bocaviurs	2.1-11.3	14	12
Rhinovirus/Enterovirus	12-45	6	5
Polyomavirus WU/K1	1-5	3	3
Parvovirus 4/5	unknown	2	2

Adapted from: Mahony JB. Expert Rev Anti Infect Ther 2010; 8:1273-1292. (Ref: 7)

Figure 1. Prevalence of various respiratory virus infections using molecular methods in studies conducted in several countries.

Our understanding of the epidemiology of each newly emerging respiratory virus has been dependent on molecular testing and the employment of molecular tests has continually compressed the time frame for acquisition of the new knowledge.

The internet has played a major role in molecular test development with the dissemination of the nucleic acid sequence of newly discovered viruses. For example, our laboratory developed a diagnostic test for SARS CoV in 5 days in 2005 after receiving our first positive clinical material and this time was improved to just 3 days following the emergence of the 2009 pandemic influenza virus. [8]

A number of excellent reviews on the epidemiology and molecular diagnosis of respiratory virus infections including RSV have recently appeared and the reader is referred to them for additional information. [9-11] In this chapter we will review the epidemiology, diagnosis, prevention and treatment of RSV infection.

RSV Epidemiology and Burden of Clinical Disease

RSV is the single most important viral etiologic agent that causes bronchiolitis and lower respiratory tract infections in infants less than two years of age which results in emergency room visits and hospitalizations. [12-16] In studies that used culture or serology, RSV was detected in 43-74% of cases of bronchiolits. [1] In a recent study of hospitalized children with bronchiolitis under the age of two years in Seattle Washington, where a virus was detected in 93% of cases, RSV was detected in 139/180 (77%) of children. [17] In this study 24%, nearly 1 in 4 children with RSV had a co-infection with at least one additional virus and RSV co-infections occurred most frequently with adenovirus (50%) followed by coronavirus (32%) hMPV (9%) and PIV (3%). This study did not include rhinovirus testing however, which has been shown to be one of the most prevalent viruses in other studies and often present as a dual infection. In two other studies in infants with acute lower respiratory tract infections that used PCR testing on nasopharyngeal aspirates, RSV was the first (43.6%) or second (28%) most commonly detected virus, with rhinovirus being the second (31.8%) or first (32%) most frequent virus, respectively. [18,19]

In North America and the USA, hospital admissions for bronchiolitis from 1997-2002 have steadily climbed and rates are highest in infants aged less than 1 year. [20,21] In Canada, for children aged 0–6 months and 6–12 months, admissions increased by 1.78 and 0.7 admissions per year respectively and were consistent over time and across all geographic regions. [20] Similarly in the USA admissions for RSV bronchiolitis have increased by 25% in infants less than 1 year of age. [12] RSV epidemics occur commonly in the late fall to early spring in cool, temperate climates while in other regions of the world the RSV season is dominant during the summer and early autumn because of the hot, humid atmospheric environment. [21-23] The duration of the season is sustained by either persisting cool or warm temperatures or low temperatures with high humidity through the year and ultraviolet radiation adversely impacts RSV activity. [24-26] Temporal and geographic RSV activity trends can be deciphered by viral surveillance based on local RSV hospital admissions and regional public or national laboratory databases and can be utilized to determine the start and end of the RSV season. [22,27,28] There are two broad serological subtypes of RSV, subtypes A and B and both may co-circulate within the community during the season. [29, 30] RSV type A may be associated with more severe disease causing both hospitalization and admission to intensive care. Re-infection is common. [31,32] In a Houston family study conducted between 1975 through 1980, which involved 345 child years of observation, there were 119 primary RSV infections in children from birth to 5 years of age with 98 further re-infections. [33] In a 10-year, prospective, longitudinal study, the attack rate was 98% for primary infections, 75% for second infections and 65% for third occurrences of infection. Immunity acquired during the primary episode did not influence the severity of RSV illness a year later. [34]

The burden of disease associated with RSV infection is equally significant. 40 - 60% of all infants are infected in the first year and by two years almost all children have had an episode of RSV-related illness of which 0.5-2% require hospitalization. [33,35,36] While the majority of infants acquire a mild upper respiratory tract infection, 50 - 90% develop bronchiolitis and 5 - 40% progress to pneumonia. [37-39] In 2005, 33.8 million new episodes of RSV lower respiratory tract infection occurred in children less than 5 years of age world-wide with estimated hospitalizations in 3.4 million (range 2.8-4.3 million) cases. [40] In a recent population based study from 2000-2004, involving 5067 children aged less than 5yrs, the overall incidence of RSV infections was 18%. [41] RSV was associated with 1 of 38 visits to the emergency room and 1 of 13 visits to a community based primary care physician. The average RSV-related hospitalization rate was 17 per 1000 for infants less than 6 months of age and 3 per1000 for children aged less than 5 years. It has been estimated in the US that 2.1 million children under 5 years of age are infected with RSV and require medical attention each year and the hospital costs in 2002 were gauged to be approximately US$1.1 billion. [41, 42] Among these children, approximately 57,527 (3%) are hospitalized, 517,747 (25%) are treated in emergency departments, and 1,534,064 (73%) are managed in pediatric practices. Of the affected outpatients, approximately 1,256,014 (61%) are between 2 and 5 years of age. [41]

There are several demographic and environmental risk factors that have an established association with RSV infection. In a comprehensive literature review Simoes examined the quality and strength of the evidence for developing severe lower respiratory tract RSV infection. [43] The strongest evidence implicated sex, age of acquisition (<1 year of age), birth early in the RSV season when maternal RSV antibody levels are low, crowding in households and siblings which facilitate viral transmission between individuals easily. Tobacco smoke exposure and daycare attendance are significant factors that contribute to the increased risk of RSV hospitalization in infants 32-25 weeks gestational age and family history of atopy has a variable role. The correlation between ethnicity, socio-economic status, malnutrition and RSV LRTI or hospitalization is relatively weak. From 1989-2007 there are approximately 10 retrospective and prospective studies evaluating independent risk factors for severe RSV disease in premature infants and an additional 5 studies that delineate the incidence of RSV hospitalization among infants and children with prematurity, chronic lung disease and congenital heart disease by chronological and gestational age. [44]

RSV is the leading cause of viral mortality with nearly nine times the mortality of influenza in infants <1 year of age. [45] Mortality from RSV infection is dependent on the health status of infected individuals. 66,000–199,000 RSV related deaths were estimated globally in children following acute lower respiratory tract infections and 99% of the deaths occurred in developing countries. [40] In the USA approximately 372-500 deaths were attributed to RSV from 1979-1999. [12,46] Death rates for male and female infants were 10.4 and 8.3 per 100,000 respectively. Risk factors that contributed to mortality from RSV bronchiolitis included race (african-american infants had a 2.3-fold higher mortality), birth weight <2500g, prematurity (≤35 weeks gestational age), young maternal age (<20 years), low maternal education level, smoking during pregnancy, poor prenatal care, single marital status, multiple birth and low five-minute Apgar score. [12,47] Underlying medical disorders are associated with a higher risk of death in hospitalized patients with RSV infection. In a cohort study conducted from 1999 to 2007 in 20 pediatric intensive care units (PICUs) in the United Kingdom, 35 out of 2009 children died following admission with serious RSV illness. [48] The overall hospital RSV mortality rate was 1.7% while the pediatric intensive care specific mortality was 8.6%. The deaths were all associated with pre-existing disease and 54% of the infants had more than 2 disorders which comprised chromosomal abnormalities (29%), cardiac lesions (27%), neuromuscular disorders (15%), chronic lung disease (12%), large airway anomalies (9%) and immunodeficiency (9%). In a comprehensive review from 1966-2009 of 36 heterogeneous studies, fatalities from RSV ranged from <1% in healthy infants without co-morbidities to 37% in infants with cardiac disease. [49] Risk factors associated with a significant mortality risk included prematurity, chronic lung disease, and congenital heart disease. Neuromuscular disease, malignancies and immunosuppression were equally important contributory factors to mortality in term infants and children aged >1 year. Higher fatality rates (0-33%) were documented for infants who acquired nosocomial infection, needed intensive care and the use of extracorporeal membrane oxygenation. There were several limitations identified in the review especially the absence of case specific causes of death and contributory factors relative to RSV disease which may have either under or over estimated the wide range of reported deaths.

RSV infection in infancy is associated with both short and long term morbidity. Hospitalization for lower respiratory tract infection involves a length of stay either in the pediatric ward or intensive care unit dependent on the severity of illness, pre-existing medical disorders and coincidental medical complications. Critically ill infants may require non-invasive ventilation or intubation with escalating strategies of mechanical ventilation and concurrent treatment and their clinical course may inadvertently terminate in death. Hospital admission imposes both a financial burden on the family and is accompanied by both significant immediate healthcare costs and downstream healthcare resource utilization following discharge from hospital. It is now established that early and severe viral lower respiratory tract infections are frequently followed by recurrent wheeze, asthma and allergy during childhood. [50,51]

The association between early onset RSV infection and subsequent wheezing and childhood asthma has been documented in case control studies over time [52-58] but the effect may steadily diminish in adolescence. The Tucson Children's Respiratory Study (a birth cohort study) reported an increased prevalence of respiratory symptoms until age 11 and residual impaired lung function at age 13 in those experiencing a relatively mild RSV LRTI (not requiring hospitalization) during the first 3 years of life. [52] Recent follow up of a cohort previously hospitalized in the first 2 years of life and followed for 18-20 years suggested that impaired lung function may persist into adulthood. [59] Similarly, in a recent study from Sweden, severe early RSV bronchiolitis in the first year of life was associated with increased prevalence of allergic asthma persisting into early adulthood. [58] These authors showed an increased prevalence of asthma/recurrent wheezing (39% versus 9%), clinical allergy (43% versus 17%) and sensitization to perennial allergens (41% versus 14%) which were present at 18 years of age in the RSV cohort compared with a control group. This study suggests that early severe RSV bronchiolitis has lifelong consequences of allergic asthma and airway remodeling. However, an active debate prevails as to whether RSV in infancy modulates immune responses or re-models airway architecture and function to produce wheeze or whether genetic predisposition and premorbid lung function pave a path for airway morbidity. [60,61] Jafri et al have clearly established through a mouse model that RSV alone induces airway hyperreactivity for 6 weeks post infection and chronic airway inflammation that persists for 6 months. [62] The model was subsequently utilized to evaluate the impact of RSV prophylaxis on the same outcomes and conclusively demonstrated reduction in lung RSV RNA loads on days 5 and 28 after RSV inoculation and significant decrease in bronchial airway hyperreactivity at 4 and 8weeks post inoculation. [63] The final answer regarding the link between RSV infection and asthma will only be resolved through a randomized, double-blind, placebo controlled trial of RSV prophylaxis which demonstrates a reduction in subsequent asthma. [60]

RSV- Description of the Agent

RSV is a single stranded, negative sense RNA virus belonging to the Group V (-ssRNA) virus within the *Pneumovirus* genus, the *Pneumovirinae* subfamily, the *Paramyxoviridae* family and the *Mononegavirales* Order. There are two genotypes or strains of RSV; RSV A and B, and infections with RSV A are thought to be more severe than RSV B. The RSV genome contains 10 genes encoding 11 proteins (there are 2 open reading frames of M2 protein). NS1 and NS2 inhibit type I interferon activity. N encodes the nucleocapsid protein that associates with the genomic RNA forming the nucleocapsid. M encodes the Matrix protein required for viral assembly. SH, G and F form the viral coat. The G protein is a surface glycoprotein that is heavily glycosylated and functions as the attachment protein. The G protein differs considerably between the two subtypes. The F protein is another important surface protein that mediates fusion of the viral membrane with the host cell membrane allowing entry of the virus into the cell cytoplasm and also allowing the formation of syncytia. Antibodies directed at the F protein neutralize infection. M2 is the second matrix protein also required for transcription, it encodes M2-1 (elongation factor) and M2-2 (transcription regulation). The L protein is the RNA polymerase and the P protein is a phosphoprotein required for transcription and genomic replication. The genome is transcribed sequentially from NS1 to L with reduction in expression levels along its length.

The development of real time polymerase chain reaction (PCR) affords the ability to determine the number of virus particles or genome equivalents present in various clinical specimens. Knowledge of the relationship between viral load and severity of disease should expand our understanding of the pathology of RSV infections and be important for determining the benefit of antiviral treatment. Early studies looking at this question in hospitalized infants involved heterogeneous populations and did not take into account possible co-infections with other viruses. More recent studies have revealed a relationship between viral load and severity of infection. In a study from The Netherlands involving 82 infants with primary respiratory virus infection (median age of 3 months) a virus was detected in 77 (94%) infants [64] and 30 of these were RSV (median age of 4 months). Disease severity was assessed using a previously published severity score by means of a standardized questionnaire and physical examination and viral loads on nasopharyngeal specimens were determined by real time PCR using the number of amplification cycles needed for a positive PCR test (cycle threshold) where the higher the cycle threshold, the lower amount of virus present.

This was the first report on viral loads in previously healthy infants with RSV infection in the community where disease severity correlated positively with viral load during primary RSV infection. Interestingly, in this study the correlation between disease severity and viral load was highest in the case of single RSV infection and was absent in RSV co-infections and rhinovirus disease severity was not correlated with viral load or the presence of co-infections. In a recent study from Germany involving 404 hospitalized patients under the age of 16 years with a LRTI, a virus was detected in 315 (78%) nasopharyngeal aspirate (NPA) specimens collected on the day of admission and a bacteria was detected in 198 (63.3%) of 311 specimens. [65] RSV strain A or B was detected in 160 (51%) followed by rhinovirus in 87 (28%). An equal number of RSV A (n=80) and B (n=80) were found. The RSV viral load significantly decreased between the first and second (day 3-4) NPA specimens ($p<0.001$). Since patients were discharged from hospital when they were clinically improved, a relationship between viral load and disease severity can be assumed. This is in agreement with a recent study in children showing a correlation between clinical improvement and a reduction in viral load after 3 days of hospitalization. [66] However, there was no correlation between viral load and disease severity including duration of hospitalization, requirement for supplemental oxygen, use of bronchodilators, systemic corticosteroids, antibiotics, chest radiography examination or presence of fever. There was a significant negative correlation between RSV viral load and blood C-reactive protein level ($p<0.005$) and leucocyte count ($p<0.001$). In contrast, Bosis et al. did not find a significant impact of RSV viral load on the disease severity in children admitted to hospital for the first episode of acute wheezing. [67]

The difference in these two studies may be related to the age at which the patients were infected with RSV, the immune status of the host or genetic factors. Further well controlled studies will be required to answer this question.

In the immunocompetent host, respiratory virus replication is limited to the respiratory epithelium. For some viruses like avian influenza (H5N1), seasonal influenza virus and SARS CoV detection of viral RNA by PCR and isolation of virus from plasma or serum has been described where these viruses may cause disseminated infection with replication outside the respiratory tract. [68,69] Among individuals with avian influenza H5N1 infection, viral RNA in blood has been detected in fatal cases and is associated with higher pharyngeal viral loads indicating dissemination, which is associated with a poor prognosis. [68] The detection of other respiratory viruses such as RSV and rhinovirus in serum or blood mononuclear cells has rarely been described in neonates or children and there has been little correlation between virus detection and disease severity. [70]

In a recent retrospective study of viral pneumonia in hematopoietic cell transplantation (HCT), respiratory viruses were detected in BAL specimens of 82 patients. [71] RSV was detected in 35 patients and the median viral load for RSV was 2.6 x 10^6copies/mL. Viral RNA was detected in serum samples of 6 of 66 patients including 4 of 41 cases of RSV pneumonia, 1 with influenza B and 1 with hMPV/influenza A virus/CoV co-infection. RSV detection in serum was associated with high viral load in bronchoalveolar lavage (BAL) specimens ($p<0.05$) and viral detection in serum was significantly associated with death (adjusted odds ratio,1.8; $p=0.02$). Detection of virus in serum samples may indicate systemic dissemination of virus, physical release of virus into the circulation from infected epithelial cells at sites of replication in the respiratory tract, or detection of virus in antigen presenting cells including pulmonary macrophages and dendritic cells that gain access to the bloodstream during severe infection.

Further studies will be required to establish whether patients with upper respiratory tract infections alone or with upper tract infections that have progressed to the lower respiratory tract also have RSV RNA in serum samples. Reverse transcriptase (RT-PCR) testing for RSV in sera may offer an adjunctive method for diagnosis of severe viral pneumonia and may offer important approaches for therapy and monitoring in immunocompromised patients. This is supported by data obtained recently with a mouse model of RSV infection, where treatment with a RSV monoclonal antibody (motavizumab) given intraperitoneally at 72 hours post infection reduced viral RNA levels in serum and improved airway obstruction. [72]

Diagnosis of Respiratory Virus Infections

The appearance of eight new respiratory viruses in the human population in the past nine years including two new pandemics (SARS coronavirus in 2003 and swine-origin influenza A/H1N1 in 2009) has tested the ability of virology laboratories to develop diagnostic tests to identify these emerging viruses. Nucleic acid based amplification tests (NATs) that first appeared two decades ago have been developed for both conventional and emerging viruses and now constitutes the backbone of the clinical laboratory. NATs provide a rapid, accurate and sensitive detection of respiratory viruses and have significantly increased our understanding of the epidemiology of these viruses. Multiplex PCR assays have recently been introduced for the detection of up to 18 different respiratory viruses in a single test and several commercial tests are now available. Quantitative RT-PCR assays are beginning to appear establishing correlations between various clinical findings and viral loads for specific viruses. The final chapter in the evolution of respiratory virus diagnosis will be the addition of allelic discrimination and detection of single nucleotide polymorphisms associated with antiviral resistance. These antiviral resistance assays together with viral load tests will enable clinical laboratories to provide physicians with new information for optimal management of patients.

Virus isolation and serology were the first methods used to diagnose respiratory virus infections. In the 1970s and 1980s virus isolation was performed using three or four cell lines and together with embryonated hens' eggs in the case of influenza, virus isolation was the major means for detecting respiratory viruses. A variety of serological tests including the hemagglutination inhibition (HAI) test, complement fixation and enzyme immunoassay (EIA) have been used for testing paired acute and convalescent phase sera to detect a four fold rise in antibody titers to specific respiratory viruses. However serology has been most useful for epidemiological studies and not for patient diagnosis. In the early 1990s shell vial culture (SVC) was introduced and together with the development of specific monoclonal antibodies, viral antigens could be detected in cell culture in 1-2 days instead of 8-10 days required for tube culture. SVC utilizing monoclonal antibodies to detect specific viral proteins provides a faster detection of virus in clinical specimens due primarily to the centrifugation assisted inoculation of the cell monolayer that facilitates virus entry and shortens the time for viral protein synthesis. RSV proteins accumulate in infected cells and can be detected with monoclonal antibodies at 24-48 hours post inoculation. Direct fluorescent antibody (DFA) staining of cells derived from nasopharyngeal swabs or NPAs became the mainstay for many laboratories in the 1990s and provided a rapid test result within 3 hours of the receipt of specimens in the laboratory. The rapid turn around time for results has provided both clinicians and infection control practitioners with important information for treatment and cohorting of patients. Clinicians could begin treatment sooner resulting in better outcomes and patient cohorting could reduce nosocomial infections. Many clinical laboratories have used a combination of DFA staining and SVC for respiratory specimens by performing DFA first on all specimens, then taking the DFA negative specimens and setting up a SVC test. The addition of the second test (SVC) has historically increased the positivity rate from 3-10% dependent on the year of the conducted study.

There is now a trend to move away from the DFA and SVC approach replacing these traditional tests with the more sensitive molecular tests (see below). Rapid EIA tests for viral antigens were introduced in the 1980s and 1990s but these point of care tests (POCTs) lacked sensitivity and although they were widely used in some settings these tests were relegated to settings with a high pre-test probability where poor test sensitivity had less of an impact. NATs and in particular multiplex PCR coupled with fluidic microarrays using microbeads or DNA chips (oligonucleotides spotted onto slide or chips) represent the latest diagnostic approach for the clinical laboratory.

Nucleic acid amplification methods including PCR, nucleic acid sequence-based amplification (NASBA), transcription mediated amplification (TMA), strand displacement amplification (SDA), loop-mediated isothermal amplification (LAMP), rolling circle amplification (RCA), and multiplex ligation-dependent probe amplification (MLPA) have been applied for most respiratory viruses and today these sensitive NATs are working their way into the routine clinical laboratory. The details of these molecular tests have been reviewed recently by Wu and Tang [73] and will not be discussed here.

DIAGNOSIS OF RSV INFECTION

Historically several diagnostic approaches have been used for the detection of RSV. Virus isolation in cell culture was the first method for diagnosing RSV infections. RSV has been more difficult to culture than other respiratory viruses because the virus is more labile and specimens need to be kept cold. A variety of cell lines have been used for RSV isolation but HEp-2, HeLa and A549 cells have been the most sensitive for primary isolation.

The sensitivity of conventional tube culture compared with rapid antigen detection by indirect immunofluorescent antibody assay (IFA) has varied from 57 to 90%. [74,75] The SVC method has shown increased sensitivity compared to tube culture and provides a shorter turn around time for reporting results. The SVC has been an important test used the majority of clinical laboratories in North America and its sensitivity for detecting RSV compared to DFA, enzyme immunoassay or conventional culture has ranged from 67% to 92%. [76-78] Commercially available R-Mix cells (Diagnostic Hybrids Inc, Athens, OH) have shortened the resulting turn around time and increased the sensitivity over conventional culture. [79-81] Many laboratories now use a combination of DFA and SVC for RSV detection. The availability of excellent monoclonal antibodies has increased the sensitivity of DFA to between 80 and 97%. [75,77,82]

Rapid EIA tests have been used for many years for RSV detection. They offer the advantage of providing results in 15 to 30 minutes but the downside to these tests is their poor sensitivity. Approximately a dozen rapid tests have been approved for RSV and for the most part their performance is similar. (Figure 2) [83] The sensitivity of these rapid tests is only 80-85 % when compared to DFA and fewer comparisons have been performed using the more sensitive RT-PCR test as the reference standard. [84-87] The sensitivity of the second version of the Directigen RSV EIA test has ranged from 61 to 86%. [88,89] It should be pointed out that the performance of these rapid tests is only as good as the reference standard to which they are compared and their sensitivity will likely be lower when they are compared to the more sensitive NATs. In addition, the specificity of these tests will be much lower when they are used during the summer because the RSV prevalence especially in temperate climates is lower. Another cautionary note is that their sensitivities will be lower in adults compared to children since adults generally shed lower titers of virus than children. [88,90,91] Although, the BinaxNOW RSV Test and the 3M Rapid Detection Test have the highest sensitivity of the rapid tests, recent evaluations of these tests have confirmed their limited overall sensitivity.

In a multi-site evaluation of 1,306 specimens comparing the performance of the 3M Rapid Detection Test and the BinaxNOW RSV Test, the 3M Rapid Detection Test had an overall sensitivity of 86.3% and the BinaxNOW RSV Test had a sensitivity of 70.8% when DFA and culture was used as the combined reference standard. [92] The specificity of the two tests was comparable. It should be noted that the BinaxNOW Test is not approved for testing of nasopharyngeal aspirates or in subjects older than 5 years of age while the 3M Rapid Detection Test is approved for use with subjects less than 22 years of age.

In a recent evaluation of the 3M Rapid Detection Test using the xTAG RVP multiplex PCR test as the gold standard involving 323 positive specimens, the 3M Rapid Detection Test had a sensitivity of 74% and a specificity of 100%. [93] The sensitivity for RSV A was higher than that for RSV B, 78% compared to 60%. In a recent study testing 311 specimens from hospitalized children with LRTI and a median age of 9 months, the performance of the BinaxNOW RSV Test was evaluated using a quantitative RT-PCR as the gold standard. [94]

Tests	Manufacturer	Sensitivity (%)	Specificity (%)
BinaxNOW® RSV	Binax,Scarborough,ME,USA	70-93	89-100
Clearview® RSV[a]	Inverness Medical Innovations,Bedford, UK	93	97
Directigen RSV	Becton-Dickinson,Cockeysville,MD, USA	93-97	90-97
Directigen EZ RSV	Becton-Dickinson,Cockeysville,MD, USA	89	93
Respi-Strip RSV	Coris Bio-Concept, Gembloux,Belgium	86-92	93-98
SAS™ RSV Alert[a]	SA Scientific,San Antonio,TX,USA	83	91
Sure-Vue RSV[a]	Thermo Fisher Scientific,Waltham,MA, USA	96	94
Xpect RSV[a]	Remel Inc,Lenexa,KS,USA	96	94

These tests were all 10-15 min tests for detection of RSV in: *BAL,* bronchoalveolar lavage; *NPA,* nasopharyngeal aspirate; *NPS,* nasopharyngeal swab; *NW,* nasal wash; *TS,* throat swab.
[a]CLIA-waived. Adapted from: Blyth et al. Methods Molec Biol 2011; 665: 415-433. (Ref:83)

Figure 2. RSV Point-of-Care Tests.

The sensitivity and specificity of the BinaxNOW Test was 72% and 97% compared with RT-PCR. The sensitivity of the BinaxNOW Test was affected by the duration of symptoms and decreased from 92% for specimens collected within one day of symptom onset versus 65% for specimens collected >5 days after the onset of symptoms ($p<0.04$). Specimens that were missed by the BinaxNOW Test and positive by RT-PCR had a median viral load of 5 x 10^7copies/mL. By comparison, the specimens that were positive by both tests had a median viral load of 1 x 10^9copies/mL indicating that rapid tests have difficulty detecting RSV when the virus is present at low levels.

A novel approach to the detection of RSV in clinical specimens involving nanoparticle-amplified immuno-PCR has recently been described. [95] In traditional immuno-PCR, a single antibody recognition event is associated with one to three DNA oligo tags which are subsequently amplified by PCR. Perez et al. developed a nanoparticle-amplified immuno-PCR that combines antibody recognition of ELISA with a 50-fold nanoparticle valence amplification step prior to the tag amplification with PCR. In this assay antibody to RSV surface proteins are coupled to 15 nm gold particles which are also tagged with DNA oligos at a DNA/antibody ratio of 50:1. The virus-antibody-nanoparticle sandwich forms a complex with magnetic particles for enrichment and after extraction DNA tags are released by heating and detected by PCR amplification. The lower limit of detection of the assay was 4 *pfu*/mL of RSV from infected HeLa cell lysates which was 4-fold more sensitive than an RT-PCR assay targeting the N gene that detected 17.9*pfu*/mL. The assay however was not been tested with clinical material and its clinical sensitivity is not known at this time. Although this assay has a higher analytical sensitivity compared with conventional RT-PCR, it required more time and reagents. The combination of highly substituted nanoparticles coupled with the specificity of an antibody-antigen reaction and signal amplification afforded by PCR is intriguing and this diagnostic approach may be worth further evaluation.

Nucleic acid detection has become the preferred diagnostic approach for RSV detection in clinical specimens owing largely to its increased sensitivity. Over the past decade a large number of NATs have been developed to address the poor sensitivity of traditional tests such as cell culture and DFA. [96-112] A variety of RT-PCR assays have been described that use gel electrophoresis, restriction fragment length polymorphism (RFLP), hybridization, sequencing, and EIA for analysis. Targets for RT-PCR have included the fusion, nucleocapsid and large polymerase subunit gene. Many assays have been developed and most are more sensitive than culture. One assay targeting the fusion gene detected 122 positives out of 668 specimens tested compared to only 47 positives by culture. [104] Freymuth et al. described an assay that detected both RSV A and B and used discordant testing to show that RT-PCR was 97.5% sensitive and 63.9% specific. [97] A commercially available NASBA assay targeting the F gene (NucliSens Easy Q RSV A and B from Biomerieux) was recently evaluated using 508 specimens.

Assay Format	Gene Target	Sensitivity (%)	Specificity (%)	Comments	Ref
RT-PCR	N (219-474 bp)	94.4	100	RT-PCR performance compared to culture using a total of 47 specimens and 18 positives.	[96]
RT-PCR	N (278 bp)	97.5	63.9	PCR detects both RSV A and B, more sensitive then IFA and culture, tested 238 specimens.	[97]
Hemi-nested RT-PCR	F (243 bp)	ND	ND	PCR more sensitive then culture and antigen detection based on testing 132 specimens	[98]
Multiplex RT-PCR		ND	ND	Hexaplex (Prodesse) detects influenza A and B, PIV I-3, RSV A and B.	[99]
Real time RT-PCR	F (242 bp) F (89 bp)	ND	ND	Real time PCR using FRET probes was more sensitive than nested PCR based on testing 71specimens, LLOD of 145 pg.	[100]
Multiplex RT-PCR	RSV A N (334 bp) RSV B N (183 bp)	ND	ND	Multiplex PCR uses 5 primer pairs, detects and subtypes influenza and RSV, LLOD <1 *pfu*, tested only 65 specimen RSV positives.	[101]
Mulitplex RT-PCR	L	100	100	Mulitplex PCR detects seven viruses including influenza A and B, PIV-1-3, RSV and Adenovirus, more sensitive then culture and IFA based on testing 598 specimens including 123 RSV positives.	[102]
Assay Format	Gene Target	Sensitivity (%)	Specificity (%)	Comments	

Figure 3 continued on next page

Multiplex RT-PCR	L (355 bp)	ND	ND	Multiplex PCR detects RSV A, B and PIV-3 using 3 primer pairs, less sensitive then IFA and culture, evaluated using 261 specimens.	[103]
RT-PCR	F (380 bp)	ND	ND	RT-PCR was twice as sensitive as culture detecting 122 vs 47 positives, evaluated using 668 specimens.	[104]
NASBA	F	99	87	NucliSens Easy Q RSV A and B (Biomerieux) was more sensitive then DFA and culture (131 vs 108), performance compared to culture - retrospective study of 508 specimens.	[105]
Multiplex quantitative RT-PCR	*pol* lb N	ND	ND	Hexaplex Multiplex PCR detects influenza A and B, RSV A and B, PIV 1-3 with a sensitivity of 5 GE.	[106]
Multiplex RT-PCR	*pol* lb N	91	98.6	Hexaplex evaluated for RSV had a sensitivity 4200 copies RSV A and 42 copies RSV B, performance based on testing 254 specimens including 44 DFA positives.	[107]
Multiplex RT-PCR	*pol* lb N	98.6	97.9	Hexaplex performance based on testing 363 specimens including 82 confirmed positives by culture or Directigen RSV EIA.	[108]
Multiplex RT-PCR	Proprietary	97.8	97.0	Compared ProFlu-1 assay to DFA and culture using 353 pediatric specimens.	[109]
	L	RSV A 100 RSV B 100	RSV A 98.4 RSV B 97.4	Multiplex RT-PCR detects 19 respiratory viruses uses fluidic microbead microarray and Luminex xMAP system, LLOD of 6 x 10^{-2} $TCID_{50}$ for RSV A and 6 $TCID_{50}$ for RSV B, positives confirmed by second PCR and amplicon sequencing, performance based on 554 specimens tested.	[110]
Multiplex RT-PCR	Proprietary	73.3	>99.1	ResPlex II detects 12 viruses, compared to culture and Taqman PCR using 360 frozen specimens.	[111]
Multipelx RT-PCR	Proprietary	ND	ND	MultiCode-PLx detects 17 viruses using Luminex xMAP system, 354 specimens tested by DFA and culture, detected all 12 DFA and culture positives.	[112]

ND, not determined; LLOD, lower limit of detection; *pfu*, plaque forming unit; L, large polymerase subunit; N, nucleocapsid protein; F, fusion protein.

Adapted from: Mahony JB. Clin Microbiol Rev 2008; 21:716-747. (Ref: 9)

Figure 3. Molecular tests for detection of respiratory syncytial virus.

NASBA was more sensitive than culture and DFA and had a sensitivity of 99% and a specificity of 87%. [105] Figure 3 describes the characteristics and performance of several molecular tests for detection of respiratory syncytial virus. [9]

A number of multiplex assays have been described that detect RSV and a number of other respiratory viruses. The first multiplex PCR assays for RSV were less sensitive than IFA and culture. The Hexaplex assay was the first multiplex PCR test and detected influenza A and B, RSV A and B, and parainfluenza 1 and 3. [106] In one study involving 254 specimens the Hexaplex assay had a sensitivity of 91% and a specificity of 98.6% for detecting RSV. [107] In a second study involving 363 specimens Hexaplex had a sensitivity of 98.6% and a specificity of 97.9%. [108] Syrmis et al. developed a multiplex assay for the detection of 7 respiratory viruses including influenza A and B, RSV A and B, PIV 1-3 and adenovirus. [102] This assay was more sensitive than culture and IFA for the detection of RSV when evaluated using 598 NPA specimens of which 123 were RSV positive. The ProFlu+ Assay (Genprobe) is a real time multiplex assay for the detection of influenza A, influenza B, RSV A and RSV B that has recently been Federal Drug Agency (FDA) cleared however, performance data for RSV is limited. Several companies (Roche Diagnositcs, Basel, Switzerland; Abbott Molecular Diagnostics, N. Chicago, IL, Cepheid, Sunnyvale, CA, and Prodesse Inc., Waukesha, WI) have developed analyte specific reagents (ASRs) consisting of primers and probes for laboratories to detect RSV. These ASRs are reagents only (not diagnostic kits with a manufacturer's protocol) and are not FDA approved; the clinical performance therefore in any one laboratory is dependent on how the reagents are used and as such carry no performance criteria.

Over the last five years a number of commercially available multiplex assays have been introduced. The ResPlex II (developed by Genaco now owned by Qiagen, Dusseldorf, Germany), the MultiCode-PLx RVP Assay (Eragen Biosciences, now owned by Luminex Corporation), the Seeplex™ RV (Seegene, Seoul, Korea), the NGEN™ RVA ASR kit (Nanogen, San Diego, CA), the RVNAT$_{SP}$ (Nanosphere Inc. Northbrook, IL) and the xTAG™ RVP Assay (Luminex Molecular Diagnostics, Toronto Canada) all detect RSV. The xTAG™ RVP Assay was the first multiplex assay cleared by the FDA for the detection of 12 respiratory viruses including RSV and uses the Luminex xMAP System. [110] The xTAG™ RVP assay consists of a multiplex PCR to amplify specific virus sequences followed by hybridization onto a micro-fluidic array consisting of differently colored microspheres which contain complimentary capture oligonucleotide probes. The fluorescently labeled microspheres are interrogated using two lasers, the first laser identifies the individual colored beads and hence virus and the second laser detects the presence or absence of amplified DNA. The xTAG™ RVP assay detects 19 different virus types and subtypes but received clearance for only 12 viruses since the number of positives for the rare viruses such as coronavirus was too low in the clinical trial. The xTAG™ RVP Assay has a reported sensitivity of 100% for RSV A and B and a specificity of 98.4% and 97.4% for RSV A and B, respectively based on clinical study data submitted to the FDA. [113] The second commercially available multiplex assay developed was the MultiCode-PLx RVP assay which detects 17 respiratory viruses including RSV and also uses the Luminex xMAP system. At the time of writing, this assay is not yet FDA cleared. In a study by Nolte et al. (2007) the sensitivity and specificity of the MultiCode-PLx RVP assay for the detection of RSV was 91.7% and 99.4%, respectively using DFA and SVC as the reference standard. [112] The Clart® PneumoVir test from Genomica (Madrid, Spain) is a recently introduced DNA microarray that detects 11 different respiratory viruses including RSV, utilizing hybridization of amplified DNA to immobilized probes set up in a microarray. [114-116] The authors indicate that this test takes approximately 8 hours to perform following nucleic acid extraction and consists of a multiplex PCR (5 hr) followed by hybridization (1.5 hr). The Clart® PneumoVir test has been used to identify a number of respiratory viruses in both children and adults presenting with upper or lower tract infections. [115,116] This test was used in a recent study of 73 children under the age of 2 years who were admitted to the ICU and at least one respiratory virus was detected in 57/73 (78%) of the children with RSV detected in 42/57 (74%). [115] In this clinical study no other tests for RSV were performed and the sensitivity and specificity of the test for RSV was not determined. In another study from France involving 95 patients (56 adults and 39 children) with influenza- like-illness, the Clart® PneumoVir test and a companion Clart® FluA Vir Test for influenza identified a respiratory virus in 65 (68.4%) patients. [116] In this study only 2 patients had RSV and no other RSV tests were performed so it was not possible to determine the sensitivity or specificity for detecting RSV. Although earlier developmental papers describe the analytical performance of the Clart® PneumoVir test [114] the clinical performance of this for RSV is largely unknown in the absence of comparative studies with large numbers of clinical specimens. Another commercially available real time RT-PCR that uses nanoparticles for the detection of four respiratory viruses including RSV has recently been FDA cleared. [117] There are two versions of this test; the manual VNAT test and the fully automated $RVNAT_{SP}$ version that both detect four respiratory viruses including influenza A and B and RSV A and B by multiplex PCR followed by hybridization to capture probes immobilized on glass slides. The test is performed with the Verigene *SP* system consisting of the Verigene *SP* processor for extraction, amplification and hybridization and the Verigene reader for reading glass slides in <1 minute. The test uses gold nanoparticle-labeled probes to detect captured target DNA. This test takes 3.5 hr to perform and has recently been FDA cleared. In a two site evaluation involving 720 nasopharyngeal swab specimens including 49 RSV positives where culture and DFA were used as the reference standard, the $RVNAT_{SP}$ test had a sensitivity and specificity of 91.7% and 98.4% respectively for RSV. [117] Performance studies involving comparisons of two or more of these commercial multiplex assays will be required to determine the "true" performance of these assays; these comparisons are eagerly awaited.

Commentary on RSV Diagnostics

Molecular testing has greatly improved the laboratory's ability to diagnose viral respiratory tract infections. NATs are the most sensitive method for detecting RSV followed by DFA, SVC, tube culture, and EIA which is the least sensitive. The increased sensitivity of molecular tests over conventional tests has necessitated the use of a combined reference standard of positivity, defining a true positive as being positive in two or more tests, and in the case of non-culturable viruses, positive results in two different molecular tests amplifying two different genomic regions. The increased sensitivity means that infected patients will be diagnosed more accurately especially at times during the course of their infection when they are shedding low levels of virus and that respiratory viruses will no longer be under diagnosed. The benefit of a more accurate diagnosis is three-fold: first, it benefits the patient in terms of receiving the appropriate anti-viral drugs such as oseltamivir in the case of influenza; second, it assists infection control practitioners in providing appropriate infection control measures such as droplet containment to minimize the risk of nosocomial spread; and third, it provides more accurate information to public health authorities regarding what viruses are circulating in the community so they can adjust public health policy accordingly. In addition, for potentially catastrophic global events such as the emergence of SARS and novel influenza strains, accurate and sensitive diagnostic tests such as NATs have played a critical role in indentifying the agent and tracking the outbreaks; these assays will likely play a key role in future pandemics.

For RSV tests that are developed in-house there is a significant need for validation of these assays before they can be used to report out results. Newly developed assays are initially evaluated using known positive and negative specimens to determine if they can accurately detect the analyte in clinical specimens. This is followed up with testing clinical specimens in parallel with a reference test (gold standard) to determine the analytical performance *viz.* sensitivity, specificity, positive and negative predictive values. Internal quality assurance should be performed on a regular basis (annually) and should include the use of external standardized specimens such as College of American Pathologists (CAP) or quality control for molecular diagnostics (QCMD) panels as part of an ongoing external quality assurance (EQA) program. Evaluation of the performance of specific molecular tests for different specimen types is also critical since interference factors may vary from one specimen type to another and the ability of commercial extraction kits to extract nucleic acid and remove interference factors will vary. For example sputum specimens are especially difficult specimens due to the presence of excess mucous and therefore the ability of a specific molecular test to detect a specific analyte such as RSV in sputum needs to be determined. In addition, natural history studies need to be performed to determine the most appropriate clinical specimen for newly discovered viruses such as SARS CoV or pandemic influenza strains.

The development and adoption of multiplex PCR tests for respiratory viruses will have an even greater benefit over the next few years since multiplex tests offer laboratories the ability to detect a wide range of viral infections not previously possible. These tests will allow laboratories to report infections with both conventional viruses such as RSV as well the newly discovered viruses such as human CoVs NL63, HKU1 and human Bocavirus, using a single test. Testing for multiple viruses in a single test may provide a savings of resources including technologist time and expendables and cost less than the aggregate cost of performing multiple uniplex PCR tests. The implementation of robotics in large volume laboratories will decrease costs further since a significant portion of the cost is technologist's labor. Dual respiratory virus infections are poorly detected using DFA and SVC methods because of subjective immunofluorescent readouts. Dual and even triple infections are routinely reported using multiplex PCR and have accounted for 8-11% positive results. [118,119] The ability to easily detect dual infections provides the means and rationale for studies to examine the clinical importance of dual infections and in particular whether certain individuals are at greater risk for dual infections or whether co infections result in poorer outcomes for patients. Finally, multiplex tests will contribute to our understanding of the epidemiology of viral respiratory tract infections as large numbers of specimens can be tested for multiple viruses providing a wealth of new information on seasonality, geographical distribution, and risk groups.

In summary, nucleic acid amplification-based methods provide a fast, accurate and sensitive diagnosis of RSV infections. NATs have increased our knowledge of the epidemiology and pathogenesis of conventional viruses such as RSV as well as newly discovered avian H5N1, pandemic H1N1, and re-emerging rhinoviruses. Reverse-transcriptase PCR is the most widely used molecular diagnostic method, although a number of other amplification methods; NASBA, ligase chain reaction (LCR), LAMP and closed circle rolling amplification (CRC) have been used for some viruses. Multiplex PCR assays have been developed to detect several different respiratory viruses including RSV in a single test, and commercial multiplex assays have recently been introduced that can detect up to 18 different viruses; some are FDA approved as *in vitro* diagnostics. Additional molecular tests for respiratory viruses including quantitative assays need to be developed and standardized for optimal patient diagnosis and treatment in health care institutions. Optimized multiplex assays can be used to better define the epidemiology of respiratory virus infections including RSV and establish the direct and indirect societal costs of conditions resulting from respiratory viral infections such as asthma and exacerbations of chronic lung disease.

Respiratory Syncytial Virus: Treatment

It is quite common for guidelines, reviews and updates of current therapies for RSV and bronchiolitis to provide itemized summaries of various interventions with the relevant literature carefully and thoughtfully presented. The take home points, distilled from large randomized controlled trials and systematic reviews, provide excellent guidance regarding whether the highlighted therapies provide benefit when used routinely in all children usually less than one year, presenting to an emergency room or admitted to an inpatient ward with a febrile viral respiratory illness. Unfortunately, RSV LRTIs can manifest as different disease presentations, and within the same patient can be extremely dynamic with alterations to the upper and lower airways competing against lung parenchyma to be the dominant physiology. [36,120,121] Much of this heterogeneity can be attributed to the equally dynamic nature of airway secretions, sloughed epithelium and mucous plugging. [36,122] Some infants, however, present with a true RSV pneumonitis or a concomitant bacterial co-infection that result in progression to hypoxic respiratory failure. [123,124] While there have been a number of very large, well conducted randomized controlled trials (RCTs) of various interventions for bronchiolitis, the clinician must apply this evidence in the context of an individual infant's physiology and with a clear understanding of the pathophysiology of the disease, weighing the potential harms and benefits of any proposed therapy.

The best illustration of this point can be made in examining the role of nasal patency in the presentation and treatment of bronchiolitis. The American Academy of Pediatrics (AAP) guidelines on the diagnosis and management of bronchiolitis published in 2006 make repeated reference to the importance of nasal suctioning and positioning in the assessment of work of breathing, as it can dramatically improve the clinical presentation, [120] reinforcing the importance of obligate nasal breathing physiology in a young infant. This relatively mundane intervention, as straight-forward as it is, begs the question; if the nasal airway of an infant presenting in an emergency room is obstructed during the course of treatment, did a trial of nebulized therapy "X" fail because of a simple drug delivery problem? While there is no clear evidence extolling the benefit of nasal suctioning, it is advocated by the AAP guidelines, and may at the very least confound clinical scoring assessments. Surprisingly this maneuver is not addressed in most reported trial protocols.

This leads to the next observation regarding aggregate effects of multiple therapies. Inherent to any trial evaluating the benefit of a single therapy is the need to control for and minimize the impact of any other potentially confounding therapies. When an infant presents with a mild to moderate respiratory illness, a sequential approach to various interventions is appropriate if the clinical usefulness and continuing need of individual therapies can be repeatedly assessed. This approach is described in the current AAP recommendation of a single trial of bronchodilator therapy with ongoing use mitigated by its effect on a patient's clinical status. [120] On the contrary, when a child presents with severe disease, where intubation and invasive ventilation is a distinct possibility, if rapid improvement in the clinical condition is not achieved, then the sequential approach is often dropped in favor of implementing multiple therapies concurrently. This latter scenario is probably more in keeping with the practical issues faced in the real world and is one that is beginning to be examined in the literature. In 2009, Plint et al published a large double-blind, RCT examining the aggregate effects of epinephrine and dexamethasone on infants with bronchiolitis and demonstrated an unadjusted improvement only with combined therapy. [125] Despite a statistically insignificant effect when adjusted for multiple comparisons, the signal was noted in the subsequent Cochrane review released in 2010, but further evidence is needed. [126] Again, subjects in the Plint et al study were only moderate ill and it is possible that the described positive treatment effects would be more pronounced in children with serious illness. The answer to this question will continue to remain elusive due to the logistic barriers of enrolling children with severe disease into clinical trials.

The effect of disease severity was highlighted in an editorial [127] that critiqued the systematic review of interventions for infants with bronchiolitis requiring intensive care admission, published by Davison et al., in 2004. [124] The authors draw attention to variability in length of mechanical ventilation in the control groups which ranges from 5.26 days to 9.91 days and may be attributed to a number different factors such as differences in illness severity, in study populations and in standard care practices. [127]

Serial examination, attention to physiologic differences in disease presentation and clinical judgment, will continue to impact decision making in infants with severe respiratory distress, where simultaneous application of multiple therapies occurs. Additionally, resource limitations inherent within emergency departments of community hospitals are important considerations in any clinical pathway or guideline, and need to be factored into clinical decisions regarding patient care. Continuous positive airway pressure, heliox and in some cases hypertonic saline are not readily available in all centers. When children present with severe respiratory distress and require inter-facility transport, trials of therapy which have questionable benefit but are easy to administer in a smaller institution, may play a vital part in determining whether some children can be safely transported without a definitive airway.

The objective of this section is to examine the evidence regarding treatment modalities for RSV infections up to and including non-invasive and invasive ventilatory strategies. While the overall structure will default to examining interventions individually and sequentially, an equally important objective is to maintain a clinical context, recognizing the heterogeneous and dynamic nature of this disease.

In keeping with this latter objective, an integrated practical approach to treatment will be incorporated into the discussion where combined therapies may achieve a greater result than might be expected from individual therapies alone.

Nebulized Therapy

Traditionally many reviews of bronchiolitis treatment begin with a category labeled 'bronchodilators', and include within it β-agonists, epinephrine and sometimes ipratropium. This classification essentially disregards what is known about the pathophysiology of bronchiolitis and that the possible benefit accrued from epinephrine in particular, may have as much to do with the upper airway as the bronchioles. [128]

From a practice perspective, therapies specifically pertaining to nebulization will be first summarized, and the proposed mechanism of action of each agent will be subsequently discussed. The agents that fall into this category include bronchodilators (β-agonists, ipratropium bromide), epinephrine, hypertonic saline, mucolytics, and steam inhalation.

Bronchodilators

The Cochrane Review of bronchodilators for bronchiolitis was recently updated as of March 2010. [129] This systematic review included 28 trials, totaling 1912 patients. Therapies were included only if they met the strict criteria as a bronchodilator, for example β-agonists and ipratropium bromide, where the mechanism of action is at the level of bronchiolar smooth muscle relaxation. The effect of adrenergic agents such as epinephrine on bronchiolitis, is discussed in a separate Cochrane publication [130] except for a small number of studies that were included in the original review. The cumulative effect of bronchodilators did not result in any differences in the rates of hospitalization, duration of hospitalization, oxygen saturation or time to resolution while at home. Many of the studies incorporated in the Cochrane review included children up to 2 years of age although more recent studies limited the age to 12 months. This observation is important because a number of studies confirm that a consistent risk factor for more serious disease progression and rate of admission to hospital and the PICU is a very young age at presentation, usually less than 2 months. [131] Excluding one study in the Cochrane review, where the data was not available, 13 studies accounted for 975 patients (51%),whose mean age was < 6 months. In only 2 of the studies, 94 patients (5%) of the total recruitment had a mean age ≤ 3months. For the front line clinician, an infant aged <3 months, presenting with RSV-related illness, represents a very different risk category than a child aged 18–24 months. Future stratification of the data into more relevant age categories will provide more useful information to facilitate clinical decision making. Caution should be exercised regarding over-generalization of the results to the youngest patients who present with RSV disease. This observation reinforces the AAP recommendation of a single trial of inhaled bronchodilator therapy, and that ongoing use should be guided by the clinical response and balanced against adverse effects in cases where the benefit is marginal. [120] It is not surprising that β-agonist therapy has failed to demonstrate any significant benefit. As a number of authors have indicated, the wheeze exhibited by most children with bronchiolitis is not the result of reversible, smooth muscle mediated bronchoconstriction, but instead due to mucosal edema, mucous plugging and epithelial debris that can lead to airway obstruction. [36,121] The physiology supporting this observation was tested in a small study of infants with mild bronchiolitis in whom the ratio of time to achieve peak tidal exploratory flow

(PTEF) over the total expiratory time (t_e), as a measure of airflow obstruction, was no different in children treated with albuterol compared to 0.9% saline. [132]

Epinephrine

A Cochrane review of epinephrine in bronchiolitis, published in 2011, pooled results of 2256 children from 19 studies. Outpatients were significantly less likely to require hospital admission during the first day following treatment in the emergency department; however, this effect did not persist to day 7. [130] Additionally in comparison to the findings of the 2004 Cochrane Review of epinephrine in bronchiolitis [133], the inclusion of several new large high quality studies demonstrated a significant benefit on hospital length of stay for inpatient populations. This enhanced clinical effect compared to the β-agonists is likely explained by the additional α-adrenergic vasoconstriction of the airway mucosa and subsequent decreased airways resistance.

It has not been well characterized whether a greater influence on respiratory mechanics by this mechanism, can be attributed to the upper or lower airways. A small study of 65 infants with bronchiolitis examined the potential role of the nasal decongestant xylometazoline compared to nebulized epinephrine and found no difference between the two therapies. [128] The authors speculate that the two therapies may act in a similar way to reduce edema in the upper airways and nasal passages, and that perhaps nebulized epinephrine is more effective in the upper rather than lower airways. It is important to note that the effect of α-adrenergic stimulation in children with more severe disease, particularly in the cohort that progresses to hypoxic respiratory failure requiring intubation, is incompletely understood and the benefit highlighted in the Cochrane Review may therefore vary. In a small study of 15 mechanically ventilated infants with confirmed RSV respiratory tract infection, 6 of the patients exhibited deterioration in their oxygenation status, following treatment with nebulized epinephrine. [134] The authors theorize that non-specific bronchodilation resulted in exacerbation of ventilation-perfusion mismatching due to simultaneous vasoconstriction of pulmonary arterial vasculature. In such cases, where the clinical picture incorporates pulmonary parenchymal disease, which may be partially quantified by chest radiography, a similar approach to the AAP recommendation for bronchodilators may be the most appropriate. A single trial of epinephrine should be administered with ongoing doses guided by the clinical response. [120]

Hypertonic Saline

The mechanism of action of hypertonic saline is likely multifactorial with effects exerted both on enhanced mucous clearance and reduction of airway mucosal edema. Osmotic fluid shifts driven by the increased tonicity may principally lead to rehydration of inspissated mucous plugs and removal of water from the mucosa and submucosa. [122,135,136] Hypertonic saline may also enhance mucociliary clearance in patients with cystic fibrosis, but it is unclear if this effect is applicable to acute respiratory illness associated with RSV bronchiolitis. [136] A recent Cochrane Review that incorporated literature up to June of 2010, examined 581 infants with mild to moderate bronchiolitis across 7 clinical trials. Admitted infants treated with 3% saline compared to 0.9% saline had significantly shorter hospital length of stay, and post-treatment clinical scores were reduced for both inpatients and outpatients. [137] Two recent RCTs included in the Cochrane Review evaluated nebulized epinephrine combined with hypertonic saline in an emergency department setting and found no difference with combination therapy. However the trials were of reasonably small size (n=46 and n=186) and the clinical scores reflected infants with mild distress in one study and moderate respiratory distress in the other. [138,139]

The most concerning potential side effect of nebulized hypertonic saline is the triggering of acute bronchospasm which the Cochrane Review was unable to appraise because most of the included studies combined the dose with a bronchodilator or epinephrine. [137] Although the authors conclude that the addition of a bronchodilator is reasonable to avoid possible bronchospasm, selecting epinephrine for this purpose to capitalize on any synergistic effect the two agents may have on bronchiolitis pathophysiology is a more valid recommendation. Finally, hypertonic saline is usually readily available in larger centers but in smaller or rural community hospitals it may be either unavailable or difficult to access because of pharmacy regulations. Transport teams should become familiar with the use of hypertonic saline, due to the high incidence of respiratory illness including bronchiolitis that require transfer to tertiary centers from community hospitals for a higher level of care. [140]

Mucolytics

Hypertonic saline is considered by some authors to be best classified as a mucolytic; however, as previously described its mechanism of action is complex with additional action on the mucosa. Therefore, this section will focus on other agents, specifically recombinant human deoxyribonuclease (rhDNase). Recombinant DNase lyses DNA molecules that remain in the airway following breakdown of inflammatory cells that contribute to a greater viscosity of mucous plugs.

In the largest study examining the effects of rhDNase on infants with bronchiolitis, 225 children were randomized to receive either 2.5 mL of rhDNase or 0.9% saline twice daily. The effect on duration of oxygen requirement, admission to the intensive care unit or hospital length of stay was insignificant. [141]

Unfortunately, the patients enrolled in the study exhibited symptom scores representative of only mild disease and were therefore less likely to have large mucous plugs on which the rhDNase could act. In another RCT involving 75 infants, significant improvement on chest radiography was achieved in the group treated with rhDNase, although no difference in symptom scores or length of stay between the two groups was detected. [142] Other case reports also describe striking improvement in some patients with volume loss on chest radiography attributed to mucous plugging. [143] Ultimately, the evidence for mucolysis using rhDNase is inconclusive. It may be considered as rescue therapy in infants with moderate to severe disease who are at risk for respiratory failure, and have airspace disease on chest radiography that can be attributed to bronchiolar obstruction from mucous plugging.

Steam or Humidified Oxygen

The current literature evaluating steam or cool mist as an effective intervention for bronchiolitis is inconclusive. A Cochrane Review published in 2011, included only one article of 156 children that failed to show a benefit from this intervention. Unfortunately there were a number of important methodological concerns with blinding and allocation during the course of the study. [144] The proposed mechanism of action is linked to hydration of mucous and improved airway clearance and the treatment strategy may have a role in under-resourced areas but further study is required.

Systemic Therapy

The agents grouped into this category have vastly different mechanisms of action, but they are therapeutically similar in that they are usually administered systemically. These include glucocorticoids, antibiotics, caffeine, leukotriene receptor antagonists, and intravenous anti-RSV monocolonal antibody. The notable exception is glucocorticoids for which both nebulized and inhaled preparations have been studied in this population. However a distinction between the routes of administration has not been made, as will be discussed later, and any potential treatment effect appears to be derived from systemic administration.

Glucocorticoids

The use of glucocorticoids in the treatment of bronchiolitis has been studied extensively. In the Cochrane Review on its use for acute viral bronchiolitis in infants and young children published in 2010, 91 studies were identified examining the use of steroids in this population, dating back to 1969. [126] An analysis of 17 RCTs, representing 2596 patients, failed to demonstrate any difference in hospital admission rates or hospital length of stay. The review included a large RCT published in 2007 that recruited 600 children with moderately severe disease and accounted for almost 25% of the total patients. [145] The infants in the treatment arm of the study received a single dose of 1mg/kg of oral dexamethasone and were no different in their rates of hospitalization, hospital length of stay, or clinical severity scores compared to the controls. A subsequent large study performed by Plint et al involving 800 patients with similar disease severity, examined the combined effects of oral dexamethasone and nebulized epinephrine using four treatment arms to separate the effects of combined therapy from steroid and epinephrine alone. [125] The study highlighted a decrease in hospital admissions at day seven following randomization only for the group of infants that received both dexamethasone and epinephrine, that was insignificant after controlling for the number of comparisons between the two groups. [125,126] The steroid intervention was different from the 2007 study because in addition to a 1mg/kg oral dose of dexamethasone administered in the emergency room, dexamethasone (0.6mg/kg dose) was continued daily for five days. The difference between single and multiple doses of dexamethasone was specifically evaluated in another study performed by Schuh et al, that randomized 125 patients to receive either a single dose of dexamethasone or a continued 4 additional daily dose regimen, and also showed no difference between the groups. [146] The uncorrected differences observed in the Plint trial are interesting, but should be viewed with caution as they were essentially insignificant. However, if they do represent a signal towards treatment benefit, it may suggest a role for synergistic treatment but further research of combination therapy is necessary to confirm positive outcomes.

Antibiotics

A number of retrospective studies have examined the relationship between bacterial co-infection in infants with bronchiolitis and observed very low incidences of bacteremia and severe bacterial infection. [147-149] In addition, a large prospective study evaluated the incidence of bacteremia and severe bacterial infections in 1248 febrile children less than 60 days of age presenting to eight pediatric emergency departments.[150] 269 infants with RSV infections had lower rates of bacteremia (1.1%), severe bacterial infection (7.0%), and urinary tract infections (5.4%) than those without RSV infection. [150] A Cochrane Review published in 2010 included only one RCT from 1966 and lead the authors to correctly conclude that no evidence exists to support the routine use of antibiotics for RSV-related illness. [151] The decision to start antibiotics lies in a clinician's assessment of the pre-test probability of an infant with bronchiolitis to possess a concomitant bacterial infection. While this assessment is influenced by prevalence data, it is also formulated based on clinical indices of bacterial infection and from previous experience in recognizing patterns of illness. It is important to appreciate the age of the population at risk and disease severity when relying on the literature to influence clinical decisions. All of the studies referred to above evaluated infants presenting to an emergency department or following admission to hospital, with one retrospective review actually excluding infants who were admitted to the PICU. [149] When studies are limited to infants admitted to an intensive care setting, the incidence of concomitant severe bacterial infection increases dramatically with rates as high as 44%. [152]

In a prospective study of 165 mechanically ventilated children admitted to a PICU over three RSV seasons, endotracheal aspirates were positive at admission for bacterial isolates in 42% and identified to be community-acquired organisms in 83%. [152] The current AAP clinical practice guideline does not recommend routine use of antibiotics in febrile infants with bronchiolitis unless there is data to suggest a high suspicion (or pretest probability) of a bacterial infection which may occur with greater frequency in patients ill enough to require intensive care management. [120]

Caffeine

Apnea and bradypnea associated with bronchiolitis are risk factors for hospital admission [127] and they also predict which infants will fail non-invasive positive pressure ventilation [153] and those that require PICU admission. [131,154] Risk factors for apnea in infants with bronchiolitis that have been reported include age <2 months at presentation [131] and a history of prematurity. [155]

Methylxanthines such as caffeine have been well demonstrated to reduce the duration of mechanical ventilation in preterm infants with apnea and is generally well tolerated in this population. [156] Caffeine inhibits adenosine which in turn increases central respiratory drive and sensitivity to carbon dioxide. [155] Unfortunately, relatively few authors have examined the use of caffeine for the treatment of bronchiolitis. [157]

One retrospective study evaluated the use of caffeine in seven infants with bronchiolitis ranging in age from 14-64 days. After administering an intravenous dose of 10mg/kg of caffeine over 30 minutes, the episodes of apnea decreased significantly and none of the infants required intubation. [158] Although this intervention mandates further study, given the safety profile of caffeine in premature infants, its use in infants with bronchiolitis and apnea who are approaching intubation, is worth considering Additionally, caffeine in combination with other therapies such as heliox or CPAP may have synergistic effects not seen individually. The cardiovascular system manifestations and other consequences of caffeine therapy such as tachycardia, tremor and feeding intolerance may be augmented if epinephrine or bronchodilators have been previously administered. [155,156]

Leukotriene Receptor Antagonists

There is no evidence supporting the administration of leukotriene receptor antagonists in the treatment of acute bronchiolitis. [135] One study evaluated the use of montelukast for a three month period following hospitalization for bronchiolitis to prevent subsequent reactive airway disease and found no benefit. [159]

Intravenous Anti-RSV Monoclonal Antibody: Palivizumab and Motavizumab

In addition to its role in prophylaxis against RSV infection in high risk infants, the anti-RSV monoclonal antibody palivizumab has been investigated as a potential therapy to prevent progression to more severe disease in infants already infected with RSV. A number of systematic reviews have summarized the existing literature [124,160], the most recent of which was published in 2010 and included 1 case report, 4 case series, and 2 RCTs involving 136 patients. [160] The included small RCTs primarily examined previously well children with RSV infection and failed to demonstrate a difference in treatment outcomes between the groups. The remaining case series and case reports included patients with underlying complex diseases or those who were immunocompromised and they cumulatively exhibited a higher mortality rate in patients who received palivizumab, likely due to the severity of their disease at the time of initiation. [160]

Motavizumab is a newer anti-RSV monoclonal antibody identified to have greater potency than palivizumab in animal studies. [161,162] In addition to human studies on its effectiveness as an agent for RSV prophylaxis [163] it has also been evaluated as a treatment modality in patients with early RSV-related infection. In a small study examining the safety and antiviral activity of motavizumab, 31 previously well children confirmed to have RSV infection requiring hospitalization less than 24 hours into their illness, were randomized to receive intravenous motavizumab or placebo. [164] Patients who received motavizumab did not experience any adverse reactions attributed to the agent and demonstrated a significant reduction in the detection of RSV on nasal washings compared to placebo. Further clinical trials of motavizumab as therapy for infants already infected with RSV are required to determine if it will have similar or greater improvements on important clinical outcomes than palivizumab.

Therapy Requiring PICU Consultation and/or Admission

Probably as important as the interventions themselves are the risk factors that may predict the need for pediatric intensive care involvement and/or respiratory support. Although the advent of RSV prophylaxis has impacted the risk profile of infants requiring intensive care, even prior to the widespread use of palivizumab, a large proportion of infants requiring PICU admission and mechanical ventilation would not have been eligible for this preventive therapy. [165] In a large prospective survey of 11 PICUs in Israel during the 2000-2001 RSV season, 84% of all admissions and 91% of ventilated infants with RSV disease were not candidates for RSV prophylaxis. [165] The majority of children in this cohort were born >36 weeks gestation, had a median age of 2.3 months and did not have chronic lung disease. Apnea was a common feature and occurred in 32% of the infants. Prematurity [154,166], low birth weight [154] and underlying medical disorders such as chronic lung disease [166] and neuromuscular impairments [167] continue to be important risk factors for PICU admission. However, in otherwise healthy infants, recurring characteristics that appear to predict a more severe outcome are young age, apnea and presence of airspace disease on chest radiography. [168] Finally, a recent 5-year study that compared risk factors between 4285 infants hospitalized for bronchiolitis with and without RSV infection in the era after widespread implementation of RSV prophylaxis. Patients with RSV infection were at greater risk for more severe disease, need for PICU admission, intubation and hospital length of stay despite a lower rate of comorbidities. [169] Congenital heart disease, neuromuscular disorders, chronic respiratory conditions, prematurity and low weight were related to an increased risk of PICU admission and young age and prematurity were associated with a greater risk of intubation. [169]

The therapies usually linked in the literature to the need for PICU admission or consultation include; heliox, high-flow nasal prong oxygen therapy, CPAP, non-invasive positive pressure ventilation (NIPPV), invasive mechanical ventilation and administration of pulmonary surfactant. These are categorized as a group because the respective treatments are generally beyond the scope of practice of a general pediatrician or emergency medicine physician, although this may vary across institutions.

Heliox

The use of heliox has been described in a variety of respiratory conditions where an obstruction to airflow occurs either in the upper or lower airways. Examples of conditions documented in the literature with positive benefit include post-extubation stridor, croup, asthma as well as bronchiolitis. [170]The helium-oxygen mixture improves laminar flow of gases through the area of airway obstruction [170-172] and this is achieved because of the lower density of helium which can be explained using the physics described by the Reynolds

Number equation. [170] The effects from the lower density of helium can only be achieved when a disproportionately high ratio of helium to oxygen is used such as an 80:20, 70:30 or 60:40 mixture and are usually observed rapidly after administration. [170] The corollary of needing such an unbalanced mixture of gases is that patients who are already in need of an inspired concentration of oxygen greater than 30%-40% will usually not tolerate a trial of heliox due to oxygen desaturation. A recent Cochrane Review examined the role of heliox in bronchiolitis. [172] Four trials, representing 84 infants, were included in the meta-analysis which found a significant improvement in respiratory distress scores but no difference in rates of intubation, need for mechanical ventilation or ICU length of stay. One of the studies was particularly interesting because it evaluated the concomitant application of continuous positive airway pressure with either heliox or an air-oxygen mixture in infants with severe bronchiolitis who were refractory to standard therapy and nebulized epinephrine. [173] The study is limited by its small sample size of 12 patients, but it demonstrated a significant improvement in carbon dioxide clearance and in clinical score in infants who received heliox. Most of the available data does not support the routine use of heliox for the treatment of bronchiolitis, but it may have a role as part of combination therapy in critically ill children who require admission to the ICU.

High Flow Nasal Prong Therapy

There is growing evidence that application of high flow rates of humidified oxygen delivered to infants using nasal prongs may obviate the need for intubation and mechanical ventilation. [174,175] Two retrospective studies have demonstrated reductions in rates of intubation over time with increased use of high-flow nasal prong therapy [174,175] and one study showed a decreased PICU length of stay. [175] This system of oxygen delivery has been reported to achieve CPAP measurements of up to 4.8 cm H_2O. A recent unpublished study [176] measured the nasopharyngeal pressures achieved using heated, humidified, high flow nasal cannula (HHHFNC) and found a significant improvement in respiratory scores at a mean nasopharyngeal pressure of 3.4 cm H_2O that was achieved at approximately 8L/min of flow. A linear correlation was found between the flow and pressure up to 6L/min which resulted in 2.7 cm H_2O of nasopharyngeal pressure and was easier to achieve when the infants' mouths were closed. High flow nasal prong therapy may represent an effective strategy to prevent intubation and stabilize children who require transfer to an ICU setting from the emergency room or from another institution and merits further evidence before adoption.

Non-Invasive Positive Pressure Support

A number of different modes of non-invasive positive pressure support have been evaluated for the treatment of bronchiolitis and include continuous positive airway pressure (CPAP), continuous negative extrathoracic pressure, and non-invasive positive pressure ventilation (NIPPV). High flow nasal prong therapy perhaps should have been included in this section because nasopharyngeal pressures similar to a more conventional CPAP device can be achieved by this method.

CPAP has been shown to dramatically reduce respiratory muscle overload in infants with bronchiolitis. [59] Direct measurement of inspiratory effort using esophageal pressure monitors was performed in twelve infants aged less than 3 months by Cambonie et al [177] and demonstrated a greater than 50% decrease in esophageal pressure swings, an almost 60% reduction in respiratory effort and a significant improvement in the degree of respiratory distress. CPAP also maintains airway patency, facilitates better secretion clearance, improves gas exchange [154] and reduces the incidence of apnea which is a known risk factor for PICU admission and mechanical ventilation. [178] Additionally, infants with bronchiolitis appear to benefit greater from CPAP when it is applied earlier in the course of illness as evidenced by improved carbon dioxide clearance. [179]

Increasing experience in the use of NIPPV in pediatric critical care and specifically in patients with bronchiolitis is being described in the literature. Essouri et al reported an increase in the use of NIPPV from 0.45% to 7% over a five year period among a denominator of 3124 patients admitted to their PICU. The intervention was most commonly used in patients with respiratory failure post extubation, community acquired pneumonia and respiratory failure in those who were immunocompromised. [180] In another study comparing NIPPV to invasive ventilation specifically in 87 infants with bronchiolitis over two RSV seasons, found a dramatically reduced need for intubation and consequently a markedly reduced rate of ventilation associated pneumonia in the NIPPV group. [181] Similarly, in a RCT of 50 children with acute respiratory failure of whom the majority had bronchiolitis, the rate of intubation was decreased by 47% although the PICU and hospital length of stays were not different. [182] Patients most likely to fail a trial of NIPPV are those of young age and lower weight, poorer early respiratory rate decrease after implementation, and infants who are hypoxic with evidence of airspace disease on chest radiography. [153]

A Cochrane Review on the use of continuous negative extrathoracic pressure (CNEP) and CPAP was published in 2010 but only included one small study on the use of CNEP in 33 infants with bronchiolitis. The authors concluded that the current literature fell short of well designed studies. While there was reported benefit on oxygenation in the study, it was compared to a control group without intervention and it is unknown if the patients receiving CNEP also received a small amount of nasal CPAP to prevent upper airway obstruction as is described in other reports. [183] This is extremely important, as described earlier in this chapter, because patency of the upper airway likely plays a key role in the pathophysiology of bronchiolitis. Some authors postulate that the improved upper airway patency results in a greater reduction in the respiratory work of breathing when CPAP is applied with a nasal device instead of a face mask. [168]

In the approach to any mode of non-invasive positive pressure, care should be exercised when deciding which patients are the best candidates for a trial of this intervention. Patients with severe potentially life threatening hypoxia, acute upper airway obstruction, loss of airway protective reflexes, significantly depressed level of consciousness, anatomic facial abnormalities or who are hemodynamically unstable may warrant proceeding directly to endotracheal intubation and mechanical ventilation. [184] Given the increased use of CPAP and NIPPV in neonatal preterm populations [185,186], many non-tertiary hospitals with level 2 care facilities will likely have access to these therapies. This may facilitate clinical stabilization and either prevent the need for intubation or at least allow for a more controlled intubation procedure if anesthetic support is required.

Invasive Mechanical Ventilation

The proportion of patients requiring mechanical ventilation is highly variable and is dependent on whether the reported rates are derived in an era before or after implementation of palivizumab prophylaxis. For example, a large prospective observational study in Canada involving nine pediatric tertiary care hospitals in the early 1990's, demonstrated a mechanical ventilation rate ranging from 3-14% and up to 21% in high risk patients with RSV bronchiolitis. [187] More recent authors report mechanical ventilation rates ranging from 1.7% [188] to 8% [154] and increases as high as 25% in patients admitted to a PICU with RSV LRTI. [189] Following ventilation, infants with a lower gestational age, a history of bronchopulmonary dysplasia, and who are colonized with bacteria endotracheally, are at risk of needing a longer duration of mechanical ventilation. [166]

Currently there is neither consensus on an optimal ventilation strategy nor is there any evidence that any particular mode of ventilation is superior to another for infants with bronchiolitis. [188] There are many reasons why this might be the case, the most obvious being related to different underlying patient comorbidities, a higher incidence of concomitant bacterial infection in infants requiring mechanical ventilation, and the degree to which different viral pathogens may progress to hypoxic respiratory failure, such as acute respiratory distress syndrome (ARDS). [190] Moreover, open lung ventilation strategies that one might use in a patient with ARDS [191,192] where pulmonary compliance is poor are counterintuitive in a patient whose underlying physiology is defined by bronchial obstruction and hyperinflation. [188,189] In light of this, high frequency oscillatory ventilation (HFOV) using moderately high initial mean airway pressures has been demonstrated to be well tolerated and result in improved oxygenation and carbon dioxide clearance in infants with RSV. [189] Ultimately, when selecting a mode of ventilation, the underlying physiology of the individual patient needs to be well understood. It is equally important to appreciate that dynamic change secondary to disease progression, mucous plugging, secondary community acquired or nosocomial bacterial infection, and adverse patient ventilator interactions, require ongoing serial reassessment.

Pulmonary Surfactant

A discussion about surfactant therapy is typically reserved for interventions involving the management of ARDS which is beyond the scope of this chapter. Surfactant has garnered special mention due to a number of studies that suggest a specific role for its use in the pathophysiology of surfactant deficiency that occurs in patients with RSV infection. [193] Surfactant proteins A and D (SP-A, SP-D) have been demonstrated to play an important part in the clearance of the virus and uptake by antigen-presenting cells such as macrophages and monocytes. [193] RSV selectively targets the destruction of type II pneumocytes causing impairment of both surfactant synthesis and release. [193] The consequence is not only an impaired immunologic defense to the virus but also a loss of surfactant that is integral to the process of alveolar collapse during expiration. [193] The potential effect of surfactant replacement therapy in pediatric acute respiratory failure has been reviewed in a meta-analysis published by Duffet et al in 2007. [194] The study included six trials totaling 314 patients, two of which recruited patients with RSV only and the remaining studies reported

RSV rates from 7-17%. Overall treatment was associated with a reduction in ventilator free days, duration of mechanical ventilation and a reduction in mortality.

Miscellaneous

The following therapies are those that did not fit neatly into any of the three categories of therapy described above and include chest physiotherapy and antiviral therapy such as ribavirine.

Chest Physiotherapy

A Cochrane Review published in 2008 examined the role of chest physiotherapy in bronchiolitis. [195] The review included 3 RCTs that enrolled 172 patients and was unable to demonstrate any combined effect favoring the use of chest physiotherapy on clinical scores or hospital length of stay. None of the children in any of the studies required mechanical ventilation and so the benefit of chest physiotherapy in this population is essentially unanswered. Since this review, one RCT of 496 non-ventilated infants was performed, evaluating an increased exhalation technique with assisted cough compared to a control intervention of gentle nasal suctioning and found no differences between the two groups except for an increased rate of respiratory destabilization and vomiting in the treatment group. [196]

Antiviral Therapy

The identification of a successful antiviral therapy against RSV has been both disappointing and promising, beginning with ribavirin. Ribavirin is a guanosine analog that provides activity against RSV and is the only approved antiviral available, although it is rarely used. [197] A systematic review of 10 RCTs of varying degrees of quality was published in 2004 and failed to find any benefit of ribavirin on any significant clinical outcomes. [198] Furthermore, the AAP recommended in their 2006 guideline that ribavirin should not be used routinely due to the lack of treatment effect and cited cumbersome delivery devices, potential risks to caregivers and high costs as additional reasons to avoid its use. [120] Ribavarin has been included in this chapter because it may have a limited role in immunocompromised patients with documented RSV infection [120] or against other selected viral pathogens. [199, 200]

The search for the next generation of antiviral agents has lead to a number of potential therapies including small interfering RNA molecules (siRNA) [162,201,202] and a novel benzodiazepine with anti-RSV activity. [162] Small interfering RNA molecules decrease the expression of viral proteins by targeted cleavage of the associated RSV messenger RNA (mRNA). [202] DeVincenzo et al evaluated a nasal spray preparation of siRNA molecules called ALN-RSV01 in a RCT in 88 healthy adults infected with RSV and found a 38% decrease in the culture identification of RSV. [202]The study was underpowered to detect any change in the viral load or clinical symptoms between groups but is encouraging for further studies using this agent. In addition to ALN-RSV01 a number of other small molecule antiviral therapies are currently in development or under investigation [201] and represent a potential paradigm shift in the treatment of RSV infection.

COMMENTARY ON RSV AND BRONCHIOLITIS TREATMENT

Bronchiolitis continues to be a major cause of acute respiratory illness requiring hospitalization for many infants. Despite the widespread adoption of prophylaxis which will be discussed in the following section on RSV prevention, rates of hospitalization and PICU admission continue to increase and may be partly related to the high proportion of young term infants who do not fulfill criteria for prophylaxis or perhaps due to changing virulence patterns of the virus. [169] The recommendation for supportive care using oxygen and fluids alone is often the conclusion provided by many reviews on the subject, citing lack of definitive evidence for other interventions combined with a low incidence of morbidity and mortality in this otherwise healthy population. [135,198] However, the results of the most recent Cochrane Reviews on epinephrine and hypertonic saline [137] were not included in these papers. Nonetheless, the underlying principle is the same; most of the existing literature is generalizable only to patients with mild or moderate illness. The question as to what frontline healthcare providers should routinely do when confronted with an infant with severe RSV-related illness remains unanswered. While navigating available therapies that one might use in this cohort, it is important to have an in-depth understanding of the respiratory physiology displayed by the patient, irrespective of whether the disease is predominantly in the upper or lower airways or parenchymal airspaces. This chapter has provided some insight into where combination therapy may be useful but these decisions need to be carefully tailored individually to the patient with an awareness of available resources if considering interventions such as hypertonic saline, heliox, high flow nasal prong therapy, or CPAP. Future research is needed into the use of combination therapies that may be more reflective of clinical practice for patients with severe bronchiolitis. A suggested practical approach to these interventions is provided in Figure 4 and is intended to provide guidance regarding the management of the patient who has severe disease and does not immediately meet criteria for invasive mechanical ventilation. An approach to infants with mild to moderate disease severity has already been well summarized by other authors [135,198] and is reflected in the existing AAP guidelines. [120]

1st Line

Supportive care including oxygen therapy and fluids
Clinical assessment before and after nasal suctioning*
Trial of nebulized epinephrine combined with hypertonic saline
Additional biochemical and radiographic assessment to evaluate risk of concurrent bacterial infection and degree of parenchymal lung disease
Start antibiotics if specific indications are present according to existing guidelines

2nd Line

Assess chest x-ray:

- If significant air-space in keeping with mucous plugging and atelectasis consider a trial of nebulized DNase

Is apnea a prominent feature of the disease presentation?

- If yes, consider a trial of intravenous caffeine if no contraindication

3rd Line **Consultation with PICU**

Trial of high flow humidified nasal prong oxygen if available

Trial of continuous positive airway pressure or non-invasive positive pressure ventilation if no contraindications

Consider heliox as an adjunct if available

Prepare for potential need for intubation and mechanical ventilation in patients with known risk factors

*Nasal suctioning with clinical reassessment should be considered in conjunction with any intervention that requires a patent nasal or nasopharyngeal airway

Figure 4. Suggested approach to patients with a severe presentation of bronchiolitis.

Respiratory Syncytial Virus: Prevention

RSV infected individuals shed large amounts of virus in saliva and nasopharyngeal secretions and the portal of entry is via the membranous linings of the respiratory mucosa. Infants with active lower respiratory tract disease may continually shed virus for up to 21 days and the virus survives on the skin, porous and non-porous surfaces for several hours, facilitating both direct and indirect transmission. [203-206] The mainstay of prevention is rigorous hand washing with soap and water or alcohol-based solutions and the evidence stems from several, cluster-randomized controlled trials involving 2077 patients. [207] A recent Cochrane review recommends a three-pronged intervention approach to reduce transmission of respiratory viruses in children; frequent hand washing, the use of gowns, gloves and masks, and hospital isolation of suspected cases. [208] In a prospective controlled study of 4 preventive strategies to control RSV nosocomial infection, the combination of rapid laboratory diagnosis, cohort nursing, and the use of gowns and gloves was highly effective. [209] Control of nosocomial transmission of RSV infection with the use of these hygienic measures has also been demonstrated to be successful and cost-effective in several other studies. [210-212]

A major breakthrough in the primary prevention of RSV infection was realized when intravenous RSV immune globulin (RSV-IGIV) became available. The product was a human-derived polyclonal immunoglobulin that was enriched with neutralizing antibody to RSV and offered passive immunity at a monthly dose of 750mg/kg. The efficacy of RSV-IGIV was shown in a large scale, randomized double-blind, placebo-controlled trial involving 510 infants who were premature or had broncho-pulmonary dysplasia (BPD). The incidence of RSV hospitalization and severity of illness was reduced by 41% with a concurrent 38% reduction in hospitalization for respiratory illness of any cause. [213] In a second study, children less than 4years of age with congenital heart disease were randomly assigned to receive RSV-IGIV or placebo. [214] There was an overall 31%reduction in RSV hospitalizations in the RSV-IGIV group but with a significantly higher occurrence of cyanotic episodes and poorer outcomes post surgery in the infants with cyanotic heart lesions (28% versus 8.5%; p=0.009). The product was never sanctioned for general use in Europe and lost favor because it was a product which posed a risk of transmitting blood-borne pathogens, had a high viscosity and required intravenous administration over 3 hours with potentially serious side-effects in children with cyanotic heart disease.

The next landmark in RSV disease prevention was established with the release of palivizumab, a humanized, genetically-engineered monoclonal antibody which was produced by recombinant DNA technology. The developed chimeric molecule involved grafting of an antigenic recognition site derived from a murine monoclonal antibody onto a human immunoglobulin framework. As addressed earlier in this chapter, RSV is composed of approximately 10 surface proteins of which the F (fusion) and G (attachment) glycoproteins are the major targets of neutralizing antibodies. [215] The F protein enables fusion with other respiratory epithelial and infected cells through syncytial formation, resulting in the pathological hallmark of the multinucleate giant cell. Palivizumab targets and binds to an epitope in the A antigenic site of the F protein and disrupts fusion of infected cells, reduces viral activity and thereby cell to cell transmission of RSV. In key laboratory studies, Johnson et al first demonstrated effective neutralization of 57 clinical isolates of RSV A and B subtypes by palivizumab and subsequently showed its efficacy in the cotton rat with a dose of 2.5mg/kg that achieved 99% reduction of lung RSV titres at an optimum serum concentration of 25-30μg/mL. [216] More importantly in a conducted series of experiments palivizumab did not augment viral replication or lung pathology during subsequent exposure to RSV. [216] This set the stage for the Phase I-II clinical trials to evaluate the tolerance, safety, immunogenicity and pharmacokinetics of monthly doses of palivizumab (15mg/kg) in premature infants ≤35 weeks gestational age (GA) and those with BPD. [217,218] These studies confirmed safety and protection against RSV with mean serum concentrations of 40μg/ml that were similar to those achieved in the cotton rat.

This was followed by a large, multicenter, randomized double-blind, placebo-controlled study (IMpact) from 1996-1997, involving 139 sites in the USA, Canada and the United Kingdom. [219] 1502 patients who were premature (≤35 weeks GA and aged <6 months) or were <2 years with BPD, were allocated to 5 monthly injections of palivizumab (15mg/kg) or placebo during the RSV season. Overall there was a statistically significant 55% reduction in the primary endpoint of RSV hospitalization (p=0.004). The overall reductions in hospitalization in the subgroups ranged from 39% in infants with BPD to 82% in 32-35weeks' GA infants without BPD. Infants who received palivizumab also had significantly fewer total days of hospitalization, days with increased oxygen and days with a lower respiratory illness score ≥3 (all p<0.001). Adverse events were similar in both the treatment and placebo arms of the clinical trial. A second, similar randomized trial was launched to investigate the efficacy of palivizumab in 1287 patients with hemodynamically significant congenital heart disease. [220] Enrolled infants were stratified by site and by cyanotic or acyanotic lesions. Treated patients experienced a 45% relative reduction in RSV hospitalizations with identical improvements in secondary endpoints as patients in the IMpact study. There was a 29% reduction in RSV hospitalizations in the cyanotic group compared to 58% in the acyanotic strata. Mean serum palivizumab levels were protective but there was a 58% reduction in serum palivizumab concentrations after bypass surgery which has implications for re-treatment following the procedure. Unlike RSV-IGIV, the tolerance, safety and protective profile of palivizumab was superior.

Data from the IMpact and congenital heart disease trials led to approval of palivizumab by the USA Food and Drug Administration and the European Medicines Evaluation Agencies (EMEA) and RSV prophylaxis was rapidly adopted and recommended in pediatric position statements in the USA, Canada and across Europe. [221-226] Indications for the use of palivizumab broadly comprise: 1) Premature infants ≤32 weeks GA who are <6 months at the start of the RSV season 2) Infants aged <2 years with hemodynamically significant cyanotic or acyanotic congenital heart disease and 3) Infants <2 years with BPD who require oxygen or medical therapy 6 months prior to the onset of the RSV season. The original IMpact study enrolled premature infants ≤35 weeks gestation and demonstrated an approximately 80% reduction in RSV hospitalizations in infants from 32-35 weeks gestational age. However, the universal use of palivizumab in this population which comprises 5-7.5% of the North American birth cohort has been restrictive because of high product costs (CAN$752.26 for 50mg vial and CAN$1504.51for 100mg). Cost-effectiveness will be discussed later in this chapter.

RSV Infection in Special Populations

33-35 Week GA Infants

Infants who are born at 33-35 completed weeks GA (33 weeks and 0 days to 35 weeks and 6 days) are not routinely targeted for RSV prophylaxis unless they have specific risk factors that make them more prone to severe RSV illness. Overall, RSV hospitalizations in premature infants are similar irrespective of gestational age. In a retrospective study of infants aged ≤3 years enrolled in the Tennessee Medicaid from July 1989-Jun 1993, hospitalizations per 1000 child-years of the RSV season were 187.5, 163.6, 159.6 for infants <28 weeks, 29-32 weeks and 33-35 weeks respectively. [227] Several studies have reported higher morbidities, healthcare resource utilization during and post RSV hospitalization and increased mortality in infants 33-35 weeks compared to term infants. [228-230]. In a retrospective analsis, Horn et al used a disease-specific comprehensive severity index to compare the outcomes of 304 premature infants hospitalized with RSV illness in 9 USA hospitals. [228] Infants who were 33-35 weeks GA had significantly higher ICU admissions (P=0.023), increased likelihood of intubation (P=0.001) and had longer ICU length of stay (P=0.003). The overall hospital length of stay for infants <32 weeks and 33-35 weeks was also significantly longer (P≤0.001). The authors concluded that the outcomes of infants 33-35 weeks GA were at best similar or worse than their counterparts <32 weeks. A second study on 684 infants in 10 USA hospitals demonstrated higher hospital resource use, costs and complication rates for infants 33-35 weeks GA admitted with RSV infection compared to premature babies <32 weeks. [229] In a Canadian nested case-control study, 2415 preterm infants 32-35 weeks GA hospitalized with proven or probable RSV infection were matched to 20,254 control infants by GA, gender and birth province and were followed for a mean duration of 2.1 years. [230] Healthcare resource utilization parameters after the index admission including number of hospitalizations, visits to the special care unit, respiratory therapist and outpatient department, physician consults and number of procedures performed were significantly higher in infected infants (P<0.001). Of note, the total mortality in RSV hospitalized infants was 5-fold higher and there was a 20-fold increase in sudden or unexplained death. While the mortality rates in the Sampalis study [230] appeared relatively high, it is important to appreciate that this cohort of infants comprises late preterm infants, a group which has become increasingly recognized to also be at a significant base-line risk for morbidity and have been documented to have 2.9-4.5 times higher neonatal and infant mortality rates than term infants. [231, 232]

Why are 33-35 week GA infants at greater risk for RSV infection and are there specific risk factors that enhance their susceptibility to disease? This group of infants is born at a critical period of lung development when the formation of alveoli accelerates with concurrent increases in bronchiolar and alveolar diameter and total lung surface area. [233] Jones et al have carefully evaluated the impact of uncomplicated prematurity on lung function. During the first year of life, healthy preterm infants show a significant reduction in forced expiratory flow compared to full-term controls and this was impacted by low GA, male gender, smoke exposure and increased weight gain. This finding was sustained in the second year of life in the presence of normal forced vital capacity implicating alterations in lung development as the root cause for lower lung function. [234-236] It is likely that the interruption of lung development coupled with inadequate adaptive immune responses, contribute significantly to RSV disease severity in these infants. Welliver et al demonstrated that infants surviving RSV LRTI had low levels of T lymphocyte specific cytokines in respiratory secretions, and lymphocytes expressing CD4 or CD8 antigen were also reduced in lung tissue. In cases of severe bronchiolitis, viral clearance is therefore relegated to suboptimal innate immune responses generated by macrophages and neutrophils instead of normal cytotoxic T lymphocyte responses which may strongly influence survival. [237] Moreover, 32-35 week GA infants are disadvantaged by an immature immune system at birth and have only half the complement of IgG levels (520mg/100mL) than term infants (1100mg/100mL). [238] Postnatally, plasma IgG levels continue to decline reaching a nadir at 3-6 months and most premature infants remain hypogamma-globulinemic at 6 months of age. This increases their propensity for infection and after discharge from the nursery 43 preterm infants followed until 10 months chronological age had a significantly higher incidence of infections than 41 term infants ($P = 0.04$). [239]

Several risk factors have been identified in 33-35 week GA infants that increase the relative risk for RSV infection and hospitalization. A multicenter, prospective, observational cohort study conducted by the **P**ediatric **I**nvestigators **C**ollaborative **N**etwork on **I**nfections in **C**anada (PICNIC) from 2001-2003 across 16 Canadian centers, analyzed 66 hospitalized infants with proven RSV infection versus 1692 infants with no respiratory tract infection. [27] Eight risk factors were independently predictive of RSV hospitalization; birth month (November, December or January; $P<0.001$), male gender ($P=0.02$), small for GA (birth weight $<10^{th}$ percentile; $P=0.019$), subject attending day care ($P=0.002$), preschool age siblings ($P=0.001$), ≥ 2 smokers in the household ($P=0.064$), >5 individuals in the household counting the subject ($P=0.088$) and eczema in 1st degree relatives ($P=0.049$), the latter of which was found to be protective. A retrospective, case-control study of the risk factors linked to RSV hospitalization in 33-35 week GA infants, was performed in 50 Spanish hospitals that enrolled 186 cases hospitalized with RSV from October 2002-April 2003 and 371 controls selected in June 2003. [240] Five variables (odds ratio; 95% confidence intervals) predicted RSV hospitalization; birth from July to December (3.95; 2.65, 5.90), breast feeding ≤ 2 months (3.26; 1.96, 5.42), ≥ 1 school age sibling (2.85; 1.88, 4.33), ≥ 4 individuals in the home (1.91; 1.19, 3.07) and history of wheezing in the family (1.90; 1.19, 3.01). The risk of hospitalization increased 3.6-fold for infants with 2 or more risk factors. Although the methodological design of these two studies [27, 240] was different, the risk factors that determined outcome were similar [241] [Figure 5]. A prospective double cohort study was subsequently conducted in Spain during the 2005-2006 and 2006-2007 RSV seasons to validate the results of their previous case-control study. The analysis comprised 202 infants hospitalized with RSV and 5239 controls. Only 3 independent risk factors were predictive of RSV infection and subsequent hospitalization; chronologic age of ≤10 weeks at the start of the RSV season, school-age siblings or day care attendance and smoking during pregnancy. [242] Several other reports that incorporate but have not specifically studied 33-35 week GA infants as a single cohort, have additionally confirmed the contribution of similar risk factors found in the Spanish and Canadian data towards RSV hospitalization. [243, 244]

Spanish Study (FLIP)[1,2]		Canadian Study (PICNIC)[3]	
Risk Factors	Odds Ratio (P-value)	Risk Factors	Odds Ratio (P-value)
*Chronological age at start of the RSV season ≤10 weeks	3.95 (p<0.001)	†Born Nov, Dec or Jan	4.88 (p<0.001)
*≥1 school-age siblings	2.85 (p<0.001)	Pre-school age siblings	2.76 (p<0.001)
≥4 residents or visitors	1.91 (p<0.007)	† ≥5 individuals in the home	1.69 (p=0.088)
*Male gender	1.43 (p=0.05)	†Male gender	1.91 (p=0.02)
*Family history (FH) of Atopy *FH of wheezing	1.90 (p=0.068)	†Eczema in 1st degree Relatives	0.42 (p=0.04)
Smoking not a risk factor. During the study Smoking decreased from 52% to 30%		† ≥2 smokers in the household	1.71 (p=0.064)
*Breast feeding <2 months	3.26 (p<0.001)	†Daycare attendance	12.32 (p=0.002)
*Birth Weight	(p=0.042)	†Small for gestational age	2.19 (p=0.019)

*Risk factors utilized in the European Model[2] and †Canadian (PICNIC) model[4]
Shaded area indicates similarities between models.

1) Figueras-Aloy J et al. Pediatr Infect Dis J 2004; 23:815-820. (Ref: 240)
2) Simoes EA. et al. Respir Res 2008; 9:78. (Ref: 246)
3) Law BJ et al. Pediatr Infect Dis J 2004; 23:806-14. (Ref: 28)
4) Sampalis J et al. Med Decis Making 2008; 28:471-480. (Ref: 245)

Figure 5. Risk Factors for RSV hospitalization in 33-35 weeks' gestational age infants – FLIP versus PICNIC studies.

The risk factors in the Canadian and Spanish studies have been used to develop robust tools to best predict RSV hospitalization and target RSV prophylaxis cost-effectively at 33-35week GA infants, who are at moderate to high risk for serious RSV infection. In the Canadian risk scoring tool, 7 dominant risk factors [Figure 5] were included in the final regression model and were each assigned a RSV hospitalization weight, which was then converted into a variable score, the sum of which totaled 100. [245] Receiver operator characteristic (ROC) curve analysis was used to determine the total score that best predicted

RSV hospitalization and cutoff values for low risk (score 0-48), moderate risk (49-64) and high risk were established. [Figure 6]

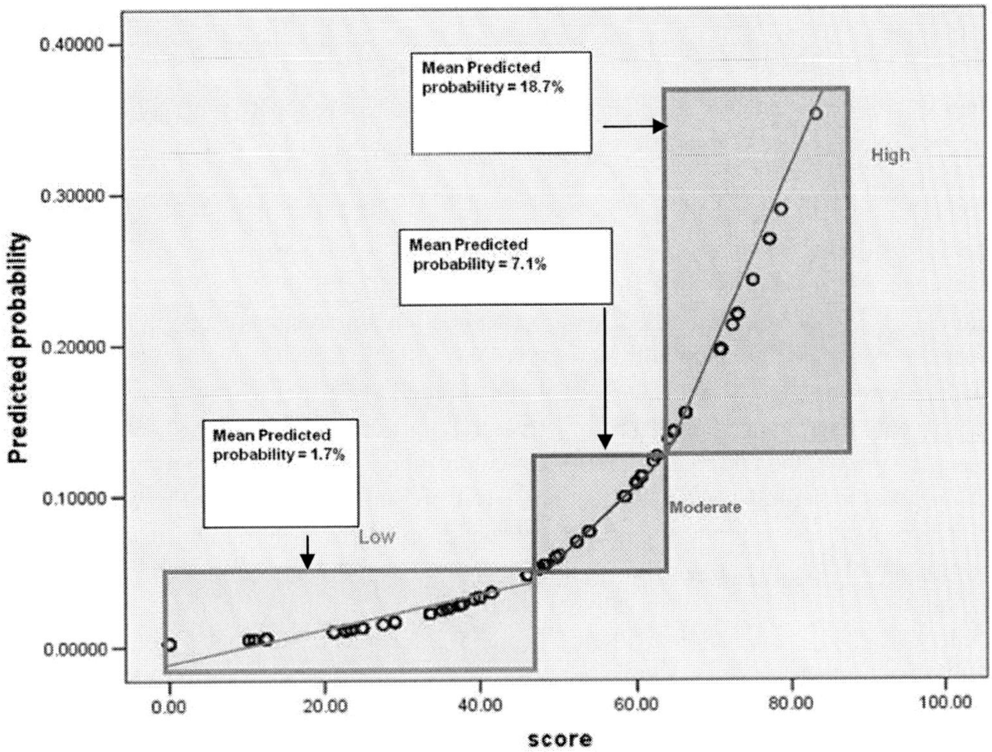

Reference: Sampalis JS et al. Med Decis Making 2008; 28:471-80. (Ref: 245)

Figure 6. Mean Predicted probability of RSV hospitalization (%) based on the Canadian Risk Scoring Tool. Low Risk (Score 0 – 48); Moderate Risk (Score 49 – 64); High Risk (Score 65 – 100).

The European risk scoring model [246] based on the Spanish FLIP (**F**actors that most **L**ikely may lead to development of RSV related respiratory **I**nfection and subsequent hospital admission among **P**remature infants) retrospective dataset [240] also consists of 7 variables. [Figure 5] The Canadian and European models have been validated against the Spanish [245], French [247] Danish [248] and Italian [249] populations with a correct 64%, 62%, 66% and 68% estimation of RSV hospitalization risk respectively. The impact of the Canadian risk scoring tool for 33-35 week GA infants has also been evaluated prospectively in a 3year study that recruited 430 infants. [250] 346 low risk infants (score 0-48) were not prophylaxed with palivizumab and 5 patients were hospitalized with RSV infection. 57 moderate risk patients (risk score 49-64) and 27 high risk infants (score 65-100) received prophylaxis and none were hospitalized. [250] The authors concluded that the risk scoring tool could be employed judiciously to single out moderate to high risk infants for palivizumab while cost-effectively avoiding prophylaxis in almost 82% of this cohort who are at low risk for RSV infection.

While the Canadian Paediatric Society recommends the use of the risk scoring tool to guide prophylaxis in 33-35week GA infants based on provincial decisions [225], in Spain the current guideline targets infants with 2 major risk factors: 1) chronological age < 10 weeks at the start of the RSV season or birth during the first 10 weeks or 2) sibling of school age or attending day-care. Infants with 1 major, and 2 minor risk factors, namely, mother smoking during pregnancy or male gender are also eligible for prophylaxis. [251] The American Academy of Pediatrics recommends prophylaxis only for infants younger than 3 months of age at the start of or birth during the RSV season with at least one of two risk factors; day care attendance or presence of siblings aged younger than five years. [226] The majority of countries worldwide are developing country-specific guidelines for RSV prophylaxis in 33-35 week GA infants based on local demographic and environmental risk factors that govern RSV hospitalization.

Cystic Fibrosis (CF)

The incidence of RSV infection in CF patients varies between 9-58% [252-254] and majority of LRTIs are associated with a decline in pulmonary function. [252,255,256] Newborns although asymptomatic may be colonized early with Staphylococcus aureus and Pseudomonas aeruginosa and have detectable inflammatory markers in their BAL profile coupled with radiological evidence of structural lung disease. [257] Synergism between respiratory viral infection and bacterial colonization is likely important in disease pathogenesis. Superimposed viral infections, occurring principally during the winter months, may correspond to the primary episode of Pseudomonas colonization and lead to recurrent exacerbations of pulmonary inflammation, increased respiratory symptoms and prolonged hospitalization. [258] In an observational study of 116 CF patients followed monthly for 8 months, 20% had exacerbations with non-bacterial infections of which 9% were due to RSV. [259] RSV infections occurred more commonly in patients who developed chronic Pseudomonas infection and was accompanied by a corresponding rise in Pseudomonas antibodies. CF mice inoculated with RSV show an amplified inflammatory response with raised neutrophils and lymphocytes in BAL fluid and decreased nitric oxide generation which may compromise RSV clearance. [260] Airway response to methacholine challenge was increased in mice infected with RSV signifying altered airway reactivity following viral exposure.

In two well conducted *in vitro* and *in vivo* experiments, RSV enhanced pseudomonas infection and this may occur asymptomatically. [261,262] Van Ewijk et al demonstrated conclusively that respiratory cell monolayers initially infected with RSV and then inoculated with pseudomonas increased Pseudomonas adherence to epithelial cells 1.2 to 8.2-fold. Simultaneous addition of RSV and pseudomonas further enhanced syncytial adherence 1.7 to 16.1-fold. [261] Vrankrijker et al infected mice intranasally with Pseudomonas some of which were co-inoculated with RSV. [262] Co-infected mice had decreased lung function manifested by reduced respiratory rates and lower minute ventilation. Histopathology of harvested lung tissue revealed a 2000-fold increase in Pseudomonas colony forming units compared to mice not infected with RSV.

RSV is also associated with similar morbidities in children with cystic fibrosis as demonstrated in the animal models. In a series of 16 children hospitalized with viral infections, predominantly RSV, 35% who were followed for 1-5 years acquired Pseudomonas compared with 6% of infants who were not hospitalized for respiratory symptoms. [263] Analysis of BAL fluid demonstrated a marked inflammatory response similar to the animal models with elevated neutrophil counts, proinflammatory cytokine IL-8, and free neutrophil elastase activity. Respiratory symptoms persisted after discharge and 71% required home oxygen therapy for 5 months. In two further CF studies, one descriptive [254] and the other case-control [256] RSV was found to pose significant short and long term morbidities. Patients who were hospitalized had prolonged lengths of hospital stay (mean duration 22 days), 43% were ventilated, 71% became newly dependent on home oxygen and developed more frequent chronic respiratory signs and lower chest radiographic scores compared to CF infants who were not infected with RSV ($P<0.05$). Following an RSV illness, 43% of CF patients developed more frequent lower respiratory tract infections, 23% were hospitalized and subsequently reduced airway function persisted for a mean of 3.2 months after the final episode of LRTI.

The evidence from bench laboratory research and theory favors the hypothesis that RSV infection early in infancy enhances pseudomonas colonization in CF patients which promotes inflammation, chronic infection, airway plugging, bronchiectasis, reduction in lung function and ultimately respiratory failure. Newborn screening for CF and early RSV immunization with palivizumab may together impact the burden of disease by reducing bacterial colonization and pulmonary CF exacerbations. Benefits in chronic lung disease (BPD) populations, not unlike CF patients, are also apparent from the IMpact trial. [219].

Down Syndrome

Children with Down syndrome are at increased risk for both upper and lower respiratory tract infections because of physiological and anatomical abnormalities. The facial structure defined by magnetic resonance imaging is characterized by mid-face and mandibular hypoplasia and the reduced upper airway size is caused by soft tissue crowding within a smaller mid- and lower face skeleton. [264,265] They have generalized hypotonia, glossoptosis, laryngomalacia and upper airway anomalies, adenoidal and tonsillar hypertrophy, swallowing dysfunction and gastroesophageal reflux which increase the risk of aspiration and subsequent pneumonia. [266-270] The lung architecture of infants with Down syndrome is also abnormal. Pathological findings include pulmonary hypoplasia with decreased terminal lung units, reduced number of alveoli in relation to acini, decreased total number of alveoli and abridged capillary and alveolar surface area which may contribute collectively to the risk of pulmonary hypertension. [271] Of note, the microscopic appearance of the alveoli reveals that they are characteristically large with dilated alveolar ducts and it is postulated that the mean radial count, an index of acinar complexity, is only 72% of the predicted value and the reduction occurs postnatally. [272] Down syndrome children are hospitalized frequently for lower respiratory tract infections, predominantly pneumonia (18%), bronchiolitis (7%) and croup (6.5%) [271,273] and incurred hospital costs for those without congenital heart disease is two to three times greater than normal children. [273] In part this may be due to abnormalities in cell numbers and function which entail innate and adaptive immunity. An increased number of proinflammatory monocytes or an intrinsic defect of the immune system may contribute to the severity of infective lung disease. [274-279] 395 Down syndrome subjects were enrolled in a retrospective (n=176) and prospective (n=219) cohort study, with 276 prospective sibling controls, that were used to estimate the relative risk of RSV hospitalization. [280] The incidence of hospitalization with RSV LRTI overall was 9.9% compared to 0.7% in controls. Premature infants < 37 weeks GA, infants with insignificant cardiac disease and those with significant cardiac disease had a 13.4-fold, 15.7 and 17-fold increased risk of RSV hospitalization respectively. Megged et al reviewed 41 RSV hospitalizations in Down syndrome patients in Jerusalem over a 9-year period. [281] The mean age at admission was 1.3 years and the mean length of hospital stay was 10.9 days. In a 7-year, matched control study conducted in Denmark of 313 pairs of infants with congenital heart disease, multivariate analysis predictors of RSV hospitalization included Down syndrome (odds ratio 3.24; 95% confidence intervals; 1.80-5.80). [282] It appears that infants with Down syndrome, irrespective of underlying congenital heart disease, have a cumulatively higher risk for RSV infection and subsequent hospitalization, based on aberrations in their anatomical and physiological profiles

Neuromuscular Disorders

Infants with neurological disorders especially those affected with serious muscle impairments, have a spectrum of gastrointestinal problems that place them at high risk for aspiration and subsequent lower respiratory tract illness. The medical conditions in this spectrum are diverse but distinctively involve either nerve, muscle or the neuromuscular junction or broadly encompass metabolic or endocrine problems that may be part of inherited chromosomal or non-chromosomal entities. In the majority, these children have oral motor dysfunction, uncoordinated swallowing, dysphagia, gut dysmotility and gastroesophageal reflux disease which impacts feeding patterns and are major risk factors for recurrent pneumonia [283,284]. Moreover, muscular weakness of the thoracic wall compromises coughing, impinges normal breathing because of impaired chest excursion, impacts expiratory airway flow and normal lung recoil and collectively enhances the potential for serious respiratory complications.

Several reports have investigated the impact of RSV infection in these children. In a Japanese survey of 756 children hospitalized with RSV infection, 16.5% had neuromuscular disease. 116 (95.1%) of the children had none or mild sequelae and there were 6 deaths (4.9%). [285] Thorburn et al [47] in their case series of 406 patients admitted to the PICU from 1999-2007, 18 deaths were reported, and 15% of the patients had neuromuscular disorders. In the Canadian PICNIC study which enrolled 156 patients with underlying pulmonary conditions, 6 patients with neurogenic disorders who had a mean age of 3.12 years were hospitalized with RSV infection, of which 50% required PICU care and 33% were ventilated. [286] An observational multicentre study conducted in Austria of RSV hospitalization in infants 29-32 weeks GA also reported that neurological disease doubled the risk of re-hospitalization (Odds ratio; 2.15; 95% confidence intervals, 0.77-5.25). [287]

In a large scale, prospective surveillance study incorporating 14 pediatric German institutions, 1541 children were admitted with RSV infection. [167] 73 (4.7%) had a neuromuscular impairment and 41 had at least one additional risk factor for severe RSV illness; prematurity (n=30), congenital heart disease (n=19), BPD (6) and immunodeficiency (8). 45.2% of the children were older than 2 years at the time of admission (median age of 14 months versus 5 months in the controls). Children with neuromuscular disorders had a higher risk of seizures (15.1% versus 1.6%) and their condition was significantly associated with PICU admission (Odds ratio 4.94; 95% Confidence intervals, 2.69, 8.94; $P < 0.001$) and need for mechanical ventilation (Odds ratio, 3.85; 95% Confidence intervals,1.28, 10.22; P=0.017). The pattern of RSV illness in patients with neuromuscular compromise, indicates that these children are at risk for severe, complicated, RSV disease beyond the first two years of life and if this finding is confirmed in future studies, prophylaxis may be warranted for a longer duration in this cohort of infants.

IMMUNODEFICIENCY

Infants with immunological disorders whether congenital or acquired, patients with cancer and those with deficiencies in cellular immunity attained during the induction phase of chemotherapy are at particular risk for severe RSV disease. In 10-year prospective study, Hall et al reviewed the course of 608 RSV positive children hospitalized in a single US institution. [288] 47 were immunocompromised; 20 (42%) were receiving chemotherapy for leukemia or tumors, 5 (11%) had congenital immunodeficiency and 22 (47%) were on chronic steroid therapy. Viral shedding was prolonged (mean 26 days; range 14-46 days) in infants with congenital immunodeficiency. Eighteen (38%) required intensive care and there were 5 deaths (3 patients on chemotherapy and 2 with congenital immunodeficiency). More severe RSV disease was not documented in children on chronic steroids and none died.

Mahdi et al evaluated RSV disease in prospective cohorts of human immunodeficiency virus (HIV) children in Soweto, South Africa. [289] The prevalence of HIV was 14.6% in children with severe RSV LRTI. Common risk factors for RSV such as prematurity, BPD and congenital heart disease were similar in HIV positive and HIV negative children. HIV positive compared to HIV negative infants were older (median age of 7 months versus 4 months) at presentation, had more frequent pneumonia (92.3% versus 68.6%, P<0.002), more concurrent bacteremia (15.4% versus 2.6%, P=0.003) and a higher relative risk of death (4.4; 95% Confidence Intervals, 1.02, 18.92). A prospective study was conducted in Maryland to determine the occurrence of moderate to severe respiratory viral illnesses in infants born to HIV mothers. [290] 29 RSV infections were detected; 10 in infants born to HIV positive mothers (attack rate 49/100 patient years) and 19 in HIV negative mothers (attack rate 19/100 patient years). Children of HIV positive mothers had a higher incidence of pneumonia, more prolonged viral shedding (median 30 days versus 6 days) and 60% were hospitalized versus none of those born to HIV negative mothers.

Sung et al retrospectively reviewed the impact of RSV infection in 2078 children enrolled in 3 multicenter chemotherapy trials for acute myeloid leukemia. [291] Thirty-five (1.7%) children developed RSV infection and 54% were aged <2.5 years. 4 children died from RSV and although the risk for RSV infection was low, the RSV-related mortality was 10% (4/40). Children undergoing solid organ transplantation are considered to be at high risk for viral infection but studies involving pediatric patients are limited. Blanchard et al reported on 2 patients who acquired RSV infection after liver transplant at ages 6 and 10 months. One required PICU admission and had pronged viral excretion. [292] RSV was similarly detected in 3.4% of children who underwent liver transplantation at a median time of 24 days post transplant. 65% acquired nosocomial infection and 2 died. [293] McCarthy et al conducted a retrospective study from 1993-1998 on 336 allogeneic stem cell transplants in Bristol. [294] 26 (6.3%) patients were RSV positive and the median age at transplant was 10.6 years (range

0.5-31 years). Five (19.2%) direct RSV-related deaths were reported and 1 further death was due to an intracranial hemorrhage during an episode of RSV infection. There were 4 graft failures attributed to RSV infection and 2 of the patients died secondary to persistent neutropenia. RSV LRTI was significantly associated with mortality (15/26; P=0.04). Unrelated donor transplants had higher RSV mortality than sibling transplants (P=0.05-0.02). Children with cancer are also seriously affected by RSV. During a 3-year study period of mortality in England and Wales, of the 734 deaths reported in children <15 years, 10 (12%) were attributed to viruses and 3 of the infection-related deaths were due to RSV bronchiolitis. [295] It is becoming increasingly recognized that RSV is emerging as a significant pathogen not only in primary immunodeficient infants but also in children of all ages undergoing chemotherapy, bone marrow and solid organ transplantation. However, majority of the studies are limited to small case series with serious sequelae, which makes it difficult to accurately gauge the overall prevalence and outcomes of RSV infection in these populations.

Aboriginal Populations

The rates of serious RSV infection in Aboriginal children are much higher than those infants residing in urban communities. RSV admission rates for preterm and term Alaska Native infants from the Yukon Delta are 317 and 178/1000 respectively compared to the average of 25-30/1000 USA children. (296,297) Inuit children in the circumpolar regions have equally high rates of admission for LRTI and bronchiolitis, ranging between 300-590/1000 live births. [297-299] In Australia from 2000-2004, the rate of community acquired RSV infection in Aboriginal versus non-Aboriginal children was 2.7-fold higher (P<0.0001). [300] The majority of children had bronchiolitis (95.4%) and 35.4% also had pneumonia. Hospital stay ranged from 4-7 days and was marginally higher in Aboriginal children. Risk factors for RSV infection in Aboriginal children globally, include difficulty in accessing medical care easily and rapidly when required, prematurity, crowded households, environmental pollutants such as cigarette smoking, low socio-economic status and rates of breast feeding, use of wood-burning stoves and genetic factors. [301-305]

Miscellaneous Disorders

The nationwide survey from Japan [285] indicates that a host of underlying medical illnesses apart from BPD and congenital heart disease make infants highly susceptible to serious RSV infection. Among 756 reported hospitalizations who did not qualify for RSV prophylaxis, 414 (55%) had respiratory disorders of which 84% were diagnosed with asthma. Chromosomal anomalies and malformations comprised 17.2% (n=130), neuromuscular disorders 16.5% (n=125), heart disorders 3.5% (n=27), immunodeficiency 1.5% (n=12), congenital metabolic disorders 1% (n=8), and other disorders 5.3% (n=40). In a population-based retrospective cohort study of 516,831 children born in Colorado from 1997-2004, there were 12,522 hospitalizations with severe RSV LRTI in children aged <2 years and 3417 (0.7%) had major congenital malformations. [306] Of the documented disorders, spina bifida without anencephaly (relative risk [RR] 2.73; 95% confidence intervals [CI] 1.9, 3.74), lung agenesis, hypoplasia or dysplasia (RR 1.42; 95% CI 1.02, 1.98) and biliary atresia (RR 3.4; 95% CI 2.2, 5.4) were statistically significant predictors of hospitalization. This preliminary data requires verification in further studies. Arnold et al [286] examined RSV hospitalizations in 156 patients with pulmonary disorders inclusive of BPD, recurrent aspiration pneumonia, tracheoesophageal fistula, CF, other respiratory disorders and pulmonary malformations. Patients were admitted at a mean age of 1.56 years (range 0.64-2.10 years), had a mean length of hospital stay of 10.6 days (range 9-13 days), 12%-50% required PICU admission and 0-30% were ventilated. Masumoto et al reviewed 21 survivors with severe congenital diaphragmatic hernia (CDH) who had a lung: thoracic ratio <0.2, for the risk of RSV infection. [307] Five contacted RSV infections within a year of discharge, 3 were hospitalized and 2 had a recurrence of their hernia which was possibly ascribed to the prosthetic sheet used for the repair. However CDH patients are usually compromised by lung hypoplasia, and respiratory distress with excessive diaphragmatic motion triggered by serious RSV infection, could potentially lead to dehiscence of the repaired diaphragm. The authors recommended that CDH patients should receive RSV prophylaxis during the season.

Nosocomial Infection

Nosocomial RSV infections on pediatric wards and neonatal intensive care units are associated with severe disease and can cause significant morbidity and mortality especially in children who are premature, immunocompromised or have underlying cardio-pulmonary disorders. Clinical presentation may be atypical, especially in neonates, leading to delayed recognition. [308] Infected infants shed virus for up to 20 days and median hospital length of stay is prolonged (10 days) compared to community acquired RSV (5 days). [309] Fatality rates range between 0-12.2%. [48] Groothuis et al in a state of the art review, describe important containment strategies which focus on rapid diagnostic screening, thorough hand washing, isolation and cohort nursing of infected patients, and limiting visitors to stop spread. [310] Other recommendations include education of healthcare personnel about relevant preventive measures such as avoidance of cross-contamination, strict surveillance , work curtailment of symptomatic staff and use of gowns, gloves, masks and goggles to reduce contact exposure when nursing infected infants. [210,211,311,312]. None of the policies or interventions has been evaluated singly or in combination in controlled trials to determine the most effective strategy for control of RSV disease. However, in a German children's hospital, adherence to a strict regimen of prospective surveillance and targeted infection control from 1999-2002 lead to a 9-fold decline in the RSV incidence density (1.67 versus 0.18/1000 patient days). [212] Similarly an enhanced seasonal infection control program within a hematology-oncology service compared to a standard targeted infection control policy decreased the cumulative nosocomial RSV incidence 11-fold from 42.8 to 3.9 cases per 1000 admissions with elimination of nosocomial RSV pneumonia attributable mortality. [313] In a comparative study, of no precautions versus 3 preventive strategies; gowns and gloves, cohorting or cohorting with gowns and gloves, the latter technique afforded the best probability of remaining uninfected. [209]

RSV Prophylaxis and Immunization of Special Populations

What is the real-world experience with the use of palivizumab and how effective is it in the reduction of RSV hospitalization? In several post-marketing studies after palivizumab became available universally, the outcomes in treated patients closely aligned with the IMpact trial. In a combined analysis of 25 studies, [314] the number needed to treat (NNT) in infants 29-32 weeks gestation and those 32-35 weeks gestation were similar. [Figure 7] However, patients with BPD had higher reductions in RSV hospitalization (NNT 8 versus 20 in the IMpact study). In the US outcomes registry [315] which enrolled 19,548 patients in 256 centers across the US from 2000-2004, there was an overall steady decline in RSV hospitalization from 2.9% in the first year to 0.7% in 2003-2004. Compared to the IMpact trial hospitalization rates were lower in all sub-populations analyzed with corresponding decreases in PICU admissions and those infants who required mechanical ventilation from 0.98% to 0.18% and 0.58% to 0.05% respectively. [Figure 8] The same results were found in other international datasets confirming the efficacy of palivizumab as determined in the pivotal randomized controlled clinical trials with reported overall rates of RSV hospitalization ranging between 1.3% -8.1%. [316-321] A single center analysis of moderate to high risk 33-35 week GA infants, who were specifically targeted for prophylaxis from 2005-2008 based on the Canadian risk scoring tool [245] indicates that none required hospitalization for RSV infection. [250] A follow-up study from 2003-2009 conducted at the same center, confirmed that none of the moderate to high risk 33-35 weeks' GA infants that received prophylaxis, developed serious RSV infection requiring PICU care. [322]

Current pediatric advisory bodies and position statements don't support the routine use of RSV prophylaxis in children with existing medical disorders e.g. airway anomalies, neuromuscular impairments, cystic fibrosis, Down syndrome or immunodeficiency unless they are considered at high risk for severe RSV infection. [225,226] This is partly related to the high cost of the product, large cohorts of children that will need passive immunization and the lack of gold standard evidence from high quality randomized controlled trials in each of the sub-populations. [323] However, it appears that healthcare professionals are moving ahead of the existing evidence and surveys such as those conducted in cystic fibrosis and neuromuscular disorders indicate that RSV immunoprophylaxis is being recommended based on perceived benefit and low risk of adverse events. [324-326]

In a North American survey of RSV prophylaxis among 73 pediatric CF center directors in the USA and 10 in Canada, during the 2007 RSV season, 70% prescribed palivizumab in the first RSV season and 38% routinely prescribed prophylaxis for their patients. [324] Interestingly, 41% stated that prophylaxis for CF patients was an accepted "standard of care". A similar survey conducted in the UK across 34 centers, identified 143 CF patients <1 year of age. [325] 11.2% of the subjects were hospitalized with RSV and none required PICU care and none died. In 3 centers, 9.8% of the infants received palivizumab and the overall likelihood of prescribing palivizumab was rated as a median of 6.5. The survey portrayed several relevant issues with regard to routine prophylaxis of this cohort of patients. Physicians feel that RSV infection contributes significantly to the burden of illness in CF patients and would prescribe palivizumab if funding was available. More importantly, large scale clinical trials examining outcomes of either reduction in RSV hospitalization or long term benefits from prophylaxis were viewed by the author as unfeasible and this has prompted healthcare professionals in the UK who advocate for treatment, to seek financial support for prophylaxis of CF patients under the category of a chronic respiratory illness.

Gestational Age in Weeks	**29-32 weeks**	**32-35 weeks**	**BPD <2 years**
Number of Patients	N=4879	N=2829	N=3712
Number of Studies	10	4	11
% Reduction in RSV hospitalization rates IMpact/Combined Analysis	81/80	79/85	38/69
Number Needed to Treat (NNT) IMpact/Combined Analysis	14/12	13/12	20/8

Adapted from Simoes EAF. Resp Med 2002; 3 Suppl 1:S26-33.

Figure 7. Comparison of the number of patients needing treatment with palivizumab to prevent one case of RSV hospitalization (NNT) in the IMpact trial versus a combined analysis of three subgroups of infants.

RSV Season	2003/04 Registry N=6050	2002/03 Registry N=6,291	2001/02 Registry N=5091	2000/01 Registry N=1,002	1996/97 IMpact*/ CHD Trial† N=1,002/639	1996/97 IMpact*/ CHD Trial† Placebo N=500/648
All Patients (%)	0.7	1.1	1.5	2.9	4.8*	10.6*
Premature without BPD (%)	0.7	1.2	1.2	2.1	1.8*	8.1*
<32 weeks' Gestational age	1.1	1.6	1.7	4.5	5.8*	11.0*
32-35 weeks Gestational age	0.2	0.7	1.3	1.6	2.0*	9.8*
BPD	1.8	1.9	2.2	5.6	7.9*	12.8*
CHD	1.5	1.4	2.8	4.3	5.3†	9.7†

Adapted from: Frogel M et al. J Perinatol 2008; 28:511-517. (Ref: 315)
*The IMpact-RSV Study Group. Pediatrics 1998; 102:531-537. (Ref: 219)
†Feltes TF et al. J Pediatr 2003; 143:532-40. (Ref: 220)

Figure 8. RSV hospitalizations in the US outcomes Registry (2000-2004) following RSV prophylaxis compared to the IMpact and Cardiac (CHD) randomized controlled trials.

Only, one randomized controlled, safety study enrolled 186 CF patients who were allocated to palivizumab or placebo and no serious adverse events were identified in either arm of the trial. [327] In the US outcomes registry, 91 CF patients received palivizumab and none were hospitalized with RSV infection. [315] Speer et al [328] compared the RSV hospitalization rates of CF patients in the US outcomes registry [315] with 80 historical controls in the Armstrong [263] and 48 patients in the Abman [254] study. There was a statistically significant reduction in hospitalization (P=0.0042; odds ratio, 18.67; 95% confidence interval, 1.048, 332.6 and P=0.0004; odds ratio, 33.07; 95% confidence interval, 1.844, 593.2) respectively. In a retrospective 8 year study of 76 CF patients diagnosed at <18 months of age who received prophylaxis, there were fewer hospitalizations for respiratory illness in palivizumab recipients (3/35 versus 7/40; P=0.05) with an insignificant reduction in length of hospital stay. [329]

With regard to chronic medical illnesses, another survey of 45 pediatric specialists who cared for 3714 children who were technology-dependent for a variety of medical disorders, 89% recommended that RSV prophylaxis should be administered to a select group of children and 51% suggested that this should be provided for children aged > 2 years. [326]

RSV poses a risk after hematopoietic or solid organ transplants. Michaels et al found in a survey of 108 solid organ transplant centers, that 97% used palivizumab for prophylaxis of which 72% administered palivizumab during the first season post transplant and 25% employed prophylaxis for 2 seasons. [330] 93% of the centers prophylaxed infants from 0-12 months and 79% from 0-24 months. RSV infection was confirmed in 27% of the centers and in 4% versus 11% (P=0.03) of the immunized and non-immunized patients respectively. 15% of the centers used palivizumab for the active treatment of RSV infection. Using a decision tree analysis, Thomas et al tried to determine whether palivizumab is effective in the prevention of RSV-induced morbidity and mortality in children who are immunosuppressed after bone marrow transplantation. [331] Probabilities were derived from available scientific literature and sensitivity analysis were performed. The authors reported a 10% increase in survival in bone marrow transplant patients who receive palivizumab and the absolute survival increased from 83% to 92% with a number needed to treat of 12.

What other subgroups of infants with underlying medical disorders are currently receiving RSV prophylaxis? Manzoni et al, in a retrospective 8-year cohort Italian study compared infants (n=461) who qualified for RSV prophylaxis in accordance with the American Academy of Pediatrics guidelines and those who received off-label prophylaxis (n=51). [332] The latter group consisted of a broad spectrum of medical conditions and was found to be more compliant with the complete prophylaxis regimen. RSV-related hospitalizations were similar in both groups (2.1% versus 2.2% respectively). Palivizumab was found to be safe without serious adverse events. In the US outcomes registry [315] during the 2002-2004 RSV seasons, 1,122 infants (9.1%) with congenital airway anomalies or severe neuromuscular disorders received prophylaxis and these infants had significantly higher rates of RSV hospitalization (2.14%) than the infants without either disorder (0.78%; n=11,219; P<0.0001). This reflects the severity of RSV in this population as addressed earlier in this section and perhaps prophylaxis may ameliorate the course of illness. A review of palivizumab utilization among Florida Medicaid patients was performed from the 1998 through the 2005 RSV seasons. [333] In 1998/1999, 18.5% of doses were administered to children extern to current indications. The proportion increased to 36.3% in 1999 and then plateaued and although the majority comprised premature infants who had exceeded the age for prophylaxis, in 2004/2005, 38 CF children (26.4%) and 18 (19.4%) with severe combined or acquired immunodeficiency also received prophylaxis. [333] Muratore et al followed 100 patients over a 9-year period that had undergone surgical repair for a congenital diaphragmatic hernia. [334] From 1997-1999, 8 patients (36%) aged <3 years who had received RSV prophylaxis required urgent assessment for RSV bronchiolitis in the emergency department. None required admission to the ICU. However, in the 2 years prior to RSV prophylaxis, 8 patients (24%) required emergency room care and 2 patients were admitted to the PICU. The authors recommended that infants less than 2 years of age with congenital diaphragmatic hernia are at risk for RSV bronchiolitis and should receive adequate prophylaxis during the RSV season. [334] In the **CA**nadian **R**SV **E**valuation **S**tudy for **S**ynagis (CARESS) from 2006-2010, there were 7,339 patients enrolled who received at least one dose of palivizumab during the respective RSV seasons. [335] 4880 were ≤35 weeks gestation without underlying medical disorders (Group 1) while 952 (Group 2) received prophylaxis for various pre-existing illnesses. [Figure 9]

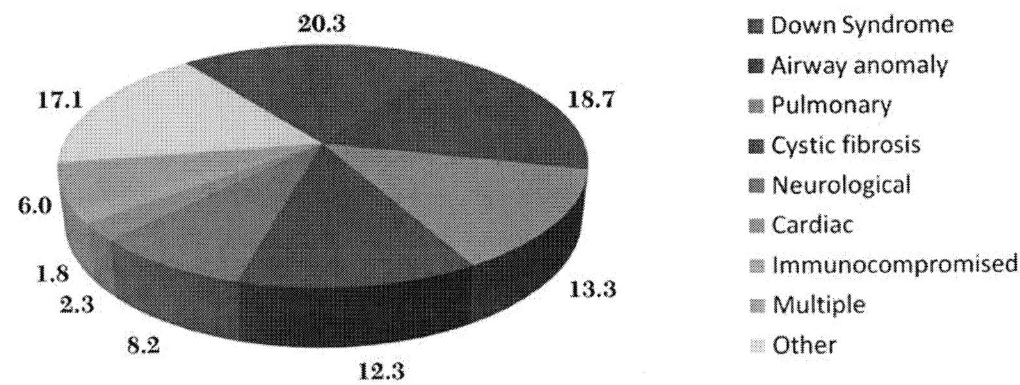

Figure 9. Sub-populations of infants (%) in the Canadian Registry for Synagis (CARESS) who received at least one dose of palivizumab during the (2006-2010) RSV seasons. (Ref: 335)

The largest proportion comprised Down syndrome without hemodynamically significant heart disease (20.3%) and airway anomalies (18.7%). There was an almost 3.5-fold increase in the proportion of infants from 5.6% (2006-2007) to 19.1% (2009-2010) who received prophylaxis for special medical indications. The overall RSV-related hospitalization rate was 1.48% and 92.0% ± 29.9% received their expected injections. Group 2 infants had higher rates of hospitalization for respiratory-related illness (9.0% versus 4.2%) and RSV infections (2.35% versus 1.32%) but neither group (P=0.102) nor compliance (P=0.702) impacted the time to first RSV hospitalization. The data once again re-affirms the findings from the US outcomes registry, that the population of infants with medical disorders is at increased risk overall for respiratory-related illnesses and that prophylaxis may steadily impact the severity of RSV-specific disease and admission to the PICU. [322]

The incidence of RSV-related hospitalization in Aboriginals, especially the Inuit and Alaskan native children is extremely high and the NNT to prevent one hospitalization ranges from 2.5 in infants < 6 months of age residing in high-risk communities to 17.8 in Iqaluit. [336] Following prophylaxis of premature infants in Alaska, Singleton et al demonstrated a decrease in hospitalization rates from 430 to 150/1000. [337]

In summary, infants with serious underlying disorders are prone to hospitalization and may merit from prophylaxis. Provincial Canadian guidelines and position statements as in Austria, USA and Canada, are gradually incorporating the use of RSV prophylaxis into existing guidelines for high-risk infants with Down syndrome, children with neuromuscular disease, cystic fibrosis and immunodeficiency syndromes. [223,225,226,338] In Canada, all full-term Inuit infants younger than six months of age at the onset of the RSV season in northern remote communities also qualify for prophylaxis based on published reports. [225, 336,337]

Is there a role for prophylaxis in outbreaks of nosocomial infection? Firstly, primary preventive measures as previously addressed, should be implemented and maintained diligently and all patients should be quickly screened for RSV. With rapidly spreading RSV infection, especially in neonatal intensive care units, palivizumab has been utilized to successfully limit ongoing disease in conjunction with stringently applied infection control policies. [339-342] Kassis et al reported on a nosocomial outbreak in an adult hematopoietic stem cell transplant unit. [339] All infected patients were placed in contact isolation and the rest of the patients underwent rapid RSV antigen screening. Intensive precautionary measures were instituted to prevent spread of RSV infection. 16 high risk patients received prophylactic palivizumab and none developed RSV infection. Four of 6 patients developed RSV pneumonia, during the outbreak and 2 died. The authors recommend that the role of palivizumab in the control of RSV hospital outbreaks should be further explored. Kurz et al reported their experience with the use of palivizumab in the control of an RSV outbreak in a neonatal intensive care unit. [340] The index case was isolated, the ward closed to admissions and infection control measures were implemented. The rest of the patients were passively immunized with palivizumab and no further cases were detected. O'Connell et al [341] and Dizdar et al [342] applied the same rapid screening technique, infection control principles and the concomitant use of palivizumab as Kassis et al [339] in high bed occupancy NICUs and successfully contained RSV spread. The effectiveness of palivizumab in the control of RSV nosocomial infection is apparent but requires high quality evidence through RCTs before acceptance into clinical practice.

Cost-Effectiveness of RSV Prophylaxis

A detailed analysis of existing studies on the cost-effectiveness of palivizumab versus no prophylaxis was conducted by Smart et al. [343] 23 articles met inclusion criteria including 11 cost-utility analyses and 12 cost-effective evaluations across all infant populations. The quality of the studies was rated fairly high with a median Quality of Health Economic Studies value of 86 (range 60-100) and all costs were calculated in Canadian dollars. In the cost utility analyses, the median score was 94 with majority of the studies documenting clear descriptions of lifetime horizons, discounting of future costs, sensitivity analyses and in some articles potential biases. Input parameters and costs included in each analysis varied. The largest sources of variability which impacted results were mortality rates and inclusion of long term outcomes such as asthma. In essence 4 studies, 3 of which were performed in the UK, Netherlands and Austria using similar models, found palivizumab to be cost-effective in premature infants $\leq$35 weeks GA, those with BPD and congenital heart disease. [344-347]

These results were further confirmed in another systematic review that compared various options for RSV prophylaxis. [348] The authors declared that the cost effectiveness of palivizumab tended to be more favorable in premature infants ≤32 weeks' GA, and infants aged < 2 years with BPD or congenital heart disease. Comparing the results of economic analyses of RSV-IGIV and palivizumab, the authors suggest that palivizumab may be the more cost-effective option. Using lower mortality rates, 2 studies conducted by Wang and Yount determined that prophylaxis was not cost-effective in the same populations. [349, 350] However in a later cost-effective re-analysis, Wang et al estimated that palivizumab would be cost-effective in infants with BPD or congenital heart disease independently, based on a threshold of £30,000/quality adjusted life-year (QALY). [351] Overall, congenital heart disease is determined to be the most cost-effective indication. Analyses conducted on specific gestational age groups such as 33-35 weeks have been uniformly positive. [352,357,358] In the Canadian study incremental cost-effective ratio (ICERs)/QALY ranged from CAN$13,029 to CAN$ 30,618 dependent on the inclusion/exclusion of direct and indirect costs and asthma. [352] Based on the risk scoring tool, palivizumab was only cost-effective in the moderate and high risk groups. [Figure 10]

Risk factors for RSV hospitalization	ICER/QALY (CAN$)
None	801,297
One	143,267
Two	81,331
Three	26,667
Four or more	808
Low Risk (Score 0-48)	179,669
Moderate Risk (Score 49-64)	34,215
High Risk (Score 65-100)	5,765
All 32-35 weeks' GA infants (including asthma)	20,924 (Direct costs)
All 32-35 weeks' GA infants (including asthma)	13,029 (Direct and indirect costs)
All 32-35 weeks' GA infants (excluding asthma)	30,618 (Direct costs)
All 32-35 weeks' GA infants (excluding asthma)	22,724 (Direct and indirect costs)

ICER, Incremental cost-effectiveness ratio; QALY, quality-adjusted life-year
*Decision threshold for adoption of interventions in Canada is usually CAN $50,000 – 75,000
Adapted from: Lanctot KL et al. Curr Med Res Opin 2008; 24:3223-3237. (Ref: 352)
*Laupacis A et al. CMAJ 1992; 146:473-481

Figure 10. Cost-effectiveness of using risk factors or the Canadian Risk Scoring Tool for 32-35 weeks' gestational age infants.

Similarly, palivizumab was deemed cost-effective in Spain for 32-35 weeks GA infants with an ICER/QALY of €13,849 from the National Health System perspective after discounting utility, and €4,605/QALY from the societal perspective which is lower than the socially acceptable threshold of €30,000 /QALY. [353] Tam et al also found palivizumab administration realized cost savings for infants < 6 months and high risk infants <1 year residing in rural regions to a CAN$153,527 ICER/QALY for those living in urban Iqaluit. [354]

The cost-effective analyses articles evaluated in the Smart et al review [343] were less robust, and in 9 studies the costs for life years gained (LYG) were approximately 50% higher than ICERs/QALY. Cost-effectiveness varied significantly based on single or multiple risk factors such as, siblings, daycare, discharge during the RSV season, gestational age, chronological age, BPD, congenital heart disease, immunodeficiency, congenital anomalies and specific sub-populations such as indigenous infants and their geographic location in urban or rural regions. Cost per hospital admission prevented with palivizumab varied from cost savings to CAN$371,569. Changing healthcare costs and palivizumab acquisition costs may also influence cost-effectiveness. Two recent studies conducted in Austria and Canada re-examined the cost-effectiveness of RSV prophylaxis in 2010. Resch et al [355] evaluated long-term epidemiological data that spanned 16 Austrian RSV seasons from 1993-2009, and re-confirmed their original results [346] that palivizumab compared with no prophylaxis had an incremental cost-utility ratio/QALY of €26,212, €26,292, €24,392, €24,654 and €8484 for all preterm infants, infants <33 weeks GA, those between 33-35 weeks GA, infants with BPD and congenital heart disease respectively, and was cost-effective in their setting. Similarly Smart et al, validated that between 2007-2010, the ICERs/QALY for palivizumab in 32-35 week GA infants in Canada remained stable, despite the changing costs of the product, and prove cost-effective with an ICER/QALY of CAN$192 for infants with four or more risk factors and CAN$ 5,274 to CAN$34,438 for moderate to high risk infants based on the Canadian risk scoring tool. [352,356]

In summary cost-effectiveness of RSV prophylaxis with palivizumab varies widely and is based on input parameters, outcomes assessed, populations studied and societal versus payer perspectives. The presence of risk factors plays a prominent role in determining cost-effectiveness and country-specific economic evaluations should be conducted to target the highest risk infant groups for prophylaxis.

New Prevention Strategies

Following the release of palivizumab for general use, new monoclonal antibodies with higher potency were sought. Motavizumab like palivizumab binds to an antigenic site of the RSV fusion (F) protein, similarly disrupting cell to cell and viral to cell transmission of the virus. [357] Motavizumab binds to RSV F-protein, 70-fold more efficiently than palivizumab and enhances neutralization of RSV in vitro 20-fold more effectively than palivizumab. [63,161,358] In cotton rats, motavizumab reduces lung RSV titres 100-fold in comparison to paliviumab and is equally superior in its inhibition of viral replication in the nasal turbinates unlike palivizumab that has no effect in the upper respiratory tract in the murine model and in children. [63,161,164,358]

The safety and efficacy of motavizumab was evaluated in a phase 3, double-blind placebo-controlled, randomized trial in healthy American Indian infants from 2004-2006 who were aged <6 months. [359] 938 infants received 5 monthly doses of motavizumab (15mg/kg) and 472 were controls. Motavizumab recipients had an 83% reduction in RSV hospitalization (1.4% motavizumab versus 8.3% placebo; p<0.001) and a 71% reduction in the incidence of RSV-specific medically attended outpatient LRTI (motavizumab 2.8% versus 9.5% placebo; p<0.001). Patients allocated to motavizumab had a 2% increase in skin and subcutaneous adverse events. A second non-inferiority RCT of motavizumab versus palivizumab was conducted which evaluated 6635 premature infants (n=3329, motavizumab; n=3306, palivizumab) aged < 6 months at study entry of which 1445 (21.8%) had BPD. [163] Patients who received motavizumab had a 26% relative reduction in RSV hospitalization and a 50% relative reduction in RSV-specific medically attended LRTIs compared to palivizumab recipients. Adverse cutaneous events were 2% higher in the motavizumab arm of the trial. 1235 hemodynamically significant congenital heart disease patients (665 cyanotic, 570 acyanotic) participated in a RCT of motavizumab (n=623) versus palivizumab (n=612). [360] Rates of RSV-related hospitalizations (1.9% versus 2.6%) and RSV-specific medically attended outpatient LRTIS (1.0% versus 1.9%) for motavizumab and palivizumab respectively, were similar among treatment groups (both P>0.05). Patients undergoing cardiac by-pass surgery received an extra dose of drug postoperatively and there were no differences in drug concentrations in these patients compared to those who did not require surgery. Similar numbers of subjects in both arms of the trial were admitted to hospital and required oxygen therapy, admission to PICU and mechanical ventilation. Once again the incidence of skin reactions were significantly higher in the motavizumab patients (1.6%) versus the palivizumab group (0.3%, P=0.038). FDA approval of motavizumab in the US is still awaited.

It is well recognized that a vaccine will offer the best protection against RSV infection. An early formalin-inactivated (F1) vaccine developed in 1961 was tested for efficacy in 4 clinical trials. The vaccine generated high RSV antibody levels but these were of low avidity, possibly due to a lack of affinity maturation, the inability to inhibit virus fusion and possibly limited neutralizing activity. [361-364] Vacinees who participated in the studies developed higher rates of RSV infection (44%) compared to controls (6%) and disease was more severe following vaccination, with a 16-fold higher rate of hospitalization, accompanied by two deaths. The F1-RSV vaccine was associated with the highest disease severity in infants < 6 months of age, a time period when maternal RSV antibodies are present. This erroneously raised questions about antibodies and their role in disease pathogenesis which was later quelled by the success of RSV-IGIV and its protective effect against RSV. [213,214] Several hypotheses evolved about the RSV vaccine failure which included; a predominant Th2 type response resulting in altered cytokine expression of IL-4 and IFN-γ, raised $CD4^{+}$T cells with eosinophilia, formalin denaturation of the F-glycoprotein and incomplete Toll-like receptor activation in B cells. [365-371] However, the exact mechanisms that jeopardized vaccine success remain elusive. Following the disastrous outcomes of the F1-RSV vaccine, major obstacles have hampered progress in the development of a new vaccine. The highest risk population is premature infants who have immature immune systems and lack the ability to mount a protective immune response in the presence of maternal antibody. The vaccine will need to be proven effective against both RSV subtypes, inhibit viral capacity to block the innate immune system, avoid enhanced disease, generate efficient cellular and humoral responses in immunosuppressed individuals, be efficacious and have a high safety profile demonstrated in both short and long term outcomes across all age groups. There are several potential vaccine candidates that can be grouped under bovine derived, RSV vectored, subunit, cold-passaged (cp) and temperature-sensitive (ts) or deletion mutant vaccines. [372] Sub-unit vaccines have undergone preliminary evaluation in young infants, 18-36 months of age and those with BPD and CF with promising results. [372-375] A recently tested recombinant vaccine has been tolerated well in infants with a potent attenuating effect and induced protective immunity. [376] In a phase-1 study, a live, attenuated RSV and parainfluenza virus type 3 intranasal vaccine was evaluated in US children aged 1-9 years and demonstrated to be safe in those who were seropositive. [377] No respiratory illnesses occurred in the 28-day period following vaccination and there were no serious adverse events over 180 days thereafter. The vaccine was described as being minimally immunogenic and no subjects shed vaccine-like virus. Further studies in seronegative infants are planned. The history of RSV-vaccine development is both interesting and intriguing and there are several comprehensive reviews outlining the many hurdles that have yet to be surmounted in the development of a safe and immunologically protective vaccine and this will likely take several years. [372, 378-382]

Conclusion

Apart from good hygiene and infection control measures, the only other non-interventional strategies to reduce the risk of RSV infection are to encourage breast feeding in infancy, avoid tobacco smoke exposure, crowded environments and contact with infected individuals during the RSV season. Highly sensitive diagnostic tests are available for rapid screening of potentially infected infants and a judicious approach to treatment based on disease severity is advocated while awaiting confirmation of more effective therapeutic modalities through randomized controlled clinical trials. Critically ill infants at risk of requiring intensive care need close observation and management should be targeted individually based on clinical presentation and ensuing complications. Currently, palivizumab offers the best protection for infants at high risk for severe RSV disease and hospitalization. The evidence supporting use in premature infants' ≤ 35 weeks gestational age and those with BPD and hemodynamically significant heart disease has been justified through well-designed, randomized, controlled studies. There is an urgent need for prospective studies of RSV prophylaxis in infants with a wide spectrum of underlying disorders before prophylaxis is adopted as standard of care in clinical practice. Research endeavors in this latter domain may be compromised by unbalanced perspectives that not unacceptably justify immunization of seriously ill children with pre-existing medical disorders versus attempts to establish efficacy, safety and improved short and long term outcomes with the use of monoclonal antibodies.

References

[1] Shay DK, Holman RC, Newman RD, Liu LL, Stout JW, Anderson LJ. Bronchiolitis-associated hospitalizations among US children, 1980-1996. *JAMA*.1999; 282:1440-1446.

[2] Weber MW, Mulholland EK, Greenwood BM. Respiratory syncytial virus infection in tropical and developing countries. *Trop Med Int Health*. 1998; 3:268-280.

[3] Bloom B, Cohen, RJ. Summary Health Statistics for U.S. Children. National Health Interview Survey. Vital and Health Statistics. *National Center for Health Statistics*.2007; Stat 10(234).

[4] Hendrickson KJ. Parainfluenza Viruses. *Clin Micro Rev*. 2003; 16:242-264.

[5] Hall CB, McCarthy CA. Respiratory syncytial virus. In: *Principles and Practice of Infectious Diseases,* Vol. 2. 2000. Mandell GL, Bennett JE, Dolin R, (Ed.), Churchill Livingstone, Philadelphia, PA. US 1782-1801.
[6] Pozzetto B, Grattard F, Pillet S. Multiplex PCR theranostics of severe respiratory infections. *Expert Rev Anti Infect Ther.* 2010; 8: 251-253.
[7] Mahony JB. Nucleic acid amplification-based diagnosis of respiratory virus infections. *Expert Rev Anti Infect Ther.* 2010; 8:1273-1292.
[8] Mahony, J. Coronavirus. In P. R. Murray, El J. Baron, J. H. Jorgensen, M. L. Landry, and M. A. Pfaller (ed.), *Manual of Clinical Microbiology, 9th edition.* 2007. pp. 1414-1423. ASM Press, Washington, D. C.
[9] Mahony JB. Detection of respiratory viruses by molecular methods. *Clin Microbiol Rev.* 2008; 21:716-747.
[10] Kehl SC, Kumar S. Utilization of nucleic acid amplification assays for the detection of respiratory viruses. *Clin Lab Med.* 2009; 29, 661-671.
[11] Beck ET, Henrickson KJ. Molecular diagnosis of respiratory viruses. *Future Microbiol.* 2010; 5: 901-916.
[12] Leader S and Kohlhase K. Recent trends in severe respiratory syncytial virus (RSV) amongst US infants, 1997 to 2000. *J Pediatr.* 2003; 143: S127-132.
[13] El-Hajje MJ, Lambe C, Moulin F, Suremain N, Pons-Catalano C, Chalumeau M, Raymond J, Lebon P, Gendrel D. The burden of respiratory viral disease in hospitalized children in Paris. *Eur J Pediatr.* 2008; 167: 435-436.
[14] Mansbach JM, McAdam AJ, Clark S, Hain PD, Flood RG, Acholonu U, Camargo CA Jr. Prospective multicenter study of the viral etiology of bronchiolitis in the emergency department. *Acad Emerg Med.* 2008; 15:111-118.
[15] Khuri-Bulos N, Williams JV, Shehabi AA, Faouri S, Al Jundi E, Abushariah O, Chen Q, Ali SA, Vermund S, Halasa NB. Burden of respiratory syncytial virus in hospitalized infants and young children in Amman, Jordan. *Scand J Infect Dis.* 2010; 42:368-374.
[16] Midulla F, Scagnolari C, Bonci E, Pierangeli A, Antonelli G, De Angelis D, Berardi R, Moretti C. Respiratory syncytial virus, human bocavirus and rhinovirus bronchiolitis in infants. *Arch Dis Child.* 2010; 95:35-41.
[17] Stempel HE, Martin ET, Kuypers J, Englund JA, Zerr DM. Multiple viral respiratory pathogens in children with bronchiolitis. *Acta Paediatr.* 2009; 98; 123-126.
[18] Freymuth F, Vabret A, Cuvillon-Nimal D, Simon S, Dina J, Legrand L, Gouarin S, Petitjean J, Eckart P, Brouard J. Comparison of Multiplex PCR Assays and Conventional Techniques for the Diagnostic of Respiratory Virus Infections in Children Admitted to Hospital With an Acute Respiratory Illness. *J Med Virol.* 2006; 78: 1498-1504.
[19] Aberle JH, Aberle SW, Pracher E, Hutter HP, Kundi M, Popow-Kraupp T. Single versus dual respiratory virus infections in hospitalized infants: impact on clinical course of disease and interferon-gamma response. *Pediatr Infect Dis J.* 2005; 24:605-610.
[20] Langley JM, LeBlanc JC, Smith B, Wang EE. Increasing incidence of hospitalization for bronchiolitis among Canadian children, 1980-2000. *J Infect Dis.* 2003; 188:1764-1767.
[21] Fry AM, Chittaganpitch M, Baggett HC, Peret TC, Dare RK, Sawatwong P, Thamthitiwat S, Areerat P, Sanasuttipun W, Fischer J, Maloney SA, Erdman DD, Olsen

SJ. The burden of hospitalized lower respiratory tract infection due to respiratory syncytial virus in rural Thailand. *PLoS One*. 2010; 5:e15098.

[22] Light M, Bauman J, Mavunda K, Malinoski F, Eggleston M. Correlation between respiratory syncytial virus (RSV) test data and hospitalization of children for RSV lower respiratory tract illness in Florida. *Pediatr Infect Dis J.* 2008; 27:512-518.

[23] MMWR Morb Mortal Wkly Rep. Respiratory syncytial virus activity - United States, July 2008-December 2009. 2010; 59:230-233.

[24] Yusuf S, Piedimonte G, Auais A, Demmler G, Krishnan S, Van Caeseele P, Singleton R, Broor S, Parveen S, Avendano L, Parra J, Chavez-Bueno S, Murguía De Sierra T, Simoes EA, Shaha S, Welliver R. The relationship of meteorological conditions to the epidemic activity of respiratory syncytial virus. *Epidemiol Infect*. 2007; 135:1077-1090.

[25] Welliver R. The relationship of meteorological conditions to the epidemic activity of respiratory syncytial virus. *Paediatr Respir Rev*. 2009; 10 Suppl 1:6-8.

[26] Meerhoff TJ, Paget JW, Kimpen JL, Schellevis F. Variation of respiratory syncytial virus and the relation with meteorological factors in different winter season. *Pediatr Infect Dis J.* 2009; 28:860-866.

[27] Panozzo CA, Stockman LJ, Curns AT, Anderson LJ. Use of respiratory syncytial virus surveillance data to optimize the timing of immunoprophylaxis. *Pediatrics*. 2010; 126:e116-123.

[28] Law BJ, Langley JM, Allen U, Paes B, Lee DS, Mitchell I, Sampalis J, Walti H, Robinson J, O'Brien K, Majaesic C, Caouette G, Frenette L, Le Saux N, Simmons B, Moisiuk S, Sankaran K, Ojah C, Singh AJ, Lebel MH, Bacheyie GS, Onyett H, Michaliszyn A, Manzi P, Parison D. The Pediatric Investigators Collaborative Network on Infections in Canada study of predictors of hospitalization for respiratory syncytial virus infection for infants born at 33 through 35 completed weeks of gestation. *Pediatr Infect Dis J.* 2004; 23:806-814.

[29] Carballal G, Videla C, Sequeira MD, Mistchenko A, Requeijo PV, Arbiza J. Respiratory syncytial virus: changes in prevalence of subgroups A and B among Argentinian children, 1990-1996. *J Med Virol.* 2000; 61:275-279.

[30] Deng J, Qian Y, Zhu RN, Wang F, Zhao LQ. Surveillance for respiratory syncytial virus subtypes A and B in children with acute respiratory infections in Beijing during 2000 to 2006 seasons]. *Zhonghua Er Ke Za Zhi*. 2006; 44:924-927.

[31] Lee JT, Chang LY, Wang LC, Kao CL, Shao PL, Lu CY, Lee PI, Chen JM, Lee CY, Huang LM. Epidemiology of respiratory syncytial virus infection in northern Taiwan, 2001-2005 -- seasonality, clinical characteristics, and disease burden. *J Microbiol Immunol Infect.* 2007; 40:293-301.

[32] Nokes DJ, Okiro EA, Ngama M, Ochola R, White LJ, Scott PD, English M, Cane PA, Medley GF. Respiratory syncytial virus infection and disease in infants and young children observed from birth in Kilifi District, Kenya. *Clin Infect Dis*. 2008 1; 46:50-57.

[33] Glezen WP, Taber LH, Frank AL, Kasel JA. Risk of primary infection and reinfection with respiratory syncytial virus. *Am J Dis Child.* 1986; 140:543-546.

[34] Henderson FW, Collier AM, Clyde WA Jr, Denny FW. Respiratory-syncytial-virus infections, reinfections and immunity. A prospective, longitudinal study in young children. *N Engl J Med*. 1979; 300:530-534.

[35] Parrott RH, Kim HW, Brandt CD, Chanock RM. Respiratory syncytial virus in infants and children. *Prev Med*. 1974; 3:473-480.

[36] Leader S, Kohlhase K. Respiratory syncytial virus-coded pediatric hospitalizations, 1997 to 1999. *Pediatr Infect Dis J.* 2002; 21:629-632.

[37] Hall CB. Respiratory syncytial virus and parainfluenza virus. *N Engl J Med.* 2001; 344:1917-1928.

[38] Glezen WP. Pathogenesis of bronchiolitis--epidemiologic considerations. *Pediatr Res.* 1977; 11:239-243.

[39] Heilman CA. From the National Institute of Allergy and Infectious Diseases and the World Health Organization. Respiratory syncytial and parainfluenza viruses. *J Infect Dis.* 1990; 161:402-406.

[40] Nair H, Nokes DJ, Gessner BD, Dherani M, Madhi SA, Singleton RJ, O'Brien KL, Roca A, Wright PF, Bruce N, Chandran A, Theodoratou E, Sutanto A, Sedyaningsih ER, Ngama M, Munywoki PK, Kartasasmita C, Simões EA, Rudan I, Weber MW, Campbell H. Global burden of acute lower respiratory infections due to respiratory syncytial virus in young children: a systematic review and meta-analysis. *Lancet.* 2010; 375:1545-1555.

[41] Hall CB, Weinberg GA, Iwane MK, Blumkin AK, Edwards KM, Staat MA, Auinger P, Griffin MR, Poehling KA, Erdman D, Grijalva CG, Zhu Y, Szilagyi P. The burden of respiratory syncytial virus infection in young children. *N Engl J Med.* 2009; 3 60:588-598.

[42] McLaurin KK, Leader S. *Pediatric Academic Societies Annual Meeting*; May 14-17; 2005, Washington, DC.

[43] Simoes EA. Environmental and demographic risk factors for respiratory syncytial virus lower respiratory tract disease. *J Pediatr.* 2003; 143:S118-126.

[44] Langley GF, Anderson LJ. Epidemiology and prevention of respiratory syncytial virus infections among infants and young children. *Pediatr Infect Dis J.* 2011; 30:510-7.

[45] Thompson WW, Shay DK, Weintraub E, Brammer L, Cox N, Anderson LJ, Fukuda K. Mortality associated with influenza and respiratory syncytial virus in the United States. *JAMA.* 2003; 289:179-186.

[46] Shay DK, Holman RC, Roosevelt GE, Clarke MJ, Anderson LJ. Bronchiolitis-associated mortality and estimates of respiratory syncytial virus-associated deaths among US children, 1979-1997. *J Infect Dis.* 2001; 183:16-22.

[47] Holman RC, Shay DK, Curns AT, Lingappa JR, Anderson LJ. Risk factors for bronchiolitis-associated deaths among infants in the United States. *Pediatr Infect Dis J.* 2003; 22:483-490.

[48] Thorburn K. Pre-existing disease is associated with a significantly higher risk of death in severe respiratory syncytial virus infection. *Arch Dis Child.* 2009; 94:99-103.

[49] Welliver RC Sr, Checchia PA, Bauman JH, Fernandes AW, Mahadevia PJ, Hall CB. Fatality rates in published reports of RSV hospitalizations among high-risk and otherwise healthy children. *Curr Med. Res Opin.* 2010; 26:2175-2181.

[50] Gelfand EW. Pediatric asthma: a different disease. *Proc Am Thorac Soc.* 2009; 6:278-282.

[51] Walton RP, Johnston SL. Role of respiratory viral infections in the development of atopic conditions. *Curr Opin Allergy Clin Immunol.* 2008; 8:150-153.

[52] Stein RT, Sherrill D, Morgan WJ, Holberg CJ, Halonen M, Taussig LM, Wright AL, Martinez FD. Respiratory syncytial virus in early life and risk of wheeze and allergy by age 13 years. *Lancet.* 1999; 354:541-545.

[53] Sigurs N, Bjarnason R, Sigurbergsson F, Kjellman B. Respiratory syncytial virus bronchiolitis in infancy is an important risk factor for asthma and allergy at age 7. *Am J Respir Crit Care Med.* 2000; 161:1501-1507.

[54] Sigurs N, Gustafsson PM, Bjarnason R, Lundberg F, Schmidt S, Sigurbergsson F, Kjellman B. Severe respiratory syncytial virus bronchiolitis in infancy and asthma and allergy at age 13. *Am J Respir Crit Care Med.* 2005; 171:137-141.

[55] Simoes EA, Groothuis JR, Carbonell-Estrany X, Rieger CH, Mitchell I, Fredrick LM, Kimpen JL; Palivizumab Long-Term Respiratory Outcomes Study Group. Palivizumab prophylaxis, respiratory syncytial virus, and subsequent recurrent wheezing. *J Pediatr.* 2007; 151:34-42, 42.e1.

[56] Pérez-Yarza EG, Moreno A, Lázaro P, Mejías A, Ramilo O. The association between respiratory syncytial virus infection and the development of childhood asthma: a systematic review of the literature. *Pediatr Infect Dis J.* 2007; 26:733-739.

[57] Simões EA, Carbonell-Estrany X, Rieger CH, Mitchell I, Fredrick L, Groothuis JR; Palivizumab Long-Term Respiratory Outcomes Study Group. The effect of respiratory syncytial virus on subsequent recurrent wheezing in atopic and nonatopic children. *J Allergy Clin Immunol.* 2010; 126:256-262.

[58] Sigurs N, Aljassim F, Kjellman B, Robinson PD, Sigurbergsson F, Bjarnason R, Gustafsson PM. Asthma and allergy patterns over 18 years after severe RSV bronchiolitis in the first year of life. *Thorax.* 2010; 65:1045-1052.

[59] Korppi M, Piippo-Savolainen E, Korhonen K, et al. Respiratory morbidity 20 years after RSV infection in infancy. *Pediatr Pulmonol.* 2004; 38:155-60.

[60] Stein RT, Martinez FD. Respiratory syncytial virus and asthma: still no final answer. *Thorax.* 2010; 65:1033-1034.

[61] Bont L, Ramilo O. The relationship between RSV bronchiolitis and recurrent wheeze: the chicken and the egg. *Early Hum Dev.* 2011; 87:S51-54.

[62] Jafri HS, Chavez-Bueno S, Mejias A, Gomez AM, Rios AM, Nassi SS, Yusuf M, Kapur P, Hardy RD, Hatfield J, Rogers BB, Krisher K, Ramilo O. Respiratory syncytial virus induces pneumonia, cytokine response, airway obstruction, and chronic inflammatory infiltrates associated with long-term airway hyperresponsiveness in mice. *J Infect Dis.* 2004; 189:1856-1865.

[63] Mejías A, Chávez-Bueno S, Ríos AM, Aten MF, Raynor B, Peromingo E, Soni P, Olsen KD, Kiener PA, Gómez AM, Jafri HS, Ramilo O. Comparative effects of two neutralizing anti-respiratory syncytial virus (RSV) monoclonal antibodies in the RSV murine model: time versus potency. *Antimicrob Agents Chemother.* 2005; 49:4700-4707.

[64] Houben ML, Coenjaerts FEJ, Rossen JWA, Belderbos ME, Hofland RW, Kimpen JLL, Bont L. Disease severity and viral load are correlated in infants with primary respiratory syncytial virus infection in the community. *J Med Vir.* 2010; 82:1266-1271.

[65] Franz A, Adams O, Willems R, Bonzel L, Neuhausen N, Schweizer-Krantz S, Ruggeberg JU, Willers R, Henrich B, Schroten H, Tenenbaum T. Correlation of viral load of respiratory pathogens and co-infections with disease severity in children hospitalized for lower respiratory tract infections. *J Clin Vir.* 2010; 48:239-245.

[66] Jansen RR, Schinkel J, Dek I, Koekkoek SM, Visser CE, de Jong MD, Molenkamp R, Pajkrt D. Quantitation of respiratory viruses in relation to clinical course in children with acute respiratory tract infections. *Pediatr Infect Dis J.* 2010; 29:82-84.

[67] Bosis S, Esposito S, Niesters HG, Zuccotti GV, Marseglia G, Lanari M, Zuin G, Pelucchi C, Osterhaus AD, Principi N. Role of respiratory pathogens in infants hospitalized for a first episode of wheezing and their impact on recurrences. *Clin Microbiol Infect.* 2008; 14:677-684.

[68] Chutinimitkul S, Bhattarakosol P, Srisuratanon S, et al. H5N1 influenza A virus and infected human plasma. *Emerg Infect Dis.* 2006; 12:1041-1043.

[69] Wang WK, Fang CT, Chen HL, et al. Detection of severe acute respiratory syndrome coronavirus RNA in plasma during the course of infection. *J Clin Microbiol.* 2005; 43:962-965.

[70] Rohwedder A, Keminer O, Foster J, Schneider K, Schneider E, Werchau H. Detection of respiratory syncytial virus RNA in blood of neonates by polymerase chain reaction. *J Med Virol.* 1998; 54:320-327.

[71] Campbell AP, Chien JW, Kuypers J, Englund JA, Wald A, Guthrie KA, Corey L, Boeckh M. Respiratory virus pneumonia after hematopoietic cell transplantation (HCT): Associations between viral load in bronchoalveolar lavage samples, viral RNA detection in serum samples, and clinical outcomes of HCT. *J Infect Dis.* 2010; 201:1404-1413.

[72] Torres JP, Gomez AM, Khokhar S, Bhoj VG, Tagliabue C, Chang ML, Kiener PA, Revell PA, Ramilo O, Mejias A. Respiratory syncytial virus (RSV) RNA loads in peripheral blood correlates with disease severity in mice. *Respir Res.* 2010; 11:125.

[73] Wu W, Tang Y-W. Emerging molecular assays for detection and characterization of respiratory viruses. *Clin Lab Med.* 2009; 29: 673-693.

[74] Halstead DC, Todd S, Fritch G. Evaluation of five methods for respiratory syncytial virus detection. *J Clin Microbiol.* 1990; 28:1021-1025.

[75] Kellogg JA. Culture vs direct antigen assays for detection of microbial pathogens from lower respiratory tract specimens suspected of containing the respiratory syncytial virus. *Arch Pathol Lab Med.* 1991; 115: 451-458.

[76] Johnston SL, Siegel CS. Evaluation of direct immunofluorescence, enzyme immunoassay, centrifugation culture, and conventional culture for the detection of respiratory syncytial virus. *J Clin Microbiol.* 1990; 28: 2394-2397.

[77] Rabalais GP, Stout GG, Ladd KL, Cost KM. Rapid diagnosis of respiratory viral infections by using a shell vial assay and monoclonal antibody pool. *J Clin Microbiol.* 1992; 30: 1505-1508.

[78] Smith MC, Creutz C, Huang YT. Detection of respiratory syncytial virus in nasopharyngeal secretions by shell vial technique. *J Clin Microbiol.* 1991; 29, 463-465.

[79] Barenfanger J, Drake C, Mueller T, Troutt T, O'Brien J, Guttman K.R-Mix cells are faster, at least as sensitive and marginally more costly than conventional cell lines for the detection of respiratory viruses. *J Clin.Virol.* 2001; 22: 101-110.

[80] Dunn JJ, Woolstenhulme RD, Langer J, Carroll KC. Sensitivity of respiratory virus culture when screening with R-Mix fresh cells. *J Clin Microbiol.* 2004; 42:79-82.

[81] St George K, Patel NM, Hartwig RA, Scholl DR, Jollick JA Jr, Kauffmann LM, Evans MR, Rinaldo CR Jr. Rapid and sensitive detection antiviral treatment using R-Mix cultures. *J Clin Virol.* 2002; 24: 107-115.

[82] Landry M L, Ferguson D. SimulFluor respiratory screen for rapid detection of multiple respiratory viruses in clinical specimens by immunofluorescence staining. *J Clin Microbiol.* 2000; 38: 708-711.

[83] Blyth CC, Booy R, Dwyer DE. Point of care testing: Diagnosis outside the virology laboratory. *Methods Molec Biol.* 2011, 665: 415-433.

[84] Slinger R, Milk R, Gaboury I, Diaz-Mitoma F. Evaluation of the QuickLab RSV test, a new rapid lateral-flow immunoassay for detection of respiratory syncytial virus antigen. *J Clin Microbiol.* 2004; 42: 3731-3733.

[85] Borek AP, Clemens SH, Gaskins VK, Aird DZ, Valsamakis A. Respiratory syncytial virus detection by Remel Xpect, Binax Now RSV, direct immuno-fluorescent staining, and tissue culture. *J Clin Microbiol.* 2006; 44: 1105-1107.

[86] Ribes JA, Seabolt JP, Overman SB. Performance characteristics of VIDAS and Directigen respiratory syncytial virus (RSV) antigen detection assays and culture for the identification or RSV in respiratory specimens. *J Clin Microbiol.* 2002; 40: 1818-1820.

[87] Zheng X, Quianzon S, Mu Y, Katz BZ. Comparison of two new rapid antigen detection assays for respiratory syncytial virus with another assays for respiratory syncytial virus with another assay and shell vial culture. *J Clin Virol.* 2004; 31: 130-133.

[88] Ohm-Smith MJ, Nassos PS, Haller BL. Evaluation of the Binax NOW, BD Directigen, and BD Directigen EZ assays for detection of respiratory syncytial virus. *J Clin Microbiol.* 2004; 42: 2996-2999.

[89] Reina J, Gonzalez Gardenas M, Ruiz de Gopegui E, Padilla E, Ballesteros F, Mari M, Munar M. Prospective evaluation of a dot-blot enzyme immunoassay (Directigen RSV) for the antigenic detection of respiratory syncytial virus from nasopharyngeal aspirates of paediatric patients. *Clin Microbiol Infect.* 2004; 10: 967-971.

[90] Falsey AR, McCann RM, Hall WJ, Criddle MM. Evaluation of four methods for the diagnosis of respiratory syncytial virus infection in older adults. *J Am Geriatr Soc.* 1996; 44: 71-73.

[91] Casiano-Colon AE, Hulbert BB, Mayer TK,Walsh EE, Falsey AR. Lack of sensitivity of rapid antigen tests for the diagnosis of respiratory syncytial virus infection in adults. *J Clin Virol.* 2003; 28: 169-174.

[92] Ginocchio CC, Swierkosz E, McAdam AJ, Marcon M, Storch GA, Valsamakis A, Juretschko S, Romero J, Yen-Lieberman B. Multicenter study of clinical performance of the 3M rapid detection RSV test. *J Clin Micro.* 2010; 48; 2337-2343.

[93] Munjal I, Gialanella P, Gross C, McKitrick JC, Avner JR, Pan Q, Litman N, Levi MH. Evaluation of the 3M rapid detection test for respiratory syncytial virus (RSV) in children during the early stages of the 2009 RSV season. *J Clin Micro.* 2011; 49:1151-1153.

[94] Miernyk K, Bulkow L, DeByle C, Chikoyak L, Boyd Hummel K, Hennessy T, Singleton R. Performance of a rapid antigen test (Binax NOW® RSV) for diagnosis of respiratory syncytial virus compared with real-time polymerase chain reaction in a pediatric population. *J Clin Vir.* 2011; 50:240-243.

[95] Perez JW, Vargis EA, Russ PK, Haselton FR, Wright DW. Detection of respiratory syncytial virus using nanoparticle amplified immuno-polymerase chain reaction. *Anal Biochem.* 2011; 410:141-148.

[96] Tang YW, Jeimgartner PJ, Tollefson SJ, Berg TJ, Rys PN, Li H, Smith TF, Persing DH, Wright PF. A colorimetric microtiter plate PCR system detects respiratory syncytial virus in nasal aspirates and discriminates subtypes A and B. Diagn. *Microbiol Infect Dis.* 1999; 34: 333-337.

[97] Freymuth F, Eugene G, Vabret A, Petitjean J, Gennetay E, Brouard J, Duhamel JF, Guillois B. Detection of respiratory syncytial virus by reverse transcription-PCR and hybridization with a DNA enzyme immunoassay. *J Clin Microbiol.* 1995; 33: 3352-3355.

[98] Henkel JH, Aberle SW, Kundi M, Popow-Kraupp T. Improved detection of respiratory syncytial virus in nasal aspriate by seminested RT-PCR. *J Med Virol.* 1997; 53: 366-371.

[99] Liolios L, Jenney A, Spelman D , Kotsimbos T, Catton M, Wesselingh S. Comparison of a multiplex reverse transcription-PCR –enzyme hybridization assay with conventional viral culture and immunofluorescence techniques for the detection of seven viral respiratory pathogens. *J Clin Microbiol.* 2001; 39: 2779-2783.

[100] Mentel R, Wegner U, Burns R, Gurtler L. Real-time PCR to improve the diagnosis of respiratory syncytial virus infection. *J Med Microbiol.* 2003; 52: 893-896.

[101] Stockton J, Ellis JS, Saville M, Clewley JP, Zambon MC. Multiplex PCR for typing and subtyping influenza and respiratory syncytial viruses. *J Clin Microbiol.* 1998; 36: 2990-2995.

[102] Syrmis MW, Whiley DM, Thomas M, Mackay IM, Williamson J, Siebert DJ, Nissen MD, Sloots TP. A sensitive specific and cost-effective multiplex reverse transcriptase-PCR assay for the detection of seven common respiratory viruses in respiratory samples. *J Mol Diagn.* 2004; 6: 125-131.

[103] Eugene-Ruellan G, Freymuth F, Bahloul C, Badrane H, Vabret A, Tordo N. Detection of respiratory syncytial virus A and B and parainfluenzavirus 3 sequences in respiratory tracts of infants by a single PCR with primers targeted to the L-polymerase gene and differential hybridization. *J Clin Microbiol.* 1998; 36: 796-801.

[104] Weinberg GA, Erdman DD, Edwards KM, Hall CB, Walker FJ, Griffin MR, Schwartz B, and the New Vaccine Surveillance Network Study Group. Superiority of reverse-transcription polymerase chain reaction to conventional viral culture in the diagnosis of acute respiratory tract infections in children. *J Infect Dis.* 2004; 189: 706-710.

[105] Moore C, Valappil M, Corden S, Westmoreland D. Enhanced clinical utility of the NucliSens EasyQ RSV A+B Assay for rapid detection of respiratory syncytial virus in clinical samples. *Eur J Clin Microbiol Infect Dis.* 2006; 25: 167-174.

[106] Fan J, Hendrickson KJ, Savatski LL. Rapid simultaneous diagnosis of infections with respiratory syncytial viruses A and B, influenza viruses A and B, and human parainfluenza virus types 1, 2, and 3 by multiplex quantitative reverse transcription-polymerase chain reaction-enzyme hybridization assay (Hexaplex). *Clin Infect Dis.* 1998; 26: 1397-1402.

[107] Hindiyeh M, Hillyard DR, Carroll KC. Evaluation of the Prodesse Hexaplex multiplex PCR away for direct detection of seven respiratory viruses in clinical specimens. *Am J Clin Pathol.* 2001; 116: 218-224.

[108] Kehl SC, Hendrickson KJ, Hua W, Fan J. Evaluation of the Hexaplex assay for detection of respiratory viruses in children. *J Clin Microbiol.* 2001; 39: 1696-1701.

[109] LeGoff J, Kara R, Moulin F, Si-Mohamed A, Krivine A, Belec L, Lebon P. Evaluation of the one-step multiplex real-time reverse-transcription-PCR ProFlu-1 Assay for detection of influenza A and influenza B viruses and respiratory syncytial viruses in children. *J Clin Microbiol.* 2008; 46:789-791.

[110] Mahony J, Chong S, Merante F, Luinstra K, Sinha T, Petrich A, Lisle C, Yaghougian S, Janeczko R. Development of a respiratory virus panel (RVP) test for the detection of twenty human respiratory viruses using multiplex PCR and a fluid Microbead-based Assay. *J Clin Microbiol.* 2007; 45: 2965-70.

[111] Li, H, McCormac MA, Estes RW, Sefers SE, Dare RK, Chappell JD, Erdman DD, Wright PF, Tang Y-W. Simultaneous detection and high-throughput identification of a panel of RNA viruses causing respiratory tract infections. *J Clin Microbiol.* 2007; 45:2105-2109.

[112] Nolte FS, Marshall DJ, Rasberry C, Schievelbein S, Banks GG, Storch GA, Arens MQ, Buller RS,Prudent JR. MultiCode-PLx system for multiplexed detection of seventeen respiratory viruses. *J Clin Microbiol.* 2007; 45, 2779-2786.

[113] Center for devices and radiological health, U.S. Food and Drug Administration, 510 (k) Premarket notification database, xTAG respiratory virus panel assay, K063765, FDA review, decision summary, database updated 03/06/2008, pp 1-39. (http://www.accessdata.fda.gov/scripts/cdrh/cfdocs/cfPMN/pmn.cfm?ID=23615)

[114] Frobert E, Escuret V, Javouhey E, Casalegno JS, Bouscambert-Duchamp M, Moulinier C, Gillet Y, Lina B, Floret D, Morfin F. Respiratory viruses in children admitted to hospital intensive care units: Evaluating the CLART® Pneumovir DNA array. *J Med Virol.* 2011; 83:150-155.

[115] Coiras MT, Lopez-Huertas MR, Lopez-Campos G, Aguilar JC, Perez-Brena P. Oligonucleotide array for simultaneous detection of respiratory viruses using a reverse-line blot hybridization assay. *J Med Vir.* 2005; 26:256-264.

[116] Renois F, Talmud D, Huguenin A, Moute L, Strady C, Cousson J, Leveque N, Anfreoletti L. Rapid detection of respiratory tract viral infections and coinfections in patients with influenza-like illnesses by use of reverse transcription-PCR DNA microarray systems. *J Clin Micro.* 2010; 48:3836-3842.

[117] Jannetto PJ, Buchan BW, Vaughan KA, Ledford JS, Anderson DK, Henley DC, Quigley NB, Ledeboer NA. Real-time detection of influenza A, influenza B, and respiratory syncytial virus A and B in respiratory specimens by use of nanoparticle probes. *J Clin Micro.* 2010; 48:3997-4002.

[118] Mahony JB, Chong S, Smieja M, Petrich A, Buracond S, Babwah J. Establishing the epidemiology of respiratory virus infections using molecular technology. *Presented at: 107th Annual Meeting of the American Society for Microbiology,* Abstr C-070, Toronto, Ontario, Canada. May 21-25. 2007

[119] Pierangeli A, Gentile M, Di Marco P, Pagnotti P, Scagnolari C, Trombetti S, Lo Russo L, Tromba V, Moretti C, Midulla F, Antonelli G. Detection and typing by molecular techniques of respiratory viruses in children hospitalized for acute respiratory infection in Rome, Italy. *J Med Virol.* 2007; 79:463-8.

[120] American Academy of Pediatrics subcommittee on diagnosis and management of bronchiolitis. Diagnosis and management of bronchiolitis. *Pediatrics.* 2006; 118:1774-1793.

[121] Zorc JJ, Hall CB: Bronchiolitis: recent evidence on diagnosis and management. *Pediatrics.* 2010; 125:342-349.

[122] Kuzik BA, Al-Qadhi SA, Kent S, Flavin MP, Hopman W, Hotte S, Gander S. Nebulized hypertonic saline in the treatment of viral bronchiolitis in infants. *J Pediatr.* 2007; 151:266-70, 270.

[123] Willwerth BM, Harper MB, Greenes DS. Identifying hospitalized infants who have bronchiolitis and are at high risk for apnea. *Ann Emerg Med.* 2006; 48:441-447.

[124] Davison C, Ventre KM, Luchetti M, Randolph AG. Efficacy of interventions for bronchiolitis in critically ill infants: a systematic review and meta-analysis. *Pediatr Crit Care Med.* 2004; 5:482-489.

[125] Plint AC, Johnson DW, Patel H, Wiebe N, Correll R, Brant R, Mitton C, Gouin S, Bhatt M, Joubert G, Black KJ, Turner T, Whitehouse S, Klassen TP. Epinephrine and dexamethasone in children with bronchiolitis. *N Engl J Med.* 2009; 360:2079-2089.

[126] Fernandes RM, Bialy LM, Vandermeer B, Tjosvold L, Plint AC, Patel H, Johnson DW, Klassen TP, Hartling L. Glucocorticoids for acute viral bronchiolitis in infants and young children. *Cochrane Database Syst Rev.* 2010; 10: CD004878.

[127] Guerguerian AM, Farrell C, Gauthier M, Lacroix J. Bronchiolitis: what's next? *Pediatr Crit Care Med. 2004*; 5:498-500.

[128] Livni G, Rachmel A, Marom D, Yaari A, Tirosh N, Ashkenazi S: A randomized, double-blind study examining the comparative efficacies and safety of inhaled epinephrine and nasal decongestant in hospitalized infants with acute bronchiolitis. *Pediatr Infect Dis J.* 2010; 29:71-73.

[129] Gadomski AM, Brower M. Bronchodilators for bronchiolitis. *Cochrane Database Syst Rev.* 2010; 12: CD001266.

[130] Hartling L, Bialy LM, Vandermeer B, Tjosvold L, Johnson DW, Plint AC, Klassen TP, Patel H, Fernandes RM. Epinephrine for bronchiolitis. *Cochrane Database Syst Rev.* 2011; 6: CD003123.

[131] Kneyber MC, Brandenburg AH, de Groot R, Joosten KF, Rothbarth PH, Ott A, Moll HA. Risk factors for respiratory syncytial virus associated apnoea. *Eur J Pediatr.* 1998; 157:331-335.

[132] Totapally BR, Demerci C, Zureikat G, Nolan B. Tidal breathing flow-volume loops in bronchiolitis in infancy the effect of albuterol [ISRCTN47364493]. *Crit Care.* 2002; 6:160-165.

[133] Hartling L, Wiebe N, Russell K, Patel H, Klassen TP. Epinephrine for bronchiolitis. *Cochrane Database Syst Rev.* 2004; 1: CD003123.

[134] Numa AH, Williams GD, Dakin CJ: The effect of nebulized epinephrine on respiratory mechanics and gas exchange in bronchiolitis. *Am J Respir Crit Care Med.* 2001; 164: 86-91.

[135] Schuh S: Update on management of bronchiolitis. *Curr Opin Pediatr.* 2011; 23:110-114.

[136] Mandelberg A, Amirav I. Hypertonic saline or high volume normal saline for viral bronchiolitis: mechanisms and rationale. *Pediatr Pulmonol.* 2010; 45:36-40.

[137] Zhang L, Mendoza-Sassi RA, Wainwright C, Klassen TP. Nebulized hypertonic saline solution for acute bronchiolitis in infants. *Cochrane Database Syst Rev.* 2008; 4: CD006458.

[138] Grewal S, Ali S, McConnell DW, Vandermeer B, Klassen TP. A randomized trial of nebulized 3% hypertonic saline with epinephrine in the treatment of acute bronchiolitis in the emergency department. *Arch Pediatr Adolesc Med.* 2009; 163:1007-1012.

[139] Anil AB, Anil M, Saglam AB, Cetin N, Bal A, Aksu N: High volume normal saline alone is as effective as nebulized salbutamol-normal saline, epinephrine-normal saline, and 3% saline in mild bronchiolitis. *Pediatr Pulmonol.* 2010; 45:41-47.

[140] Gregory CJ, Nasrollahzadeh F, Dharmar M, Parsapour K, Marcin JP. Comparison of critically ill and injured children transferred from referring hospitals versus in-house admissions. *Pediatrics.* 2008; 121:e906-e911.

[141] Boogaard R, Hulsmann AR, van VL, Vaessen-Verberne AA, Yap YN, Sprij AJ, Brinkhorst G, Sibbles B, Hendriks T, Feith SW, Lincke CR, Brandsma AE, Brand PL, Hop WC, de HM, Merkus PJ. Recombinant human deoxyribonuclease in infants with respiratory syncytial virus bronchiolitis. *Chest.* 2007; 131:788-795.

[142] Nasr SZ, Strouse PJ, Soskolne E, Maxvold NJ, Garver KA, Rubin BK, Moler FW. Efficacy of recombinant human deoxyribonuclease I in the hospital management of respiratory syncytial virus bronchiolitis. *Chest.* 2001; 120:203-208.

[143] Merkus PJ, de HM, van GR, de Jongste JC. DNase treatment for atelectasis in infants with severe respiratory syncytial virus bronchiolitis. *Eur Respir J.* 2001; 18:734-737.

[144] Umoren R, Odey F, Meremikwu MM. Steam inhalation or humidified oxygen for acute bronchiolitis in children up to three years of age. *Cochrane Database Syst Rev.* 2011; 1: CD006435.

[145] Corneli HM, Zorc JJ, Mahajan P, Shaw KN, Holubkov R, Reeves SD, Ruddy RM, Malik B, Nelson KA, Bregstein JS, Brown KM, Denenberg MN, Lillis KA, Cimpello LB, Tsung JW, Borgialli DA, Baskin MN, Teshome G, Goldstein MA, Monroe D, Dean JM, Kuppermann N. A multicenter, randomized, controlled trial of dexamethasone for bronchiolitis. *N Engl J Med.* 2007; 357:331-339.

[146] Schuh S, Coates AL, Dick P, Stephens D, Lalani A, Nicota E, Mokanski M, Khaikin S, Allen U. A single versus multiple doses of dexamethasone in infants wheezing for the first time. *Pediatr Pulmonol.* 2008; 43:844-850.

[147] Purcell K, Fergie J. Concurrent serious bacterial infections in 912 infants and children hospitalized for treatment of respiratory syncytial virus lower respiratory tract infection. *Pediatr Infect Dis J.* 2004; 23:267-269.

[148] Greenes DS, Harper MB. Low risk of bacteremia in febrile children with recognizable viral syndromes. *Pediatr Infect Dis J.* 1999; 18:258-261.

[149] Antonow JA, Hansen K, McKinstry CA, Byington CL. Sepsis evaluations in hospitalized infants with bronchiolitis. *Pediatr Infect Dis J.* 1998; 17:231-236.

[150] Levine DA, Platt SL, Dayan PS, Macias CG, Zorc JJ, Krief W, Schor J, Bank D, Fefferman N, Shaw KN, Kuppermann N. Risk of serious bacterial infection in young febrile infants with respiratory syncytial virus infections. *Pediatrics.* 2004; 113:1728-1734.

[151] Spurling-Geoffrey KP, Fonseka K, Doust J, Del-Mar CB: Antibiotics for bronchiolitis in children. *Cochrane Database Syst Rev.* 2007; 1:CD005189.

[152] Thorburn K, Harigopal S, Reddy V, Taylor N, van Saene HK. High incidence of pulmonary bacterial co-infection in children with severe respiratory syncytial virus (RSV) bronchiolitis. *Thorax.* 2006; 61:611-615.

[153] Mayordomo-Colunga J, Medina A, Rey C, Diaz JJ, Concha A, Los AM, Menendez S: Predictive factors of non invasive ventilation failure in critically ill children: a prospective epidemiological study. *Intensive Care Med.* 2009; 35:527-536.

[154] Greenough A. Role of ventilation in RSV disease: CPAP, ventilation, HFO, ECMO. *Paediatr Respir Rev.* 2009; 10 Suppl 1:26-28.

[155] McNamara DG, Nixon GM, Anderson BJ. Methylxanthines for the treatment of apnea associated with bronchiolitis and anesthesia. *Paediatr Anaesth.* 2004; 14:541-550.

[156] Henderson-Smart DJ, De-Paoli AG. Methylxanthine treatment for apnoea in preterm infants. *Cochrane Database Syst Rev*. 2010; 12: CD000140.

[157] Sajit NT, Steggall M, Padmakumar B. Apnoeas in bronchiolitis: is there a role for caffeine? *Arch Dis Child.* 2005; 90:438.

[158] Tobias JD. Caffeine in the treatment of apnea associated with respiratory syncytial virus infection in neonates and infants. *South Med J.* 2000; 93:294-296.

[159] Proesmans M, Sauer K, Govaere E, Raes M, De Bilderling G, De Boeck K. Montelukast does not prevent reactive airway disease in young children hospitalized for RSV bronchiolitis. *Acta Paediatr*. 2009; 98:1830-1834.

[160] Hu J, Robinson JL. Treatment of respiratory syncytial virus with palivizumab: a systematic review. *World J Pediatr*. 2010; 6:296-300.

[161] Wu H, Pfarr DS, Johnson S, Brewah YA, Woods RM, Patel NK, White WI, Young JF, Kiener PA. Development of motavizumab, an ultra-potent antibody for the prevention of respiratory syncytial virus infection in the upper and lower respiratory tract. *J Mol Biol*. 2007; 368:652-665.

[162] Nokes JD, Cane PA. New strategies for control of respiratory syncytial virus infection. *Curr Opin Infect Dis*. 2008; 21:639-643.

[163] Carbonell-Estrany X, Simoes EA, Dagan R, Hall CB, Harris B, Hultquist M, Connor EM, Losonsky GA. Motavizumab for prophylaxis of respiratory syncytial virus in high-risk children: a noninferiority trial. *Pediatrics*. 2010; 125:e35-e51.

[164] Lagos R, DeVincenzo JP, Munoz A, Hultquist M, Suzich J, Connor EM, Losonsky GA. Safety and antiviral activity of motavizumab, a respiratory syncytial virus (RSV)-specific humanized monoclonal antibody, when administered to RSV-infected children. *Pediatr Infect Dis J*. 2009; 28:835-837.

[165] Prais D, Schonfeld T, Amir J. Admission to the intensive care unit for respiratory syncytial virus bronchiolitis: a national survey before palivizumab use. *Pediatrics*. 2003; 112:548-552.

[166] Flamant C, Hallalel F, Nolent P, Chevalier JY, Renolleau S. Severe respiratory syncytial virus bronchiolitis in children: from short mechanical ventilation to extracorporeal membrane oxygenation. *Eur J Pediatr*. 2005; 164:93-98.

[167] Wilkesmann A, Ammann RA, Schildgen O, Eis-Hubinger AM, Muller A, Seidenberg J, Stephan V, Rieger C, Herting E, Wygold T, Hornschuh F, Groothuis JR, Simon A. Hospitalized children with respiratory syncytial virus infection and neuromuscular impairment face an increased risk of a complicated course. *Pediatr Infect Dis J*. 2007; 26:485-491.

[168] Tasker RC: CPAP and HFOV: different guises of the same underlying intensive care strategy for supporting RSV bronchiolitis. *Intensive Care Med*. 2008; 34:1560-1561.

[169] Garcia CG, Bhore R, Soriano-Fallas A, Trost M, Chason R, Ramilo O, Mejias A. Risk factors in children hospitalized with RSV bronchiolitis versus non-RSV bronchiolitis. *Pediatrics*. 2010; 126:e1453-e1460.

[170] Frazier MD, Cheifetz IM. The role of heliox in paediatric respiratory disease. *Paediatr. Respir Rev*. 2010; 11:46-53.

[171] Kneyber MC, van HM, Twisk JW, Plotz FB, Markhors DG. Heliox reduces respiratory system resistance in respiratory syncytial virus induced respiratory failure. *Crit Care*. 2009; 13:R71.

[172] Liet JM, Ducruet T, Gupta V, Cambonie G. Heliox inhalation therapy for bronchiolitis in infants. *Cochrane Database Syst Rev.* 2010; 4:CD00 2010.

[173] Martinon-Torres F, Rodriguez-Nunez A, Martinon-Sanchez JM. Nasal continuous positive airway pressure with heliox versus air oxygen in infants with acute bronchiolitis: a crossover study. *Pediatrics.* 2008; 121:e1190-e1195.

[174] Schibler A, Pham TM, Dunster KR, Foster K, Barlow A, Gibbons K, Hough JL: Reduced intubation rates for infants after introduction of high-flow nasal prong oxygen delivery. *Intensive Care Med.* 2011; 37:847-852.

[175] McKiernan C, Chua LC, Visintainer PF, Allen H. High flow nasal cannulae therapy in infants with bronchiolitis. *J Pediatr.* 2010; 156:634-638.

[176] Arora B, Mahajan P, Zidan M, Sethuraman U. Nasopharyngeal Airway Pressures with Heated, Humidified, High Flow Nasal Cannula (HHHFNC). *Oxygen Therapy in Patients with Bronchiolitis - A Pilot Study.* 2011.

[177] Cambonie G, Milesi C, Jaber S, Amsallem F, Barbotte E, Picaud JC, Matecki S. Nasal continuous positive airway pressure decreases respiratory muscles overload in young infants with severe acute viral bronchiolitis. *Intensive Care Med* 2008; 34:1865-1872.

[178] McNamara F, Sullivan CE. Nasal CPAP treatment in an infant with respiratory syncytial virus-associated apnea. *Pediatr Pulmonol.* 1997; 24:218-221.

[179] Thia LP, McKenzie SA, Blyth TP, Minasian CC, Kozlowska WJ, Carr SB. Randomised controlled trial of nasal continuous positive airways pressure (CPAP) in bronchiolitis. *Arch Dis Child.* 2008; 93:45-47.

[180] Essouri S, Chevret L, Durand P, Haas V, Fauroux B, Devictor D. Noninvasive positive pressure ventilation: five years of experience in a pediatric intensive care unit. *Pediatr Crit Care Med.* 2006; 7:329-334.

[181] Javouhey E, Barats A, Richard N, Stamm D, Floret D. Non-invasive ventilation as primary ventilatory support for infants with severe bronchiolitis. *Intensive Care Med.* 2008; 34:1608-1614.

[182] Yanez LJ, Yunge M, Emilfork M, Lapadula M, Alcantara A, Fernandez C, Lozano J, Contreras M, Conto L, Arevalo C, Gayan A, Hernandez F, Pedraza M, Feddersen M, Bejares M, Morales M, Mallea F, Glasinovic M, Cavada G. A prospective, randomized, controlled trial of noninvasive ventilation in pediatric acute respiratory failure. *Pediatr Crit Care Med.* 2008; 9:484-489.

[183] Hartmann H, Jawad MH, Noyes J, Samuels MP, Southall DP. Negative extrathoracic pressure ventilation in central hypoventilation syndrome. *Arch Dis. Child.* 1994; 70:418-423.

[184] Calderini E, Chidini G, Pelosi P. What are the current indications for noninvasive ventilation in children? *Curr Opin Anaesthesiol.* 2010; 23:368-374.

[185] Lista G, Castoldi F, Fontana P, Daniele I, Cavigioli F, Rossi S, Mancuso D, Reali R. Nasal continuous positive airway pressure (CPAP) versus bi-level nasal CPAP in preterm babies with respiratory distress syndrome: a randomised control trial. *Arch Dis Child Fetal Neonatal Ed.* 2010; 95:F85-F89.

[186] Morley CJ, Davis PG, Doyle LW, Brion LP, Hascoet JM, Carlin JB. Nasal CPAP or intubation at birth for very preterm infants. *N Engl J Med.* 2008; 358:700-708.

[187] Wang EE, Law BJ, Boucher FD, Stephens D, Robinson JL, Dobson S, Langley JM, McDonald J, MacDonald NE, Mitchell I. Pediatric Investigators Collaborative Network on Infections in Canada (PICNIC) study of admission and management variation in

patients hospitalized with respiratory syncytial viral lower respiratory tract infection. *J Pediatr.* 1996; 129:390-395.

[188] Leclerc F, Scalfaro P, Noizet O, Thumerelle C, Dorkenoo A, Fourier C: Mechanical ventilatory support in infants with respiratory syncytial virus infection. *Pediatr Crit Care Med.* 2001; 2:197-204.

[189] Berner ME, Hanquinet S, Rimensberger PC. High frequency oscillatory ventilation for respiratory failure due to RSV bronchiolitis. *Intensive Care Med.* 2008; 34:1698-1702.

[190] Kneyber MC, Brouwers AG, Caris JA, Chedamni S, Plotz FB. Acute respiratory distress syndrome: is it underrecognized in the pediatric intensive care unit? *Intensive Care Med.* 2008; 34:751-754.

[191] Meade MO, Cook DJ, Guyatt GH, Slutsky AS, Arabi YM, Cooper DJ, Davies AR, Hand LE, Zhou Q, Thabane L, Austin P, Lapinsky S, Baxter A, Russell J, Skrobik Y, Ronco JJ, Stewart TE. Ventilation strategy using low tidal volumes, recruitment maneuvers, and high positive end-expiratory pressure for acute lung injury and acute respiratory distress syndrome: a randomized controlled trial. *JAMA.* 2008; 299:637-645.

[192] Briel M, Meade M, Mercat A, Brower RG, Talmor D, Walter SD, Slutsky AS, Pullenayegum E, Zhou Q, Cook D, Brochard L, Richard JC, Lamontagne F, Bhatnagar N, Stewart TE, Guyatt G. Higher vs lower positive end-expiratory pressure in patients with acute lung injury and acute respiratory distress syndrome: systematic review and meta-analysis. *JAMA.* 2010; 303:865-873.

[193] Barreira ER, Precioso AR, Bousso A. Pulmonary surfactant in respiratory syncytial virus bronchiolitis: The role in pathogenesis and clinical implications. *Pediatr Pulmonol.* 2010. [E-Pub ahead of print]

[194] Duffett M, Choong K, Ng V, Randolph A, Cook DJ. Surfactant therapy for acute respiratory failure in children: a systematic review and meta-analysis. *Crit Care.* 2007; 11:R66.

[195] Perrotta C, Ortiz Z, Roque M. Chest physiotherapy for acute bronchiolitis in paediatric patients between 0 and 24 months old. *Cochrane Database Syst Rev.* 2007; 1:CD004873.

[196] Gajdos V, Katsahian S, Beydon N, Abadie V, de PL, Larrar S, Epaud R, Chevallier B, Bailleux S, Mollet-Boudjemline A, Bouyer J, Chevret S, Labrune P. Effectiveness of chest physiotherapy in infants hospitalized with acute bronchiolitis: a multicenter, randomized, controlled trial. *PLoS Med.* 2010; 7:e1000345.

[197] Guerguerian AM, Gauthier M, Lebel MH, Farrell CA, Lacroix J. Ribavirin in ventilated respiratory syncytial virus bronchiolitis. A randomized, placebo-controlled trial. *Am J Respir Crit Care Med.* 1999; 160:829-834.

[198] King VJ, Viswanathan M, Bordley WC, Jackman AM, Sutton SF, Lohr KN, Carey TS. Pharmacologic treatment of bronchiolitis in infants and children: a systematic review. *Arch Pediatr Adolesc Med.* 2004; 158:127-137.

[199] Hu J, Doucette K, Hartling L, Tjosvold L, Robinson J. Treatment of hepatitis C in children: a systematic review. *PLoS One.* 2010; 5:e11542.

[200] Soares-Weiser K, Thomas S, Thomson G, Garner P. Ribavirin for Crimean-Congo hemorrhagic fever: systematic review and meta-analysis. *BMC Infect Dis.* 2010; 10:207.

[201] Ramilo O. Evolution of prophylaxis: MoAb, siRNA, vaccine, and small molecules. *Paediatr Respir Rev.* 2009; 10 Suppl 1:23-25.

[202] DeVincenzo J, Lambkin-Williams R, Wilkinson T, Cehelsky J, Nochur S, Walsh E, Meyers R, Gollob J, Vaishnaw A. A randomized, double-blind, placebo-controlled study of an RNAi-based therapy directed against respiratory syncytial virus. *Proc Natl Acad Sci USA.* 2010; 107:8800-8805.

[203] Hall CB, Douglas RG Jr, Geiman JM. Respiratory syncytial virus infections in infants. quantitation and duration of shedding. *J Pediatr*. 1976; 89:11-15.

[204] Hall CB, Douglas RG Jr, Geiman JM. Possible transmission by fomites of respiratory syncytial virus. *J Infect Dis*. 1980; 141:98-102.

[205] Hall CB, Douglas RG Jr, Schnabel KC, Geiman JM. Infectivity of respiratory syncytial virus by various routes of inoculation. *Infect Immun.* 1981; 33:779-783.

[206] Hall CB, Douglas RG Jr. Modes of transmission of respiratory syncytial virus. *J Pediatr.* 1981; 99:100-103.

[207] Cruz AT. Review: physical interventions may reduce the transmission of respiratory viruses. *Arch Dis Child Educ Pract Ed.* 2011; 96:160.

[208] Jefferson T, Del Mar C, Dooley L, Ferroni E, Al-Ansary LA, Bawazeer GA, van Driel ML, Nair S, Foxlee R, Rivetti A. Physical interventions to interrupt or reduce the spread of respiratory viruses. *Cochrane Database Syst. Rev*. 2010; 1:CD006207.

[209] Madge P, Paton JY, McColl JH, Mackie PL. Prospective controlled study of four infection-control procedures to prevent nosocomial infection with respiratory syncytial virus. *Lancet.* 1992; 340:1079-1083.

[210] Leclair JM, Freeman J, Sullivan BF, Crowley CM, Goldmann DA. Prevention of nosocomial respiratory syncytial virus infections through compliance with glove and gown isolation precautions. *N Engl J Med.* 1987; 317:329-334.

[211] Macartney KK, Gorelick MH, Manning ML, Hodinka RL, Bell LM. Nosocomial respiratory syncytial virus infections: the cost-effectiveness and cost-benefit of infection control. *Pediatrics*. 2000; 106:520-526.

[212] Simon A, Khurana K, Wilkesmann A, Müller A, Engelhart S, Exner M, Schildgen O, Eis-Hübinger AM, Groothuis JR, Bode U. Nosocomial respiratory syncytial virus infection: impact of prospective surveillance and targeted infection control. *Int J Hyg Environ Health*. 2006; 209:317-324.

[213] Reduction of respiratory syncytial virus hospitalization among premature infants and infants with bronchopulmonary dysplasia using respiratory syncytial virus immune globulin prophylaxis. The PREVENT Study Group. *Pediatrics*. 1997; 99:93-99.

[214] Simoes EA, Sondheimer HM, Top FH Jr, Meissner HC, Welliver RC, Kramer AA, Groothuis JR. Respiratory syncytial virus immune globulin for prophylaxis against respiratory syncytial virus disease in infants and children with congenital heart disease. The Cardiac Study Group. *J Pediatr*. 1998; 133:492-499.

[215] Murphy BR, Hall SL, Kulkarni AB, Crowe JE Jr, Collins PL, Connors M, Karron RA, Chanock RM. An update on approaches to the development of respiratory syncytial virus (RSV) and parainfluenza virus type 3 (PIV3) vaccines. *Virus Res*. 1994; 32:13-36.

[216] Johnson S, Oliver C, Prince GA, Hemming VG, Pfarr DS, Wang SC, Dormitzer M, O'Grady J, Koenig S, Tamura JK, Woods R, Bansal G, Couchenour D, Tsao E, Hall WC, Young JF. Development of a humanized monoclonal antibody (MEDI-493) with potent in vitro and in vivo activity against respiratory syncytial virus. *J Infect Dis*. 1997; 176: 1215-1224.

[217] Subramanian KN, Weisman LE, Rhodes T, Ariagno R, Sánchez PJ, Steichen J, Givner LB, Jennings TL, Top FH Jr, Carlin D, Connor E. Safety, tolerance and pharmacokinetics of a humanized monoclonal antibody to respiratory syncytial virus in premature infants and infants with bronchopulmonary dysplasia. MEDI-493 Study Group. *Pediatr Infect Dis* J. 1998; 17:110-115.

[218] Sáez-Llorens X, Castaño E, Null D, Steichen J, Sánchez PJ, Ramilo O, Top FH Jr, Connor E. Safety and pharmacokinetics of an intramuscular humanized monoclonal antibody to respiratory syncytial virus in premature infants and infants with bronchopulmonary dysplasia. The MEDI-493 Study Group. *Pediatr Infect Dis J.* 1998; 17:787-791.

[219] Palivizumab, a humanized respiratory syncytial virus monoclonal antibody, reduces hospitalization from respiratory syncytial virus infection in high-risk infants. The IMpact-RSV Study Group. *Pediatrics.* 1998; 102:531-537.

[220] Feltes TF, Cabalka AK, Meissner HC, Piazza FM, Carlin DA, Top FH Jr, Connor EM, Sondheimer HM. Cardiac Synagis Study Group. Palivizumab prophylaxis reduces hospitalization due to respiratory syncytial virus in young children with hemodynamically significant congenital heart disease. *J Pediatr.* 2003; 143:532-540.

[221] Canadian Paediatric Society. Use of palivizumab in children with congenital heart disease. *Paediatr Child Health.* 2003; 8:631-633.

[222] Rondini G, MacagnoF, Barberi I. Raccomandazioni della Societa Italiana di Neonatologia per la prevenzione delle malattie da virus respiratorio sinciziale (VRS). *Acta Neonatal.* 2004; 1:1-11.

[223] Resch B, Berger A, Bernert G, Eber E, Frischer T, Simma B, et al. Konsensuspapier zur Prophylaxe der RSV-Infektion mit Palivizumab und Post-RSV-Atemwegserkrankung. *Monatsschr Kinderheilkd.* 2008; 156:381–383.

[224] Figueras Aloy J, Quero J, Doménech E, López Herrera MC, Izquierdo I, Losada A, Perapch J, Sánchez-Luna M; Comité de Estándares de la Sociedad Española de Neonatología.[Recommendations for the prevention of respiratory syncytial virus infection]. *An Pediatr.* (Barc) 2005; 63:357-362.

[225] Samson L. The Canadian Paediatric Society, Infectious Diseases and Immunization Committee. *Paediatr Child Health.* 2009; 14:521-26.

[226] Committee on Infectious Diseases. From the American Academy of Pediatrics: Policy statements--Modified recommendations for use of palivizumab for prevention of respiratory syncytial virus infections. *Pediatrics.* 2009; 124:1694-1701.

[227] Boyce TG, Mellen BG, Mitchel EF Jr, Wright PF, Griffin MR. Rates of hospitalization for respiratory syncytial virus infection among children in medicaid. *J Pediatr.* 2000; 137:865-870.

[228] Horn SD, Smout RJ. Effect of prematurity on respiratory syncytial virus hospital resource use and outcomes. *J Pediatr.* 2003; 143:S133-141.

[229] Willson DF, Landrigan CP, Horn SD, Smout RJ. Complications in infants hospitalized for bronchiolitis or respiratory syncytial virus pneumonia. *J Pediatr.* 2003; 143:S142-9.

[230] Sampalis JS. Morbidity and mortality after RSV-associated hospitalizations among premature Canadian infants. *J Pediatr.* 2003; 143:S150-156.

[231] Kramer MS, Demissie K, Yang H, Platt RW, Sauvé R, Liston R. The contribution of mild and moderate preterm birth to infant mortality. Fetal and Infant Health Study Group of the Canadian Perinatal Surveillance System. *JAMA.* 2000; 284:843-849.

[232] Khashu M, Narayanan M, Bhargava S, Osiovich H. Perinatal outcomes associated with preterm birth at 33 to 36 weeks' gestation: a population-based cohort study. *Pediatrics*. 2009; 123:109-113.

[233] Hislop AA, Haworth SG. Airway size and structure in the normal fetal and infant lung and the effect of premature delivery and artificial ventilation. *Am Rev Respir Dis*. 1989; 140:1717-126.

[234] Friedrich L, Stein RT, Pitrez PM, Corso AL, Jones MH. Reduced lung function in healthy preterm infants in the first months of life. *Am J Respir Crit Care Med*. 2006; 173:442–447.

[235] Friedrich L, Pitrez PM, Stein RT, Goldani M, Tepper R, Jones MH. Growth rate of lung function in healthy preterm infants. *Am J Respir Crit Care Med*. 2007; 176:1269–1273.

[236] Jones M. Effect of preterm birth on airway function and lung growth. *Paediatr Respir Rev*. 2009; 10:S9-11.

[237] Welliver TP, Garofalo RP, Hosakote Y, Hintz KH, Avendano L, Sanchez K, Velozo L, Jafri H, Chavez-Bueno S, Ogra PL, McKinney L, Reed JL, Welliver RC Sr. Severe human lower respiratory tract illness caused by respiratory syncytial virus and influenza virus is characterized by the absence of pulmonary cytotoxic lymphocyte responses. *J Infect Dis*. 2007; 195:1126-1136.

[238] Yeung CY, Hobbs JR. Serum-gamma-G-globulin levels in normal premature, post-mature, and "small-for-dates" newborn babies. *Lancet*. 1968; 1:1167-1170.

[239] Ballow M, Cates KL, Rowe JC, Goetz C, Desbonnet C. Development of the immune system in very low birth weight (less than 1500 g) premature infants: concentrations of plasma immunoglobulins and patterns of infections. *Pediatr Res*. 1986; 20:899-904.

[240] Figueras-Aloy J, Carbonell-Estrany X, IRIS Study Group. Case–control study of the risk factors linked to respiratory syncytial virus infection requiring hospitalization in premature infants born at a gestational age of 33–35 weeks in Spain. *Pediatr Infect Dis J*. 2004; 23:815–820.

[241] Carbonell-Estrany X, Figueras-Aloy J, Law BJ; Infección Respiratoria Infantil por Virus Respiratorio Sincitial Study Group; Pediatric Investigators Collaborative Network on Infections in Canada Study Group. Identifying risk factors for severe respiratory syncytial virus among infants born after 33 through 35 completed weeks of gestation: different methodologies yield consistent findings.*Pediatr Infect Dis J*. 2004; 23:S193-201.

[242] Figueras-Aloy J, Carbonell-Estrany X, Quero-Jiménez J, et al. IRIS Study Group. FLIP-2 Study: risk factors linked to respiratory syncytial virus infection requiring hospitalization in premature infants born in Spain at a gestational age of 32 to 35 weeks.*Pediatr Infect Dis J*. 2008; 27:788-793.

[243] Doering G, Gusenleitner W, Belohradsky BH, Burdach S, Resch B, Liese JG. The risk of respiratory syncytial virus-related hospitalizations in preterm infants of 29 to 35 weeks' gestational age. *Pediatr Infect Dis J*. 2006; 25:1188-1190.

[244] Rossi GA, Medici MC, Arcangeletti MC, Lanari M, Merolla R, Paparatti UD, Silvestri M, Pistorio A, Chezzi C; Osservatorio RSV Study Group. Risk factors for severe RSV-induced lower respiratory tract infection over four consecutive epidemics. *Eur J Pediatr*. 2007; 1166:1267-1272.

[245] Sampalis JS, Langley J, Carbonell-Estrany X, et al. Development and validation of a risk scoring tool to predict respiratory syncytial virus hospitalization in premature

infants born at 33 through 35 completed weeks of gestation. *Med Decis Making.* 2008; 28:471-480.

[246] Simões EA, Carbonell-Estrany X, Fullarton JR, et al. European RSV Risk Factor Study Group. A predictive model for respiratory syncytial virus (RSV) hospitalisation of premature infants born at 33-35 weeks of gestational age, based on data from the Spanish FLIP Study. *Respir Res.* 2008; 9:78.

[247] Carbonell-Estrany X, Simões EA, Fullarton JR, Ferdynus C, Gouyon JB; European RSV Risk Factor Study Group. Validation of a model to predict hospitalization due to RSV of infants born at 33-35 weeks' gestation. *J. Perinat Med.* 2010; 38:411-417.

[248] Stensballe LG, Fullarton JR, Carbonell-Estrany X, Simões EA. Population based external validation of a European predictive model for respiratory syncytial virus hospitalization of premature infants born 33 to 35 weeks of gestational age. *Pediatr Infect Dis J.* 2010; 29:374–376.

[249] Simões EA, Carbonell-Estrany X, Fullarton JR, Rossi GA, Barberi I, Lanari M; European RSV Risk Factor Study Group. European risk factors' model to predict hospitalization of premature infants born 33-35 weeks' gestational age with respiratory syncytial virus: validation with Italian data. *J Matern Fetal Neonatal Med.* 2011; 24:152-157.

[250] Paes B, Steele S, Janes M, Pinelli J. Risk-scoring tool for respiratory syncytial virus prophylaxis in premature infants born at 33–35 completed weeks' gestational age in Canada. *Curr Med Res Opin.* 2009; 25:1585–1591.

[251] Figueras Aloy J, Carbonell Estrany X; Comité de Estándares de la Sociedad Española de Neonatología. Recommendations for the use of palivizumab in the prevention of respiratory syncytial virus infection in late preterm infants (32(1) to 35(0) weeks of gestation)]. *An Pediatr.* (Barc) 2010; 73:98.e1-4.

[252] van Ewijk BE, van der Zalm MM, Wolfs TF, van der Ent CK. Viral respiratory infections in cystic fibrosis. *J Cyst Fibros.* 2005; 4:S31-6.

[253] Smyth AR, Smyth RL, Tong CY, Hart CA, Heaf DP. Effect of respiratory virus infections including rhinovirus on clinical status in cystic fibrosis. *Arch Dis Child.* 1995; 73:117-120.

[254] Abman SH, Ogle JW, Butler-Simon N, Rumack CM, Accurso FJ. Role of respiratory syncytial virus in early hospitalizations for respiratory distress of young infants with cystic fibrosis. *J Pediatr.* 1988; 113:826-830.

[255] Wang EE, Prober CG, Manson B, et al. Association of respiratory viral infections with pulmonary deterioration in patients with cystic fibrosis. *N Engl J Med.* 1984; 311:1653–1658.

[256] Hiatt PW, Grace SC, Kozinetz CA, et al. Effects of viral lower respiratory tract infection on lung function in infants with cystic fibrosis. *Pediatrics.* 1999; 103:619-626.

[257] Sly PD, Brennan S, Gangell C, de Klerk N, Murray C, Mott L, et al. Lung disease at diagnosis in infants with cystic fibrosis detected by newborn screening. *Am J Respir Crit Care Med.* 2009; 180:146–152.

[258] Johansen HK, Høiby N. Seasonal onset of initial colonisation and chronic infection with Pseudomonas aeruginosa in patients with cystic fibrosis in Denmark. *Thorax.* 1992; 47:109-11.

[259] Petersen NT, Høiby N, Mordhorst CH, Lind K, Flensborg EW, Bruun B. Respiratory infections in cystic fibrosis patients caused by virus, chlamydia and mycoplasma--

possible synergism with Pseudomonas aeruginosa. *Acta Paediatr Scand.* 1981; 70:623-628.

[260] Colasurdo GN, Fullmer JJ, Elidemir O, Atkins C, Khan AM, Stark JM. Respiratory syncytial virus infection in a murine model of cystic fibrosis. *J Med Virol.* 2006; 78:651-8.

[261] Van Ewijk BE, Wolfs TF, Aerts PC, Van Kessel KP, Fleer A, Kimpen JL, Van der Ent CK. RSV mediates Pseudomonas aeruginosa binding to cystic fibrosis and normal epithelial cells. *Pediatr Res.* 2007; 61:398-403.

[262] de Vrankrijker AM, Wolfs TF, Ciofu O, Høiby N, van der Ent CK, Poulsen SS, Johansen HK. Respiratory syncytial virus infection facilitates acute colonization of Pseudomonas aeruginosa in mice. *J Med Virol.* 2009; 81:2096-2103.

[263] Armstrong D, Grimwood K, Carlin JB, Carzino R, Hull J, Olinsky A, Phelan PD. Severe viral respiratory infections in infants with cystic fibrosis. *Pediatr Pulmonol. 1998*; 26:371–379.

[264] Uong EC, McDonough JM, Tayag-Kier CE, Zhao H, Haselgrove J, Mahboubi S, Schwab RJ, Pack AI, Arens R. Magnetic resonance imaging of the upper airway in children with Down syndrome. *Am J Respir Crit Care Med.* 200; 163:731-736.

[265] Fink GB, Madaus WK, Walker GF. A quantitative study of the face in Down's syndrome. *Am J Orthod.* 1975; 67:540-553.

[266] Frazier JB, Friedman B. Swallow function in children with Down syndrome: a retrospective study. *Dev Med. Child Neurol.* 1996; 38:695-703.

[267] Weir K, McMahon S, Barry L, Ware R, Masters IB, Chang AB. Oropharyngeal aspiration and pneumonia in children. *Pediatr Pulmonol.* 2007; 42:1024-1031.

[268] Moore SW. Down syndrome and the enteric nervous system. *Pediatr Surg Int.* 2008 ; 24:873-883.

[269] Macchini F, Leva E, Torricelli M, Valadè A. Treating acid reflux disease in patients with Down syndrome: pharmacological and physiological approaches. *Clin Exp Gastroenterol.* 2011; 4:19-22.

[270] Bertrand P, Navarro H, Caussade S, Holmgren N, Sánchez I. Airway anomalies in children with Down syndrome: endoscopic findings. *Pediatr Pulmonol.* 2003; 36:137-141.

[271] Cooney TP, Thurlbeck WM. Pulmonary hypoplasia in Down's syndrome. *N Engl J Med.* 1982; 307:1170-1173.

[272] Cooney TP, Wentworth PJ, Thurlbeck WM. Diminished radial count is found only postnatally in Down's syndrome. *Pediatr Pulmonol.* 1988; 5:204-209.

[273] Hilton JM, Fitzgerald DA, Cooper DM. Respiratory morbidity of hospitalized children with Trisomy 21. *J Paediatr. Child Health.* 1999; 35:383-386.

[274] Bloemers BL, Broers CJ, Bont L, Weijerman ME, Gemke RJ, van Furth AM. Increased risk of respiratory tract infections in children with Down syndrome: the consequence of an altered immune system. *Microbes Infect.* 2010; 12:799-808.

[275] Bloemers BL, van Bleek GM, Kimpen JL, Bont L. Distinct abnormalities in the innate immune system of children with Down syndrome. *J Pediatr.* 2010; 156:804-9, 809.e1-809.e5.

[276] de Hingh YC, van der Vossen PW, Gemen EF, Mulder AB, Hop WC, Brus F, de Vries E. Intrinsic abnormalities of lymphocyte counts in children with down syndrome. *J Pediatr.* 2005; 147:744-747.

[277] Ram G, Chinen J. Infections and immunodeficiency in Down syndrome. *Clin Exp Immunol.* 2011; 164:9-16.

[278] Kusters MA, Verstegen RH, Gemen EF, de Vries E. Intrinsic defect of the immune system in children with Down syndrome: a review. *Clin Exp Immunol.* 2009; 156:189-193.

[279] Kusters MA, Gemen EF, Verstegen RH, Wever PC, DE Vries E. Both normal memory counts and decreased naive cells favor intrinsic defect over early senescence of Down syndrome T lymphocytes. *Pediatr Res.* 2010; 67:557-562.

[280] Bloemers BL, van Furth AM, Weijerman ME, Gemke RJ, Broers CJ, van den Ende K, Kimpen JL, Strengers JL, Bont LJ. Down syndrome: a novel risk factor for respiratory syncytial virus bronchiolitis--a prospective birth-cohort study. *Pediatrics.* 2007; 120:e1076-1081.

[281] Megged O, Schlesinger Y. Down syndrome and respiratory syncytial virus infection. *Pediatr Infect Dis J.* 2010; 29:672-673.

[282] Kristensen K, Stensballe LG, Bjerre J, Roth D, Fisker N, Kongstad T, Svendsen AL, Nielsen BW Risk factors for respiratory syncytial virus hospitalisation in children with heart disease. *Arch Dis Child.* 2009; 94:785-789.

[283] Sullivan PB. Gastrointestinal disorders in children with neurodevelopmental disabilities. *Dev Disabil Res Rev.* 2008; 14:128-136.

[284] de Veer AJ, Bos JT, Niezen-de Boer RC, Böhmer CJ, Francke AL. Symptoms of gastroesophageal reflux disease in severely mentally retarded people: a systematic review. *BMC Gastroenterol.* 2008; 8:23.

[285] Mori M, Kawashima H, Nakamura H, Nakagawa M, Kusuda S, Saji T, Tsutsumi H, Yokota S, Itoh S; Surveillance Committee for Severe RSV Infection. Nationwide survey of severe respiratory syncytial virus infection in children who do not meet indications for palivizumab in Japan. *J Infect Chemother.* 2011; 17:254-263.

[286] Arnold SR, Wang EE, Law BJ, et al. Variable morbidity of respiratory syncytial virus infection in patients with underlying lung disease: a review of the PICNIC RSV database. Pediatric Investigators Collaborative Network on Infections in Canada. *Pediatr Infect Dis J.* 1999; 18:866-869.

[287] Resch B, Gusenleitner W, Müller WD, Haas J. Observational study of respiratory syncytial virus-associated hospitalizations and use of palivizumab in premature infants aged 29-32 weeks. *Eur J Cli. Microbiol Infect Dis.* 2006; 25:120-122.

[288] Hall CB, Powell KR, MacDonald NE, Gala CL, Menegus ME, et al. Respiratory syncytial viral infection in children with compromised immune function. *N Engl J Med.* 1986; 315:77–81.

[289] Madhi SA, Venter M, Madhi A, Petersen MK, Klugman KP. Differing manifestations of respiratory syncytial virus-associated severe lower respiratory tract infections in human immunodeficiency virus type 1-infected and uninfected children. *Pediatr Infect Dis J.* 2001; 20:164-170.

[290] King JC Jr, Burke AR, Clemens JD, Nair P, Farley JJ, Vink PE, Batlas SR, Rao M, Johnson JP. Respiratory syncytial virus illnesses in human immunodeficiency virus- and noninfected children. *Pediatr Infect Dis J.* 1993; 12:733-739.

[291] Sung L, Alonzo TA, Gerbing RB, Aplenc R, Lange BJ, Woods WG, Feusner J, Franklin J, Patterson MJ, Gamis AS; Children's Oncology Group. Respiratory syncytial

virus infections in children with acute myeloid leukemia: a report from the Children's Oncology Group. *Pediatr Blood Cancer.* 2008; 51:784-786.

[292] Blanchard SS, Gerrek M, Siegel C, Czinn SJ. Significant morbidity associated with RSV infection in immunosuppressed children following liver transplantation: case report and discussion regarding need of routine prophylaxis. *Pediatr Transplant.* 2006; 10:826-829.

[293] Pohl C, Green M, Wald ER, Ledesma-Medina J. Respiratory syncytial virus infections in pediatric liver transplant recipients. *J Infect Dis.* 1992; 165:166-169.

[294] McCarthy AJ, Kingman HM, Kelly C, Taylor GS, Caul EO, Grier D, Moppett J, Foot AB, Cornish JM, Oakhill A, Steward CG, Pamphilon DH, Marks DI. The outcome of 26 patients with respiratory syncytial virus infection following allogeneic stem cell transplantation. *Bone Marrow Transplant.* 1999; 24:1315-1322.

[295] Bate J, Ladhani S, Sharland M, Chisholm J, Lamagni T, Ramsay M, Johnson A, Pebody R. Infection-related mortality in children with malignancy in England and Wales, 2003-2005. *Pediatr Blood Cancer.* 2009; 53:371-374.

[296] Singleton RJ, Bruden D, Bulkow LR, Varney G, Butler JC. Decline in respiratory syncytial virus hospitalizations in a region with high hospitalization rates and prolonged season. *Pediatr Infect Dis J.* 2006; 25:1116-1122.

[297] Young M, Kandola K, Mitchell R, et al. Hospital admission rates for lower respiratory tract infections in infants in the Northwest Territories andKitikmeot region of Nunavut for 2000–2004. *Paediatr Child Health.* 2007; 12:563–566.

[298] Carson JB, Postl BD, Spady D, et al. Lower respiratory tract infections among Canadian Inuit Children. *Int J Circumpolar Health.* 1984; 84:226–228.

[299] Banerji A. High rates of hospitalisation for bronchiolitis in Inuit children on Baffin Island. *Int. J. Circumpolar Health.* 2001; 60:375–379.

[300] Dede A, Isaacs D, Torzillo PJ, Wakerman J, Roseby R, Fahy R, Clothier T, White A, Kitto P. Respiratory syncytial virus infections in Central Australia. *J Paediatr Child Health.* 2010; 46:35-39.

[301] Banerji A, Greenberg D, White LF, et al. Risk factors and viruses associated with hospitalization due to lower respiratory tract infections in Canadian Inuit children: a case-control study. *Pediatr Infect Dis J.* 2009; 28:697-701.

[302] Moore H, Burgner D, Carville K, Jacoby P, Richmond P, Lehmann D. Diverging trends for lower respiratory infections in non-Aboriginal and Aboriginal children. *J Paediatr Child Health.* 2007; 43:451-457.

[303] Banerji A, Bell A, Mills EL, et al. Lower respiratory tract infections in Inuit infants on Baffin Island. *CMAJ.* 2001; 164:1847-1850.

[304] Reeve CA, Whitehall JS, Buettner PG, Norton R, Reeve DM, Francis F. Predicting respiratory syncytial virus hospitalisation in Australian children. *J Paediatr Child Health.* 2006; 42:248-252.

[305] Lowther SA, Shay DK, Holman RC, Clarke MJ, Kaufman SF, Anderson LJ. Bronchiolitis-associated hospitalizations among American Indian and Alaska Native children. *Pediatr Infect Dis J.* 2000; 19:11-17.

[306] Zachariah P, Ruttenber M, Simões EA. Hospitalizations due to respiratory syncytial virus in children with congenital malformations. *Pediatr Infect Dis J.* 2011; 30:442-5.

[307] Masumoto K, Nagata K, Uesugi T, Yamada T, Kinjo T, Hikino S, Hara T, Taguchi T. Risk of respiratory syncytial virus in survivors with severe congenital diaphragmatic hernia. *Pediatr Int.* 2008; 50:459-463.

[308] Hall CB. Nosocomial respiratory syncytial virus infections: the "Cold War" has not ended. *Clin Infect Dis.* 2000; 31:590-596.

[309] Langley JM, LeBlanc JC, Wang EE, Law BJ, MacDonald NE, Mitchell I, Stephens D, McDonald J, Boucher FD, Dobson S. Nosocomial respiratory syncytial virus infection in Canadian pediatric hospitals: a Pediatric Investigators Collaborative Network on Infections in Canada Study. *Pediatrics.* 1997; 100:943-946.

[310] Groothuis J, Bauman J, Malinoski F, Eggleston M. Strategies for prevention of RSV nosocomial infection. *J Perinatol.* 2008; 28:319-323.

[311] Karanfil LV, Conlon M, Lykens K, Masters CF, Forman M, Griffith ME, Townsend TR, Perl TM. Reducing the rate of nosocomially transmitted respiratory syncytial virus. *Am J Infect Control.* 1999; 27:91-96.

[312] Krasinski K, LaCouture R, Holzman RS, Waithe E, Bonk S, Hanna B. Screening for respiratory syncytial virus and assignment to a cohort at admission to reduce nosocomial transmission. *J Pediatr.* 1990; 116:894-898.

[313] Lavergne V, Ghannoum M, Weiss K, Roy J, Béliveau C. Successful prevention of respiratory syncytial virus nosocomial transmission following an enhanced seasonal infection control program. *Bone Marrow Transplant.* 2011; 46:137-142.

[314] Simoes EA. Immunoprophylaxis of respiratory syncytial virus: global experience. *Respir Res.* 2002; 3:S26-33.

[315] Frogel M, Nerwen C, Cohen A, VanVeldhuisen P, Harrington M, Boron M; Palivizumab Outcomes Registry Group. Prevention of hospitalization due to respiratory syncytial virus: results from the Palivizumab Outcomes Registry. *J Perinatol.* 2008; 28:511-517.

[316] Oh PI, Lanctĵt KL, Yoon A, Lee DS, Paes BA, Simmons BS, Parison D, Manzi P; Composs Investigators. Palivizumab prophylaxis for respiratory syncytial virus in Canada: utilization and outcomes. *Pediatr Infect Dis J.* 2002; 21:512-518.

[317] Romero JRPalivizumab prophylaxis of respiratory syncytial virus disease from 1998 to 2002: results from four years of palivizumab usage. *Pediatr Infect Dis J.* 2003; 22:S46-54.

[318] Pedraz C, Carbonell-Estrany X, Figueras-Aloy J, Quero J; IRIS Study Group. Effect of palivizumab prophylaxis in decreasing respiratory syncytial virus hospitalizations in premature infants. *Pediatr Infect Dis J.* 2003; 22:823-827.

[319] Lacaze-Masmonteil T, Rozé JC, Fauroux B; French Pediatricians' Group of Sunagis Patients' Name-Based Programs. Incidence of respiratory syncytial virus-related hospitalizations in high-risk children: follow-up of a national cohort of infants treated with Palivizumab as RSV prophylaxis. *Pediatr Pulmonol.* 2002; 34:181-188.

[320] Simon A, Nowak H, Sterz R. Use of Palivizumab in Germany: Data from 2002-2007. *Klin Padiatr.* 2011; 223:292-298.

[321] Mitchell I, Paes BA, Li A, Lanctôt KL; the CARESS investigators. CARESS: The Canadian Registry of Palivizumab. *Pediatr Infect Dis J.* 2011; 30:651-655.

[322] Butt ML, Symington A, Janes M, Elliott L, Steele S, Paes BA. The impact of prophylaxis on paediatric intensive care unit admissions for RSV infection: a retrospective, single-centre study. *Eur J Pediatr.* 2011; 170:907-913.

[323] Paes B, Manzoni P. Special populations: do we need evidence from randomized controlled trials to support the need for respiratory syncytial virus prophylaxis? *Early Hum Dev.* 2011; 87:S55-58.

[324] Giusti R. North American synagis prophylaxis survey. *Pediatr Pulmonol* 2009; 44:96–98.

[325] McCormick J, Southern KW. A survey of palivizumab for infants with cystic fibrosis in the UK. *Arch Dis Child.* 2007; 92:87–88.

[326] Panitch HB, Cohen A, Boron M, Van Veldhuisen P, Ciesla G. Physician survey on viral pathogens and respiratory disease in technology-dependent children. *Pediatr Res.* 2004; 55: Abstract 603A.

[327] Cohen AH, Boron ML, Dingivan C. A phase IV study of the safety of synagis (Palivizumab) for prophylaxis of respiratory syncytial virus disease in children with cystic fibrosis. Paper presented at: International Conference of the American Thoracic Society; May 20–25, 2005; San Diego, CA. Abstract-A53.

[328] Speer ME, Fernandes CJ, Boron M, Groothuis JR. Use of Palivizumab for prevention of hospitalization as a result of respiratory syncytial virus in infants with cystic fibrosis. *Pediatr Infect Dis J.* 2008; 27:559-561.

[329] Giebels K, Marcotte JE, Podoba J, Rousseau C, Denis MH, Fauvel V, Laberge S. Prophylaxis against respiratory syncytial virus in young children with cystic fibrosis. *Pediatr Pulmonol.* 2008; 43:169-174.

[330] Michaels MG, Fonseca-Aten M, Green M, Charsha-May D, Friedman B, Seikaly M, Sánchez PJ. Respiratory syncytial virus prophylaxis: a survey of pediatric solid organ transplant centers. *Pediatr Transplant.* 2009; 13:451-456.

[331] Thomas NJ, Hollenbeak CS, Ceneviva GD, Geskey JM, Young MJ. Palivizumab prophylaxis to prevent respiratory syncytial virus mortality after pediatric bone marrow transplantation: a decision analysis model. *J Pediatr Hematol Oncol.* 2007; 29:227-232.

[332] Manzoni P, Leonessa M, Galletto P, Gallo E, Sala U, Gomirato G, Farina D. Use of palivizumab in neonates who not meet the American Academy of Pediatrics Guidelines for respiratory syncytial virus prophylaxis. *Early Human Dev.* 2009;85:S93

[333] Hampp C, Saidi AS, Winterstein AG. Palivizumab utilization and compliance: trends in respiratory syncytial virus prophylaxis in Florida. *J Pediatr.* 2010; 156:953-959, 959.e1.

[334] Muratore CS, Kharasch V, Lund DP, Sheils C, Friedman S, Brown C, Utter S, Jaksic T, Wilson JM. Pulmonary morbidity in 100 survivors of congenital diaphragmatic hernia monitored in a multidisciplinary clinic. *J Pediatr Surg.* 2001; 36:133-140.

[335] Paes B, Li A, Lanctot KL, Mitchell I. Respiratory syncytial virus prophylaxis in special populations. Abstract #43. *Paediatr Child Health.* 2011; 16 Suppl A: 24A.

[336] Banerji A, Lanctôt KL, Paes BA, Masoud ST, Tam DY, Macdonald WA, Roberts A. Comparison of the cost of hospitalization for respiratory syncytial virus disease versus palivizumab prophylaxis in Canadian Inuit infants. *Pediatr Infect Dis J.* 2009; 28:702-706.

[337] Singleton R, Dooley L, Bruden D, Raelson S, Butler JC. Impact of palivizumab prophylaxis on respiratory syncytial virus hospitalizations in high risk Alaska Native infants. *Pediatr Infect Dis J.* 2003; 22:540-545.

[338] Ontario Ministry of Health and Long-Term Care. Synagis. Respiratory Syncytial Virus Prophylaxis for High-Risk Infants Program. 2009. Available at www.transfusionontario.org.

[339] Kassis C, Champlin RE, Hachem RY, Hosing C, Tarrand JJ, Perego CA, Neumann JL, Raad II, Chemaly RF. Detection and control of a nosocomial respiratory syncytial virus outbreak in a stem cell transplantation unit: the role of palivizumab. *Biol Blood Marrow Transplant.* 2010; 16:1265-1271.

[340] Kurz H, Herbich K, Janata O, Sterniste W, Bauer K. Experience with the use of palivizumab together with infection control measures to prevent respiratory syncytial virus outbreaks in neonatal intensive care units. *J Hosp Infect.* 2008; 70:246-252.

[341] O'Connell K, Boo TW, Keady D, Niriain U, O'Donovan D, Commane M, Faherty C, Cormican M. Use of palivizumab and infection control measures to control an outbreak of respiratory syncytial virus in a neonatal intensive care unit confirmed by real-time polymerase chain reaction. *J Hosp Infect.* 2011; 77:338-342.

[342] Dizdar EA, Aydemir C, Erdeve O, Sari FN, Oguz S, Uras N, Dilmen U. Respiratory syncytial virus outbreak defined by rapid screening in a neonatal intensive care unit. *J Hosp Infect.* 2010; 75:292-294.

[343] Smart KA, Lanctôt KL, Paes BA. The cost effectiveness of palivizumab: a systematic review of the evidence. *J Med Econ.* 2010; 13:453-463.

[344] Nuijten MJC, Wittenberg W, Lebmeier M. Cost effectiveness of palivizumab for respiratory syncytial virus prophylaxis in high-risk children. *Pharmacoeconomics.* 2007;25:55-71

[345] Nuijten M, Lebmeier M, Wittenberg W. Cost effectiveness of palivizumab for RSV prevention in high-risk children in the Netherlands. *J Med Econ.* 2009; 12:291-300.

[346] Resch B, Gusenleitner W, Nuijten MJC, et al. Cost-effectiveness of palivizumab against respiratory syncytial viral infection in high-risk children in Austria. *Clin Ther.* 2008; 30:749-760.

[347] Chirico G, Ravasio R, Sbarigia U. Cost-utility analysis of palivizumab in Italy: results from a simulation model in the prophylaxis of respiratory syncytialvirus infection (RSV) among high-risk preterm infants. *Ital J Pediatr.* 2009; 35:4.

[348] Prescott WA Jr, Doloresco F, Brown J, Paladino JA. Cost effectiveness of respiratory syncytial virus prophylaxis: a critical and systematic review. *Pharmacoeconomics.* 2010; 28:279-293.

[349] Wang D, Cummins C, Bayliss S, et al. Immunoprophylaxis against respiratory syncytial virus (RSV) with palivizumab in children: a systematic review and economic evaluation. *Health Technol Assess.* 2008; 12.2008; 12:iii, ix-x, 1-86.

[350] Yount LE, Mahle WT. Economic analysis of palivizumab in infants with congenital heart disease. *Pediatrics.* 2004; 114:1606-1611.

[351] Wang D, Bayliss S, Meads C. Palivizumab for immunoprophylaxis of respiratory syncytial virus (RSV) bronchiolitis in high-risk infants and young children: a systematic review and additional economic modelling of subgroup analyses. *Health Technol Assess.* 2011; 15: iii-iv, 1-124.

[352] Lanctôt KL, Masoud ST, Paes BA, Tarride JE, Chiu A, Hui C, Francis PL, Oh PI. The cost-effectiveness of palivizumab for respiratory syncytial virus prophylaxis in premature infants with a gestational age of 32-35 weeks: a Canadian-based analysis. *Curr Med Res Opin.* 2008; 24: 3223-3237.

[353] Carbonell-Estrany X, Lázaro y de Mercado P. Health economics and RSV. *Paediatr Respir Rev*. 2009; 10:S12-13.

[354] Tam DY, Banerji A, Paes BA, Hui C, Tarride JE, Lanctôt KL. The cost effectiveness of palivizumab in term Inuit infants in the Eastern Canadian Arctic. *J Med Econ*. 2009; 12:361-370.

[355] Resch B, Sommer C, Nuijten MJC, Seidinger S, Walter E, Schoellbauer V, Mueller D. Cost-effectiveness of palivizumab for respiratory syncytial virus in high-risk children, based on long-term epidemiologic data from Austria. *Pediatr Infect Dis J*. 2011; September 28. [E-pub ahead of print].

[356] Smart KA, Paes BA, Lanctot KL. Changing costs and the impact on RSV prophylaxis. *J Med Econ*. 2010; 4:705-708.

[357] Huang K, Incognito L, Cheng X, Ulbrandt ND, Wu H. Respiratory syncytial virus-neutralizing monoclonal antibodies motavizumab and palivizumab inhibit fusion. *J Virol*. 2010; 84:8132-8140.

[358] Wu H, Pfarr DS, Losonsky GA, Kiener PA. Microbiol Immunol. Immunoprophylaxis of RSV infection: advancing from RSV-IGIV to palivizumab and motavizumab. *Curr Top Microbiol Immunol*. 2008; 317:103-123.

[359] Chandran A, Millar EV, Weatherholtz R, Campbell JJ, Perilla MJ, Moulton LH, Reid R, Harris B, Connor EM, Losonsky GA, Griffin MP, Karron R, Santosham M, O'Brien KL. Abstract 4460.5. Presented at the Pediatric Academic Societies Meeting in Hawaii. May 4. 2008.

[360] Feltes TF, Sondheimer HM, Tulloh RM, Harris BS, Jensen KM, Losonsky GA, Griffin MP; for The Motavizumab Cardiac Study Group.A Randomized Controlled Trial of Motavizumab Versus Palivizumab for the Prophylaxis of Serious Respiratory Syncytial Virus Disease in Children With Hemodynamically Significant Congenital Heart Disease. *Pediatr Res*. 2011 Apr 25. [Epub ahead of print]

[361] Kapikian AZ, Mitchell RH, Chanock RM, Shvedoff RA, Stewart CE. An epidemiologic study of altered clinical reactivity to respiratory syncytial (RS) virus infection in children previously vaccinated with an inactivated RS virus vaccine. *Am J Epidemiol*. 1969; 89:405- 421.

[362] Fulginiti VA, Eller JJ, Sieber OF, Joyner JW, Minamitani M, Meiklejohn G. Respiratory virus immunization. I. A field trial of two inactivated respiratory virus vaccines; an aqueous trivalent parainfluenza virus vaccine and an alum-precipitated respiratory syncytial virus vaccine. *Am J Epidemiol*. 1969; 89:435- 448.

[363] Chin J, Magoffin RL, Shearer LA, Schieble JH, Lennette EH. Field evaluation of a respiratory syncytial virus vaccine and a trivalent parainfluenza virus vaccine in a pediatric population. *Am J Epidemiol*. 1969; 89:449-463.

[364] Kim HW, Canchola JG, Brandt CD, Pyles G, Chanock RM, Jensen K, Parrott RH. Respiratory syncytial virus disease in infants despite prior administration of antigenic inactivated vaccine. *Am J Epidemiol*. 1969; 89:422-434.

[365] Alwan WH, Record FM, Openshaw PJ. CD4+ T cells clear virus but augment disease in mice infected with respiratory syncytial virus. Comparison with the effects of CD8+ T cells. *Clin Exp Immunol*. 1992; 88:527-536.

[366] Murphy BR, Walsh EE. Formalin-inactivated respiratory syncytial virus vaccine induces antibodies to the fusion glycoprotein that are deficient in fusion-inhibiting activity. *J Clin Microbiol*. 1988; 26:1595-1597.

[367] Connors M, Giese NA, Kulkarni AB, Firestone CY, Morse HC 3rd, Murphy BR. Enhanced pulmonary histopathology induced by respiratory syncytial virus (RSV) challenge of formalin-inactivated RSV-immunized BALB/c mice is abrogated by depletion of interleukin-4 (IL-4) and IL-10. *J Virol.* 1994; 68:5321-5325.

[368] Delgado MF, Coviello S, Monsalvo AC, Melendi GA, Hernandez JZ, Batalle JP, Diaz L, Trento A, Chang HY, Mitzner W, Ravetch J, Melero JA, Irusta PM, Polack FP. Lack of antibody affinity maturation due to poor Toll-like receptor stimulation leads to enhanced respiratory syncytial virus disease. *Nat Med.* 2009; 15:34-41.

[369] Stevens WW, Sun J, Castillo JP, Braciale TJ. Pulmonary eosinophilia is attenuated by early responding CD8(+) memory T cells in a murine model of RSV vaccine-enhanced disease. *Viral Immunol.* 2009; 22:243-251.

[370] Sparer TE, Matthews S, Hussell T, Rae AJ, Garcia-Barreno B, Melero JA, Openshaw PJ. Eliminating a region of respiratory syncytial virus attachment protein allows induction of protective immunity without vaccine-enhanced lung eosinophilia. *J Exp Med.* 1998; 187:1921-1926.

[371] Moghaddam A, Olszewska W, Wang B, Tregoning JS, Helson R, Sattentau QJ, Openshaw PJ. A potential molecular mechanism for hypersensitivity caused by formalin-inactivated vaccines. *Nat Med.* 2006; 12:905-907.

[372] Schickli JH, Dubovsky F, Tang RS. Challenges in developing a pediatric RSV vaccine. *Hum Vaccin.* 2009; 5:582-591.

[373] Tristram DA, Welliver RC, Mohar CK, Hogerman DA, Hildreth SW, Paradiso P. Immunogenicity and safety of respiratory syncytial virus subunit vaccine in seropositive children 18-36 months old. *J Infect Dis.* 1993; 167:191-195.

[374] Piedra PA, Cron SG, Jewell A, Hamblett N, McBride R, Palacio MA, Ginsberg R, Oermann CM, Hiatt PW; Purified Fusion Protein Vaccine Study Group. Immunogenicity of a new purified fusion protein vaccine to respiratory syncytial virus: a multi-center trial in children with cystic fibrosis. *Vaccine.* 2003; 21:2448-2460.

[375] Groothuis JR, King SJ, Hogerman DA, Paradiso PR, Simoes EA. Safety and immunogenicity of a purified F protein respiratory syncytial virus (PFP-2) vaccine in seropositive children with bronchopulmonary dysplasia. *J Infect Dis.* 1998; 177:467-469.

[376] Karron RA, Wright PF, Belshe RB, Thumar B, Casey R, Newman F, Polack FP, Randolph VB, Deatly A, Hackell J, Gruber W, Murphy BR, Collins PL. Identification of a recombinant live attenuated respiratory syncytial virus vaccine candidate that is highly attenuated in infants. *J Infect Dis.* 2005; 191:1093-1104.

[377] Gomez M, Mufson MA, Dubovsky F, Knightly C, Zeng W, Losonsky G. Phase-I study MEDI-534, of a live, attenuated intranasal vaccine against respiratory syncytial virus and parainfluenza-3 virus in seropositive children. *Pediatr Infect Dis J.* 2009; 28:655-658.

[378] Murata Y. Respiratory syncytial virus vaccine development. *Clin Lab Med.* 2009; 29:725-739.

[379] Blanco JC, Boukhvalova MS, Shirey KA, Prince GA, Vogel SN. New insights for development of a safe and protective RSV vaccine. *Hum Vaccin.* 2010; 6:482-492.

[380] Groothuis JR, Hoopes JM, Jessie VG. Prevention of serious respiratory syncytial virus-related illness. I: Disease pathogenesis and early attempts at prevention. *Adv Ther.* 2011; 28:91-109.

[381] Chang J. Current progress on development of respiratory syncytial virus vaccine. *BMB Rep.* 2011; 44:232-237.

[382] Graham BS. Biological challenges and technological opportunities for respiratory syncytial virus vaccine development. *Immunol Rev.* 2011; 239:149-166.

In: Respiratory Syncytial Virus
Editors: Haneul Nam and Gippeum Kun, pp. 79-121
ISBN 978-1-62100-835-4

Chapter 2

RESPIRATORY SYNCYTIAL VIRUS: PREVENTION, DIAGNOSIS AND TREATMENT

Young Yoo
Department of Pediatrics, College of Medicine,
Korea University, Seoul, South Korea

1. EPIDEMIOLOGY

1) Respiratory Syncytial Virus (RSV)

RSV is a leading cause of viral respiratory tract infections (LRI) during infancy and early childhood. By age 2, nearly all children will have had exposure to RSV manifesting as an upper or lower airway infection. RSV is identified as the etiologic agent in approximately 40-90% of patients with bronchiolitis and in 30-50% of those with pneumonia. [1, 2] From a prospective study conducted on children, admitted with an acute wheezing episode, viruses were detected in nasopharyngeal aspirates. RSV was the most frequently detected, followed by rhinovirus, adenovirus, human bocavirus and human metapneumovirus especially under 2 years of age. [1](Table 1) RSV respiratory infections are usually mild in healthy toddlers, older children, and adolescents because they mainly involve the upper respiratory tract or cause only transient wheezing. However, during the first 2 years of life, most children with RSV infection manifest bronchiolitis whose particular clinical picture includes upper and lower respiratory tract involvement, respiratory distress, a harsh cough, bilateral crepitations, air trapping, and wheezing. [3]

2) Global RSV Burden

RSV is one of the major respiratory tract viral pathogens throughout the world, causing acute lower respiratory tract infection (LRI). World Health Organization (WHO) has estimated the global RSV disease burden at 64 million cases and 160,000 deaths every year. According to the global incidence of acute LRI attributable to RSV in children in 2005, an estimated 33.8 million new episodes of RSV LRI occurred worldwide in children younger than 5 years (22% of LRI episodes), with at least 3.4 million episodes representing severe RSV LRI necessitating hospital admission. Globally, RSV is the most common cause of childhood LRI and a major cause of admission to hospital. [4]

Table 1. Respiratory viruses identified in 626 acute wheezing episodes during a 3-year study period

Virus	Single infection, N	Dual or multiple infection, N
Respiratory syncytial virus	102	68
Rhinovirus	84	73
Adenovirus	47	63
Human bocavirus	33	67
Human metapneumovirus	15	15
Parainfluenza virus type 1–4	8	21
Influenza A, B, and C viruses	8	8
Coronavirus types OC43 and 229E	1	8
Enterovirus	4	6
Total	302	269

Adapted from Pediatr Pulmonol 2010;45:585-91.

3) Fatality Rates of RSV Infection

Among all children younger than 5 years in industrialized countries, 0.3% of RSV-associated severe LRI resulted in fatalities. The majority of mortality (99%) was observed in developing countries.

Table 2. Range of RSV case-fatality rate by comorbidity

Comorbidity	RSV case-fatality rate range, %
Chronic lung disease	3.5–23
Congenital heart disease	2–37
Premature infants (≤36 weeks' gestational age)	0–6.1
Nosocomial RSV infection	0–12.2
Intensive care support	1.1–33
No comorbidity or risk factors	<1
Mixed population or undefined risk factors	0–5.9

RSV, respiratory syncytial virus

Adapted from CMRO 2010;26:2175-81.

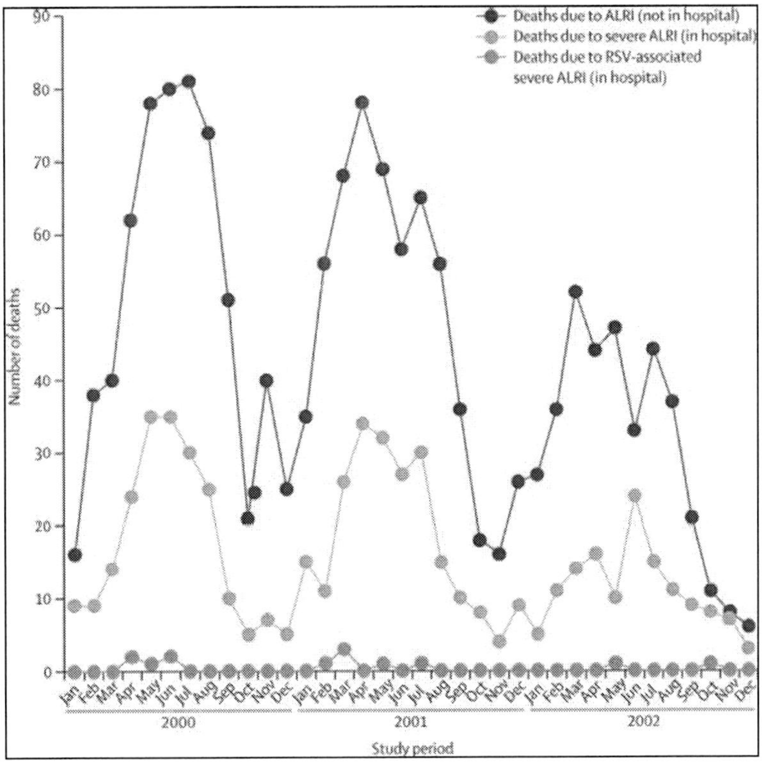

Adapted from Lancet 2010;375:1545-55.

Figure 1. LRI (including RSV)-associated mortality pattern in children younger than 2 years in Lombok, Indonesia.

Based on a literature review for death among children hospitalized for RSV (1966-2009), case fatality rates ranged from 0 to 33%. It was estimated that 66,000~199,000 children younger than 5 years died from RSV-associated LRI in 2005, with 99% of these deaths occurring in developing countries. [4] In general, subgroups of high-risk children such as chronic lung disease (CLD), congenital heart disease (CHD), or prematurity, had higher fatality rates than older or otherwise healthy children. [5](Table 2)

Mortality data suggest that RSV is an important cause of death in childhood from LRI, after pneumococcal pneumonia and *Haemophilus influenza* type b. A study in Indonesia reported LRI-associated mortality pattern in children younger than 2 years. [4](Figure 1)

4) RSV LRI among High-Risk Infants

A recent data revealed that outpatient RSV LRI visits increase with younger age and prematurity. The incidence of outpatient, non-hospitalized, RSV LRI visits are highest among infants, especially high-risk infants such as those with chronic lung disease of prematurity, CHD or immune deficiency. They estimated that approximately 1 in every 5 high-risk infants develops outpatient RSV LRI infection during their first RSV season. [2]

Outpatient RSV LRI represents an unrecognized aspect of the burden of RSV. Given this high burden, more attention should be paid toward RSV prevention. [2](Table 3).

Table 3. RSV-related outpatient visits per 1,000 population

Data source	Time interval	Infant group[1]	N	Rate per 1,000 children		
				Emergency	Ambulatory	All outpatient
MEDSTAT MarketScan	October–April	Infants with CLD	497	23.1–31.6	189.1–241.0	212.2–272.6[2]
		Infants <31 weeks	450	18.7–23.3	140.0–186.7	158.7–210.0[2,3]
		Infants 31–32 weeks	618	12.8–16.7	188.8–240.8	201.6–257.5[2,3]
		Infants 33–34 weeks	1,509	23.6–28.6	159.6–204.6	183.2–233.2[2,3]
		Infants 35–36 weeks	2,762	19.4–23.7	167.1–222.0	186.5–245.7[2,3]
		Infants without GA code	6,004	19.8–23.7	145.9–193.1	165.7–216.8[2,3]
		Full-term infants	84,290	13.5–16.5	115.3–154.8	128.8–171.3[2,3]

Adapted from Pediatr Pulmonol 2010;45:578-84.

5) RSV LRI versus non-RSV LRI

In a study with large number of young children (n=4,800) for assessing differences in disease severity between children with RSV and non-RSV LRI, RSV LRI were younger at hospitalization and had a lower percentage of underlying medical conditions than children hospitalized with non-RSV LRI. However, disease severity defined by length of hospitalization and requirement of supplemental oxygen, intensive care, and mechanical ventilation was significantly worse in children with RSV LRI. RSV infection and prematurity, regardless of etiology, were identified as independent risk factors for severe LRI. [6](Figure 2, Table 4)

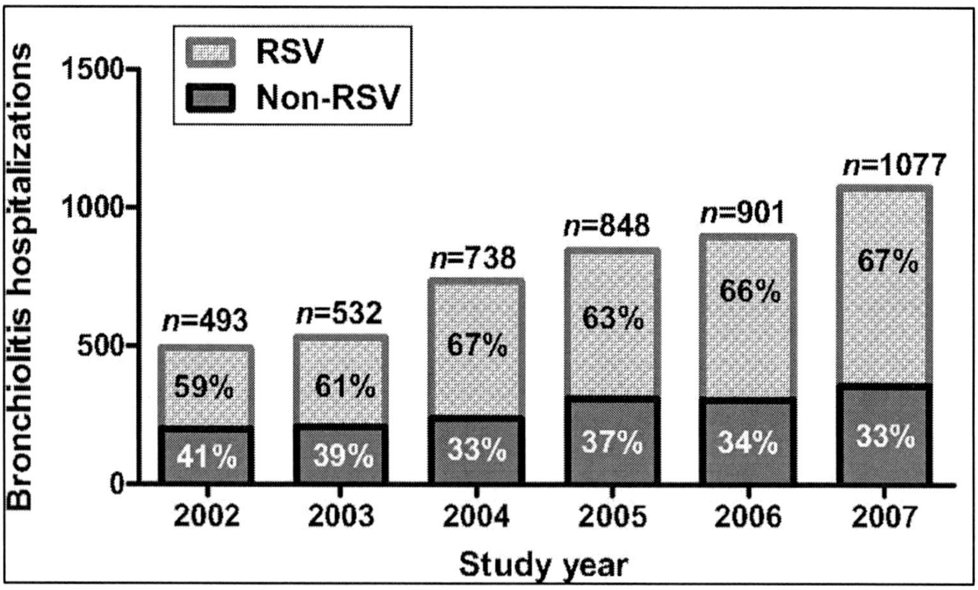

Adapted from Pediatrics 2010;26:e1453.

Figure 2. RSV and non-RSV bronchiolitis hospitalizations.

Table 4. Disease characteristics in children hospitalized with RSV and non-RSV bronchiolitis

Parameters of Disease Severity	RSV Bronchiolitis (N = 2840)	Non-RSV Bronchiolitis (N = 1445)	P
Length of stay, median (IQR [25th–75th percentile]), d	3 (2–5)	2 (2–4)	<.001
Supplemental oxygen			
Requirement, n (%)	1600 (56.3)	675 (46.7)	<.001
Duration, median (IQR [25th–75th percentile]), d	2 (1–4)	2 (1–4)	.239
ICU			
Requirement, n (%)	329 (11.6)	119 (8.2)	<.001
Duration, median (IQR [25th–75th percentile]), d	4 (2–7)	2 (1–5)	<.001
Ventilatory support			
Requirement, n (%)	171 (6)	46 (3.2)	<.001
Duration, median (IQR [25th–75th percentile]), d	6 (4–9)	4 (1–7)	.003

Adapted from Pediatrics 2010;26:e1453.

2. Clinical Characteristics

1) Clinical Characteristics Of RSV Infection

The clinical manifestations vary from mild disease of the upper respiratory tract to severe bronchiolitis or pneumonia. The 1st signs of infection of the infant with RSV are rhinorrhea and pharyngitis. Cough may appear simultaneously but more often after an interval of 1-3 days, at which time there may also be sneezing and a low grade fever. Soon after the cough develops, the child begins to wheeze audibly. If the disease is mild, the symptoms may not progress beyond this stage. Auscultation often reveals diffuse rhonchi, fine rales or crackles, and wheezes. Clear rhinorrhea usually persists throughout the illness, with intermittent fever. Chest x-rays at this stage are frequently normal. If the illness progresses, cough and wheezing increase and air hunger ensues, with increased respiratory rate, intercostal and subcostal retraction, hyperexpansion of the chest, restlessness, and peripheral cyanosis develop. Signs of severe, life-threatening illness are central cyanosis, tachypnea of > 70 breaths/min, listlessness, and apneic spells. At this stage, the chest may be greatly hyperexpanded and almost silent to auscultation because of poor air movement. [7] In some infants, the course of the illness may resemble pneumonia with the prodromal rhinorrhea and cough followed by dyspnea, poor feeding, and listlessness, with a minimum of wheezing and hyperexpansion. Although the clinical diagnosis is pneumonia, wheezing is often present intermittently and the chest x-ray may show air trapping. In this population, perhaps more prominently in the developing world, superinfection with pneumococcus or other pathogenic bacteria may occur, and the clinical picture merges with that of bacterial pneumonia. [7]

2) Chest X-Rays

Chest x-rays of infants hospitalized with RSV bronchiolitis are normal in 10-30% of cases, and show hyperexpansion of the chest in 20-40%, peribronchial thickening or central pneumonia in 35-50%, and segmental or lobar consolidation in 8-20%. Pleural effusion is unusual. [7]

3) *RSV Infection in Immunocompromised Hosts*

RSV infection in profoundly immunocompromised hosts may be severe at any age. The mortality associated with RSV pneumonia in the 1st few weeks after bone marrow or solid organ transplantation in both children and adults is > 50%. RSV infection does not seem to be more severe in HIV-infected patients. [7]

4) *Post-RSV Bronchiolitis Obliterans (BO)*

Post-infectious BO is an unusual consequence of epithelial injury of the lower respiratory tract, but may be more common than previously thought. [8] BO, described by Lange in 1901, [9] results from extensive necrosis of the entire bronchiolar tissue, extending as far as but sparing, the cartilage plaque. In the acute stage, hyaline membranes, denuded epithelium and inflammatory cells fill the bronchial lumen. Then, a proliferation of fibroblasts and collagen occurs and polyp-like masses obliterate the lumen. [10] Its clinical and X-ray characteristics cannot be distinguished from other viral infections. Wheezing, respiratory distress and oxygen requirements persist and chest X-rays often show bronchopneumonic infiltrates and persistent atelectasis. [11]

Criteria for suspecting BO include: 1) absence of respiratory illness during the perinatal period and up to the onset of the viral illness, 2) Severe bronchiolitis in a previously healthy infant, requiring hospital admission, needing additional oxygen and demonstrating low oxygen saturation levels for more than 1 month, 3) following the acute phase of the illness, persistence for more than 3 months of respiratory distress, signs of bronchial obstruction and air trapping with arterial oxygen saturation < 95%. [11] Chest X-rays show air trapping and, less frequently, atelectasis and honeycombing. Chest computed tomography (CT) scans show mosaic patterns of perfusion with air trapping adjacent to areas of bronchiectasis and atelectasis. [12] Airway hyperresponsiveness (AHR) in patients with post-infectious BO was frequent but not similar to that in asthmatic patients. [8] Treatment of BO is supportive. There may be limited response to bronchodilators during acute exacerbations. Corticosteroids are used empirically but yet no studies have confirmed their efficacy. [11]

5) *Neurologic Complications in RSV Infection*

In approximately 1.2-1.8% of hospitalized patients with RSV infection is known to be associated with symptoms of the central nervous system. [13, 14] The number of case reports on RSV encephalopathy has also recently increased. The suggested pathogenesis of acute encephalopathies with RSV infection were metabolic error, cytokine storm, or excitotoxicity. [15]

3. Pathogenesis

RSV is the leading cause of respiratory disease in infants and young children worldwide. Direct viral cytopathology may play only a minor role in the pathogenesis of RSV induced disease and it appears that much of the injury caused by RSV infection may be the result of the host immune response. [16, 17]

1) Recognition of RSV by Cytoplasmic Sensors

The immune response to virus infection begins with the recognition of viral pathogen-associated molecular patterns (PAMPs) as 'non-self' signatures. This recognition occurs through host pattern recognition receptors (PRRs). Toll-like receptors (TLRs) are a class of PRRs that recognize viral motifs presented at the cell surface or within the endosomal compartment but are not known for mediating cytosolic pathogen recognition. [18] On the other hand, once in the cell, RSV can be recognized by RNA helicases that include retinoic acid inducible gene 1 (RIG-1), melanoma differentiation associated gene 5 (MAD5), and laboratory of genetics and physiology 2 (LGP2). (19) RNA recognition by RIG-1 requires the presence of a free 5'-triphosphate structure and this allows for differentiation of non-self viral RNA versus self-RNA, as host RNA is either capped or post-translationally modified to remove the 5'-triphosphate. [18] RIG-1 and MAD5 contain two N-terminal caspase activation and recruitment domains (CARDS) which are essential for their signaling activity. [19] Figure 3 shows RLR structure diagram showing positions of functional domains (upper) and 3-step model of RIG-1 activation from a monomeric resting from (lower left) to RNA-ligand bound, dimeric form (center) and the final active form (lower right). [18, 20]

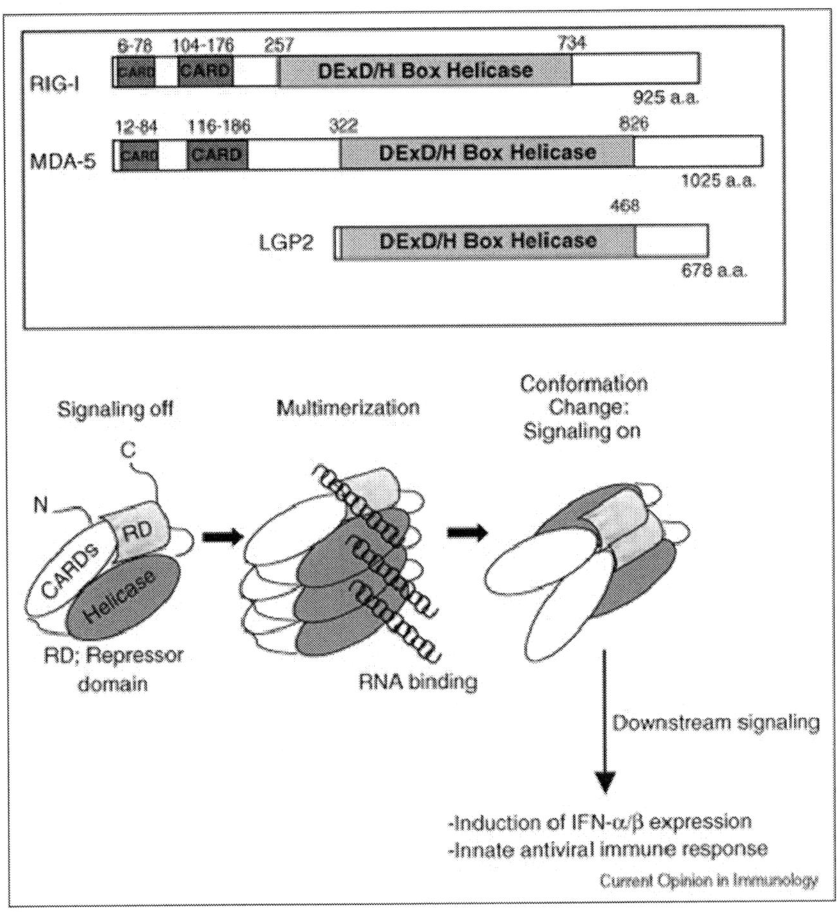

Adapted from Curr Opin Immunol 2010;22:41-7.

Figure 3. RLR structure diagram and 3-step model of RIG-1 activation.

The positions of the CARDs, helicase domain, and repressor domain (RD) are indicated. Ligand binding by RIG-1 facilitates a conformation change that releases it from autorepression by the RD, thus driving downstream signaling of innate antiviral immunity. [20] After binding nonself-ligand, RIG-1 and MAD5 interact via these CARD domains with the signaling-adaptor molecule IFN-β promoter stimulator 1 (IPS-1) which is present in the outer mitochondrial membrane. [19] These events lead to the induced expression of IFN-β, IRF3-target genes, and NF-κB target genes to drive antiviral and inflammatory responses against infection. [21-24](Figure 4)

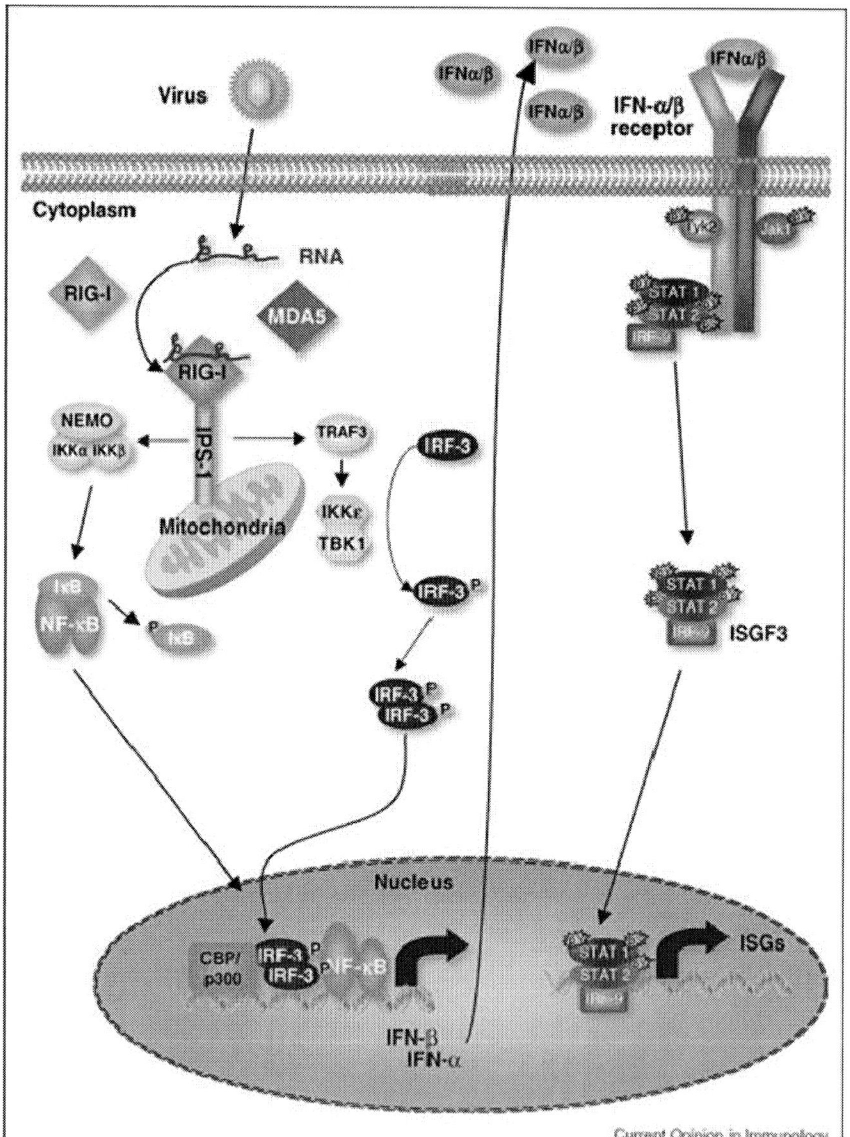

Adapted from Curr Opin Immunol 2010;22:41-7.

Figure 4. RLR signaling pathway.

The RLR signaling pathway showing RIG-1 bound to ligand RNA and signaling downstream to IRF3 and NF-κB to induce IFN-α/β production from a virus-infected cell. IFN-α/β is then shown signaling through the IFN-α/β receptor and the Jak-STAT pathway to drive ISG expression and an innate immune response.

After the Type 1 IFNs are produced by the cell, they can act in either an autocrine or paracrine fashion to stimulate cellular antiviral defense by binding to the same heterodimeric IFN-α/β receptor, resulting in activation of Tyk2, and Jak 1 and phosphorylation of the cytoplasmic transcription factors STAT 1 and 2. [18] The phenotypic response to RSV infection, both at the molecular, cellular and the individual subject level can be explained at least in part by the immunologic milieu of the host at the time of infection which is dependent on host gene environment interactions. RSV has unique qualities to subvert host antiviral responses and understanding these mechanisms may provide novel therapeutic targets against this very important pathogen.

2) Innate Immune Responses

RSV has a variety of different mechanisms by which it can suppress the host anti-viral immune response and therefore aid its own survival. RSV binds to the epithelial cell membrane through its G protein, which is the attachment protein. The RSV F protein is the fusion protein which allows for the virus to penetrate the cell membrane. [25]

2.1. Epithelial Cell Responses

Primary target in RSV infection are the respiratory epithelial cells. In mild cases of bronchiolitis, inflammation may consist only of a sparse collection of lymphocytes surrounding bronchioles, but in severe RSV disease the bronchioles are plugged by necrotic cell debris and mucus. Airway obstruction is a critical problem in the very small infant in addition to the epithelial cell necrosis and virus-mediated immunopathology. [26] Table 5 shows the chemokines induced from respiratory epithelial cells by RSV infection.

Table 5. Chemokines induced by RSV infection of respiratory epithelial cells

Chemokine (122)	*Receptor*	*Function (79)*
RANTES (CCL5)	CCR1	Effector T cells (Th1)
MIP-1α (CCL3)		
MCP-1 (CCL2)	CCR2	Effector T cells, monocytes, macrophages, immature DCs
Eotaxin-1 (CCL11)	CCR3	Effector T cells (Th2), eosinophils
RANTES (CCL5)		
RANTES (CCL5)	CCR5	Effector T cells (Th1)
MIP-1α (CCL3)		
MIP-1β (CCL4)		
I309 (CCL1)	CCR8	Effector T cells (Th2), NK cells
IL-8 (CXCL8)	CXCR1	PMNs
IL-8 (CXCL8)	CXCR2	PMNs and mast cells
GROα (CXCL1)		
GROβ (CXCL2)		
GROγ (CXCL3)		
ENA-78 (CXCL5)		
I-TAC (CXCL11)	CXCR3	Effector T cells (Th1)
MIG (CXCL9)		
IP10 (CXCL10)		
Fractalkine (CX3CL1)	CX3CR1	Effector T cells

Adapted from Viral Immunol 2004;17:370-80.

2.2. Type 1 Interferon (IFN)s

The earliest responses to viral pathogens begin with virus entry into susceptible cells. One of these is the production of type 1 IFNs, which play critical roles not only in the fate of the infected cell itself, but also in the immediate protection of neighboring cells and in the shaping of subsequent adaptive immune responses. [27, 28] RSV is also known to resist the antiviral effects of IFNs. [29] Mechanisms by which IFN signaling is disrupted have been intensively studied in several of viruses among the Paramyxoviridae family, in which multiple strategies to defeat IFN signaling have been found. [30-32] Interestingly, the viral genes responsible for these activities are absent in RSV. Recent work has demonstrated, however, that NS1 and NS2, two genes found in pneumoviruses such as RSV but absent in other paramyxoviruses, function cooperatively both to disrupt the activity and to prevent the induction of IFNs in infected cells. [33-35] Surprisingly, unlike other paramyxoviruses, RSV apparently does not disrupt the function of the primary IFN signal transduction pathway, the Jak/STAT pathway. [16]

2.3. Responses to Glycoproteins F and G

In addition to the anti-IFN activities of NS1 and NS2, it has been suggested that RSV glycoproteins, F and G, may affect aspects of innate immunity. It has been reported that glycoprotein F binds to and activates Toll-like receptor (TLR) 4, [36] the receptor mediating innate immune responses to LPS. Activation of TLR4 triggers a signaling cascade that results in the activation of transcription factor NF-κB, and consequently the activation of multiple mediators of innate immunity. [37] The RSV glycoprotein, G, is thought to be primarily responsible for the recognition of, and attachment to target cell surfaces by virions. [38] Unlike the analogous protein in other paramyxoviruses, however, the deletion of G from RSV is of only modest consequence to viral replication in culture. [39] In vivo, however, absence of the G glycoprotein results in significant attenuation of RSV infectivity. [40] Thus, F glycoprotein is sufficient for both viral attachment and penetration of target cells, though G glycoprotein may significantly enhance the avidity of virion-cell recognition.

2.4. Other Antiviral Factors

In addition to the induction of type 1 IFNs by virus, a number of anti-viral factors and immunoregulatory chemokines are produced by the respiratory epithelium. Surfactant proteins A and D appear to play a antiviral defense role by binding to the viral surface glycoproteins F and G. [41-43] Once bound, surfactant proteins have been reported to neutralize virus and to increase virus uptake by macrophages and neutrophils. This protective effect is also seen in vivo with increased viral replication and inflammation in surfactant deficient mice. [44, 45]

3) T Cell Response

T cells are essential for virus clearance, but also appear to mediate RSV immunopathology. [46-48] In mice lacking both CD4+ and CD8+ T cell subsets, RSV was very slowly cleared but produced essentially no disease. Conversely, both T cell subsets are important to clearance, but also correlate with pathology and illness. [16]

The importance of Th2 cytokines in the course of a natural RSV infection is much more complex and more controversial. In mice lacking a normal IFN response, primary infection is associated with Th2 cytokines and lung eosinophils. [49] CTLs have a major role in the clearance of virus infection, and there is a robust expansion of RSV specific CD8+ cells in the lungs. [16] Cytokine profiles of RSV infection in children demonstrate variable results. Infants with RSV infection elicit a predominant Th2 response such as IL-4, IL-5. However, in addition to Th2 cytokines, Th1 cytokine such as IFN-γ is also elevated during RSV infection. [50]

3.1. Role of CD4+ T Cells

CD4+ T cells play an important role in antiviral immunity by providing help for B cells in generating antiviral antibodies as well as secreting cytokines such as IFN-γ and TNF-α. [17] The CD4+ T cell immune response to RSV has been most extensively studied in BALB/c mice. Studies using the BALB/c model have demonstrated that CD4+ T cells can provide detrimental to the host by mediating immunopathology and exacerbating disease. [48, 51, 52]. For example, transfer of RSV G-specific Th2 CD4+ T cell lines into naïve recipients has been shown to induce lung eosinophilia following intranasal RSV infection, [53] a phenotype similar to that exhibited by the subset of children who received the FI-RSV vaccine and later developed enhanced disease following natural RSV infection. In contrast, BALB/c mice sensitized with vv expressing the F or matrix (M2) proteins also develop extensive pulmonary inflammation, characteristic of a memory T cell response, but without lung eosinophilia following RSV challenge infection. [54] These results can be explained in part because the G protein does not generate a detectable MHC class I restricted CD8+ T cell response but does induce a strong memory G protein-specific CD4+ T cell response in the lungs characterized by a mixture of Th1 and Th2 cytokine-secreting cells. [55-57] In contrast, the F protein induces MHC class I restricted CTL as well as Th1, but not Th2, cytokine-producing CD4+ T cells. [56] Thus these observations suggest that lung pathology and pulmonary eosinophilia induced by F1-RSV or vvG immunization may result from the selective priming of virus-specific CD4+ T cells and implicate Th2 cytokine production (i.e., IL-4, IL-5, and IL-13) as an important factor in this disease process. [17, 58](Figure 5).

3.2. Role of CD8+ T Cells

Although there is not a detectable CD8+ T cell response to the G protein of RSV, strong CD8+ T cell responses are elicited to several other proteins including M, N, and F. [51, 59, 60] Several studies have demonstrated that CD8+ T cells play an important role in the lungs of G protein-sensitized mice challenged with RSV. As mentioned above, adoptive transfer of RSV G-specific T cell lines into BALB/c mice infected with RSV can reproduce the pathology observed in mice sensitized with vvG. [53] Interestingly, cotransfer of M2-specific CD8+ T cells reduced the degree of pulmonary eosinophilia induced by transfer of Th2-like G-specific CD4+ T cells. [53] Similarly, insertion of a MHC class I restricted CD8+ T cell epitope derived from the M2 protein into the G protein used to prime a memory CD4+ T cell response prevented the development of pulmonary eosinophilia following sensitization and RSV challenge infection. [55] Deletion of CD8+ T cells in F-sensitized mice leads to the development of pulmonary eosinophilia following live RSV challenge infection. [17] The examination of the CD8+ T cell response during RSV infection has demonstrated that the M2-specific CD8+ T cells within the RSV infected lung are impaired in their expression of effector activity, including cytokine production and ex vivo cytolytic activity. [61].

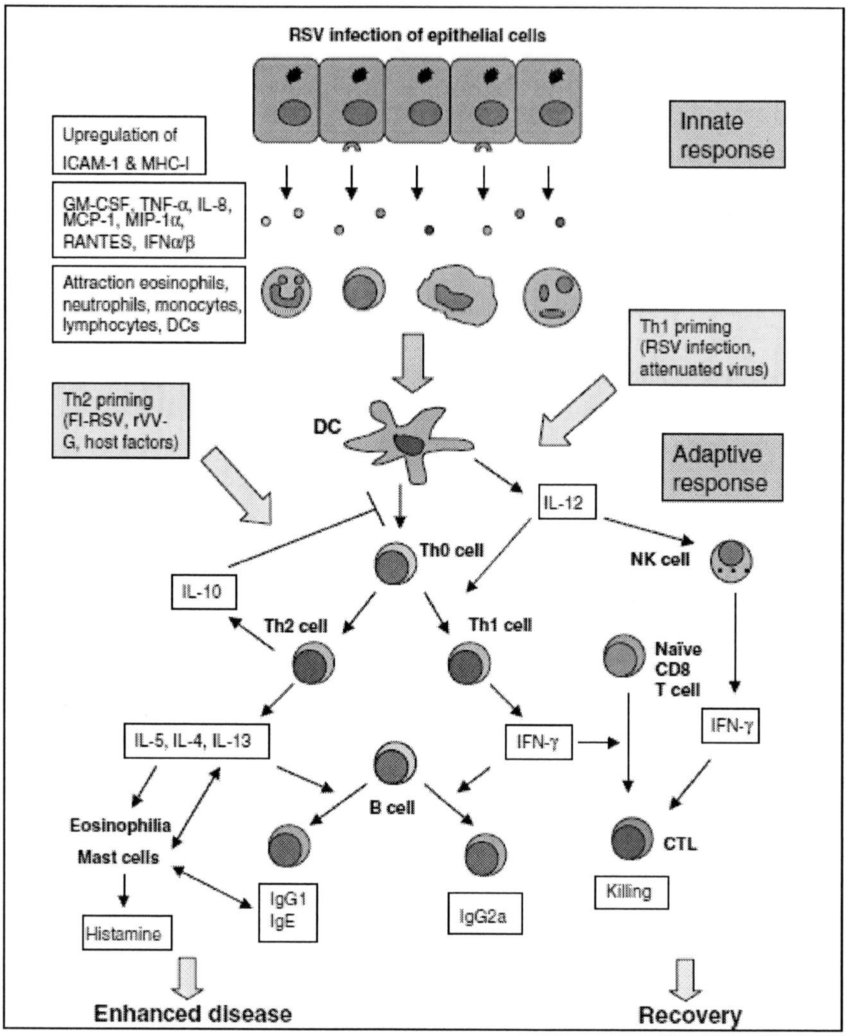

Adapted from Rev Med Virol 2007;17:5-34.

Figure 5. Innate and adaptive responses to RSV infection.

Furthermore, in vitro incubation of the CD8+ T cells in IL-2 prior to antigenic stimulation restored the ability of the CD8+ T cells to make IFN-γ. [61] These results suggest that the inhibition of CD8+ T cell effector activity is due to interference with T cell receptor signaling of the RSV M2-specific CD8+ T cells by one or more RSV gene products. [17]

4) B Cell Response

4.1. Antibody Response

With most viral pathogens cell mediated immunity is essential for virus clearance following acute infection, but it is generally the antibody response that protects against reinfection. [16] Unlike the T cell response, serum antibody titers will increase following RSV reinfection, and there is a gradual acquisition of protective antibodies. [62, 63]

Patients of any age with a low titer of serum neutralizing antibody are at greater risk for developing severe RSV LRI than those with high antibody titers. [64, 65] In the absence of any effective vaccine, prophylactic treatment of high risk infants with antibody to RSV has been shown to decrease hospitalization for severe disease. [66] Weakness of the B cell response to RSV allows continual reinfection and requires repeated activation of virus specific T cells. While the basis for the poor B cell response to RSV is not known, a reported role for IFN-α/β in the generation of a robust antibody response [67] would suggest that poor IFN-α/β induction by virus is at least partly responsible.

The role of Th2 cells in RSV immunopathology remains a central question. It is not yet clear whether RSV antigens stimulate Th2 responses in the course of natural infection, or whether Th2 differentiation occurs only in atopic individuals. [16] Figure 6 depicts a model showing how individual differences in chemokine and/or cytokine induction could influence disease outcome following RSV infection. Development of robust Th1 immunity to virus infection depends upon α/β IFNs secreted by epithelial and dendritic cells, IL-12 secreted by dendritic cells, and IFN-γ secreted by activated NK cells. [16] These cytokines will promote both the differentiation of Th1 lymphocytes and the induction of chemokines that will attract them to the site of infection. [68]

Nearly 98% of all infants become infected with RSV by the age of 2 years and experience severe bronchiolitis because their small airways easily become occluded [69].

Recurrent infections with RSV are common, and the pulmonary pathology is known to persist long after the virus has been cleared efficiently. RSV disease pathology is clinically characterized by AHR, increased mucus production, and inflammation. [70-72] An altered immune environment due to an imbalance in the Th1 and Th2 responses is thought to underlie this disease phenotype. [73]

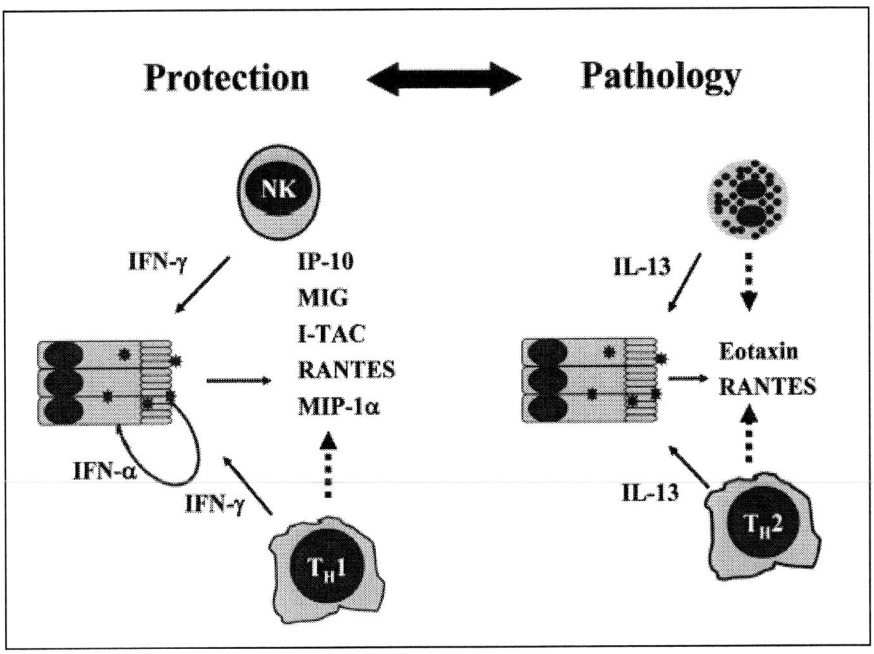

Adapted from Viral Immunol 2004;17:370-80.

Figure 6. Model of inflammatory mediators induced by RSV infection of the respiratory tract.

4.2. RSV-Specific Antibody

Although severe RSV LRI usually occurs in children during primary infections, symptomatic reinfections are frequent in healthy individuals. [74] These reinfections can occur with the same RSV strain, indicating that acquired immunity is not effectively established or does not completely protect against reinfection. [75] Precise correlates of protection for RSV-induced LRI are not defined, and the reason for incomplete immune protection is not clear. Antibodies provide partial protection against severe RSV LRI. [76, 77] The role of RSV-specific antibodies is likely diverse. Neutralizing antibodies can contribute to the reduction of viral load and, as a result, decrease innate immune responses. [75] Non-neutralizing antibodies might enhance infection and might cause immune complex deposition, leading to enhanced respiratory disease. [78] Antibodies play a role in the uptake of immune complexes by APCs via FcRs or complement receptors and influence CD4+ and CD8+ T cell activation. [79-82] In addition, antibodies might alter innate immune activation by targeting viral particles to endosomal compartments where TLRs get activated or by interacting with viral proteins or carbohydrates that bind to immune receptors that play regulatory roles during innate and adaptive immune responses. [75].

Virus-specific antibodies play a crucial role in the regulation of RSV-specific T cell responses. Polyclonal virus-specific antibodies generated in vivo are a complex mixture of neutralizing and non-neutralizing antibodies. [75] The ratio of neutralizing and non-neutralizing RSV-specific antibodies in serum may affect the efficacy of antigen presentation to virus-specific CD4+ and CD8+ T cells. Both neutralizing and non-neutralizing antibodies enhanced antigen presentation to RSV-specific CD4+ T cells, whereas neutralizing antibodies lowered RSV-specific CD8+ T cell response. Therefore, the presence of virus-specific maternal antibodies in neonates before natural RSV infection, or induced by a RSV vaccination, might affect the activation of virus-specific T cells in vivo. [75]

5) IL-17

Recently, it was reported that IL-17, produced by a subset of CD4+ T cells (Th17 cells), was regulated by STAT-1 during RSV infections in rodents. (83) Three important underlying mechanisms by which IL-17 modulates immune response to RSV infection were speculated: 1) hypermucus production in the airways, 2) alteration of effector CD8+ T cell responses, and 3) viral clearance. [73] Each of these mechanisms may contribute to RSV-induced pulmonary pathology. [73] In addition, IL-17 produced during RSV infection appears to participate in RSV-induced exacerbation of allergic lung disease. [84]

IL-17 has also been associated with increased neutrophilic infiltration at the site of infection during host responses to bacterial and fungal infections through induction of CXC chemokines. [85, 86]

Current evidence indicates that viral infection of epithelial cells increases neutrophil chemoattractants, which induce neutrophil migration into the inflammatory sites. [87-89] CD8+ T cell antiviral responses confer protective immunity during viral infection. [73] RSV-induced IL-17 augments increasing mucus production, inhibiting CD8+ T cell activation, and reducing viral clearance. [73] The negative regulatory effects of IL-17 on cytotoxic CD8+ T cells during both RSV infection and the exacerbated allergic response contribute to the viral associated pathology. [73]

6) Impaired Immune Response in Severe RSV Infection

There was evidence that severe RSV infection is associated with an impaired immune response. Severe RSV infection in infants younger than 6 months of age is associated with low numbers of circulating lymphocytes, NK cells, and low concentrations of plasma cytokines, which could be related to an impaired immune response. [90] Severe RSV infection is associated with a peripheral impaired immune response, especially during the first days of illness, that is characterized by low T cell counts compared with healthy infants, particularly CD8+ T cells, a poor expression of certain circulating proinflammatory mediators such as IFN-γ, TNF-α, and IL-17 and high concentration of IL-8 chemokine in plasma, that could not effectively control the infection. [90] Infants with severe RSV infection have low natural killer (NK) cell counts in blood, particularly those expressing the CD94 antigen, while another group of activated NK cells that did not express the CD94 antigen were in higher percentage, especially in patients with severe disease. [90] The lack of regulation of the NK system, mediated by a poor expression of CD94-NKG2 receptors could lead to increases of lung damage, either through increased direct RSV damage on epithelial cells in the absence of an effective immune response or through apoptotic signals in the lung. [91, 92]

It is becoming increasingly clear that RSV infection of the respiratory tract uniquely affects the host response in the airways. Studies in experimental models suggest that RSV can affect both the expression and the type of effector activity of T cells responding to RSV infection in the milieu of respiratory tract. It is also becoming increasingly clear that the complex interplay of the innate and adaptive immune systems in response to RSV plays a pivotal role in the development of severe acute pulmonary disease during RSV infection. [93]

Immunopathology following subsequent infections will depend upon both the ability of the antibody response to limit their severity, allergic responses in the host, and the nature of the T cell memory. [16]

4. Diagnosis

Effective diagnosis of viral respiratory infections, as well as recognition and understanding of the benefits and limitations of diagnostic laboratory testing, is essential. [94] A variety of laboratory methods are available to aid in the diagnosis of RSV infection in children and adults. [94] These tests typically detect the presence of RSV in respiratory secretions. In general, children have higher concentrations of RSV in their secretions (several logs) than adults. Immunocompromised individuals and the elderly often have lower concentrations. [94] Immunocompromised children may have intermittently high titers depending on their degree of immunosuppression, but tend to have prolonged shedding at lower titers. [95, 96] Currently available methods for diagnosis of RSV infections include cell (tissue) culture, serology, indirect and direct immunofluorescent antibody tests, enzyme-linked immunoassays (EIAs), and nucleic acid amplification (PCR). [94]

1) Cell Culture

For many years, RSV culture was considered the gold standard for diagnosing respiratory viral infections. Advantages of culture are its ability to detect viral coinfection and the isolated virus can be stored for future diagnostic studies. [94] However, RSV culture has disadvantages, including requirements for special specimen handling procedures to maintain viral viability, a long assay time, (average 2-5 days), greater financial and labor costs, and relatively poor sensitivity compared with molecular assays. [94] Even though recently developed diagnostic methods are more widely used, RSV culture will remain important for analyzing a subset of each year's viral strains for genetic and antigenic change and for discovering unknown viruses. [94]

2) Serology

Serology usually is not helpful for diagnosis of acute respiratory virus infections because 10-30% of patients with documented respiratory viral infections will remain serologically negative. However, research-based serologic techniques do provide useful seroepidemiologic information. [97, 98]

3) Antigen-Based Assays

Rapid test for the identification of virus in the respiratory secretions of infants and children are useful in improving the diagnosis of RSV infection. Most clinical laboratories use antigen detection assays to diagnose RSV infection, and several tests are available that will provide clinicians with the means for rapid diagnosis. [99] Antigen-based assays, which have been available for more than 30 years, include indirect and direct immunofluorescent antibody tests, EIA, and optical immunoassays. [94] Of the commercially available rapid diagnostic assays, EIAs usually have the best combination of sensitivity, specificity, and ease of use. [94] However, the sensitivity and specificity of these tests vary according to the manufacturer, virus, and strain being detected, and adequacy of the specimen. [94](Table 7)

Antigen-based methods are widely used because they are inexpensive, easy to perform, and easy to interpret. However, the assays currently approved by the Food and Drug Administration (FDA) continue to lack adequate sensitivity and specificity, especially when the prevalence of the virus is low (off-season) or in special populations, such as the immunocompromised or the elderly. [94] Their sensitivity and specificity mean that they are most reliable when the prevalence of infection is high, which suggests that their routine use should be limited to the peak periods of viral circulation. (Table 6). Recent advances in laboratory diagnostic methods enable rapid multiplex point of care antigen detection for RSV. The benefits associated with rapid tests are the reduced number of ancillary tests and antibiotic uses, and possibility of avoiding blood cultures to diagnoses serious bacterial infections in younger children with sourceless fever.

Table 6. Antigen-based rapid diagnostic assays compared to tissue culture or other FDA-approved assays for RSV

	Sensitivity (%)	Specificity (%)
IFA/DFA	93–98	92–97
EIA	59–97	75–100
DIA	93	91
OIA	88–95	97–100

IFA/DFA indicates indirect and direct immunofluorescent antibody tests; EIA, enzyme-linked immunoassay; DIA, direct immunoassay; OIA, optical immunoassay.

Adapted from Pediatr Infect Dis J 2007;26:3S36-S40.

4) Molecular Assays

Molecular assays have become the new gold standards for respiratory virus detection. They offer the advantage of being highly sensitive and highly specific (approaching 100%), when compared with culture or antigen assays. [98, 100] Studies comparing molecular assays to culture assays demonstrate significantly better sensitivity (12-50%) if a method for determining true positives is included in the assay. (Figure 7)

PCR technology has evolved to include novel chemistry and detection methods. [98, 100] Most of these methods are single- or dual-agent assays detected by gel analyses, enzyme hybridization, or real-time (RT)-PCR. Although these assays are rapid (3-4 hours) and sensitive, their inability to be highly multiplexed (only 3 or 4 analytes) has limited their use for the diagnosis of common community-acquired respiratory viruses. [94]

Recently, 3 highly multiplex assays were developed as research use only kits (EraGen Biosciences, TM Bioscience, and AutoGenomics Inc). [94] All 3 assays rely on multiplex PCR for amplification of 16, 19, or 27 different respiratory viruses including RSV. [94] EraGen Biosciences and TM Bioscience assays are partially open-format assays where different nucleic acid isolation platforms can be chosen if desired. Multiplex PCR followed by micro bead detection is performed on a cell sorting machine (Luminex Corporation). [94] The technology is available, but additional work is required to create assays with improved sensitivity and specificity. [94] Current research use only assays are being used for epidemiologic studies in many laboratories around the world but require an 8-9 hour turnaround time, use expensive equipment, and have sensitivities that are logarithmically less than those achieved with multiplex RT-PCR, enzyme hybridization, or single analyte real-time assays. [94]

Accurate and timely diagnosis of the cause of LRTI in children has potential benefits, including improved treatment of the individual child, decreasing the overall costs of care and reducing selection for antimicrobial organisms due to excessive antibiotic use. [101, 102]

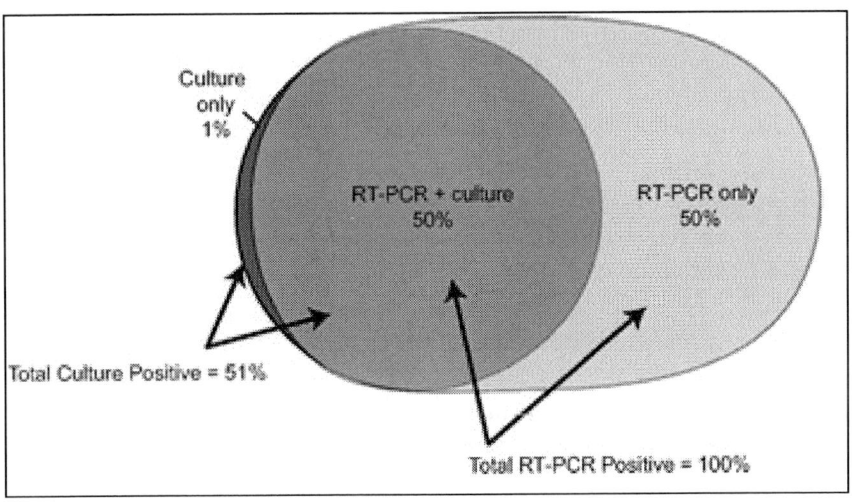

Adapted from Pediatr Infect Dis J 2007;26:3S36-S40.

Figure 7. Diagnosis of RSV infection by RT-PCR compared with tissue culture among 983 nasopharyngeal swab specimens from children in Rochester, NY.

5) Factors Affecting Sensitivity and Specificity of the Assays

A number of factors may affect the sensitivity and specificity of an assay for viral detection. These include quality of the specimen, transport conditions of the specimen, quality of the reagents, laboratory technician experience, inter- and intra-laboratory standardization, suitability of the assay to specific populations (eg, rapid antigen test in elderly versus young people) and prevalence of the agent in the community. [94]

6) Comparison of RSV Detection Methods

Accurate and rapid diagnosis of the cause of LRI is essential. Serology is not useful for diagnosing acute respiratory illness. Antigen-based assays are widely available, easy to use, provide rapid results, and are inexpensive; however, they are less sensitive than cell culture utilizing good specimen collection and processing techniques. Cell culture, which was previously considered the gold standard for identification of respiratory viruses, in many settings is being replaced by nucleic acid amplification assays that have even greater sensitivity and provide more rapid results. [94]

During the height of the RSV season, rapid antigen detection tests may be helpful in diagnosing RSV as the cause of LRI in children. [94] Among hospitalized children these tests may be useful adjuncts for infection control procedures. [94] However, they are not routinely recommended by the American Academy of Pediatrics (AAP) for use among children with bronchiolitis. [103] The value and reliability of these tests for diagnosis among children with upper respiratory tract infections (URI) is not clear. As previously noted, the advantages of these rapid antigen tests are their practicality and availability. They have good sensitivity and specificity, especially if used among normal children, and only if used during the peak of the virus season. [94]

The value of RT-PCR as a detection method for RSV has now been demonstrated. However, there are no standardized FDA-approved assays, and variation among laboratories remains a problem. [94] The sensitivity and specificity, as well as the predictive value of a positive or negative test must be established for each laboratory. [94] Other disadvantages of RT-PCR include expense and its correlation with clinical findings. This is particularly problematic among immunocompromised patients. [94] If a non-immunocompromised child is RSV-positive by RT-PCR, it means that this child is acutely infected with RSV, has been ill recently with RSV, or is about to become ill with RSV. [94] Almost all children are negative for RT-PCR after 14-21 days; but occasionally a child will remain positive for up to 4 weeks. During these longer periods of shedding detected by RT-PCR, the chance increases that another undetected viral infection may be present, especially among young children who have frequent viral infections during the respiratory season. [94] Differentiation as to which is the cause of the acute illness may be aided in the future by the development of more readily available, practical, and cost-effective methods of quantitative RT-PCR. [94]

Future developments in diagnostic tests should enhance our ability to rapidly, inexpensively, and easily determine the causative agent in suspected viral respiratory infections. Rapid diagnosis allows prompt implementation of the most effective and appropriate management to reduce morbidity, mortality, and healthcare costs. [94]

The clinical interpretation of the detection of a virus from nasopharyngeal secretions in a child with LRI can be challenging. It is possible that the virus is from a resolving upper respiratory infection and not the cause of the lower respiratory tract diseases. Detection of RSV can generally be assumed to correlate with LRI, but coinfection or superinfection with bacteria is not rare. [101] Viral quantification may prove helpful to determine when an isolate is associated with severe disease. [101] In evaluating new diagnostic platform, it is not enough to demonstrate that the new test correctly identifies the presence of a number of respiratory pathogens. The clinician must be able to interpret a positive test result in the context of the clinical illness and determine the appropriate management. [101]

5. RSV Infection and Wheezing, Asthma

1) Preschool Asthma after RSV Infection

Wheezing illnesses are associated with viral respiratory infections in patients of all ages. In infants, RSV bronchiolitis has many similarities to acute asthma: wheezing, rapid breathing, small airway inflammation, and, in some children, respiratory compromise. [104] About a third of children with an initial wheezing episode due to bronchiolitis will have recurrent episodes of wheezing. [105] This association has prompted speculation that severe episodes of RSV bronchiolitis in infancy initiate the development of asthma. [104]

On the basis of a systematic review of studies of the association between RSV infection in the first 36 months of life and the subsequent development of asthma in preschool children, there is an association between RSV infection and the emergence of different asthma phenotypes, with a clear gradient effect and progress disappearance of this effect with increasing age. [106]

2) Asthma and Allergy Patterns after RSV Infection

In a prospective controlled follow-up from Sweden, hospitalization for RSV bronchiolitis at less than 12 months of age was a significant risk factor for both asthma and atopy at 7-8 and 13-14 years of age. [106]

Sigurs et al., [107] explored the association between an RSV infection sufficient to cause admission to hospital and the eventual development of asthma. Beginning in 1989, they identified 52 infants who were receiving treatment in hospital for RSV bronchiolitis and assessed their disease progression until they were 13 years old. The patients were matched 93 healthy individuals of similar age and sex. When the children were 13 years old, the occurrence of asthma/recurrent wheezing was significantly higher in the RSV group (43%) than among the control subjects (8%). Data from this study suggest that severe RSV infections together with a family history of asthma increase the likelihood of an individual developing asthma. Recently, they reported longitudinal wheeze and allergy patterns at 18 years after severe RSV bronchiolitis in their first year of life. [108] They showed that severe RSV bronchiolitis in the first year of life is frequently followed by allergic asthma persisting into early adulthood. (Figure 8, Figure 9) Subjects with RSV infection with and without current asthma have reduced airway function as measured by spirometry. They suggested that early severe RSV bronchioltis has lifelong consequences of allergic asthma and airway remodeling.

These findings accord with the widespread idea that both genetic (a family history of asthma) and environmental (RSV infection) factors combine to determine expression of disease (asthma). [104]

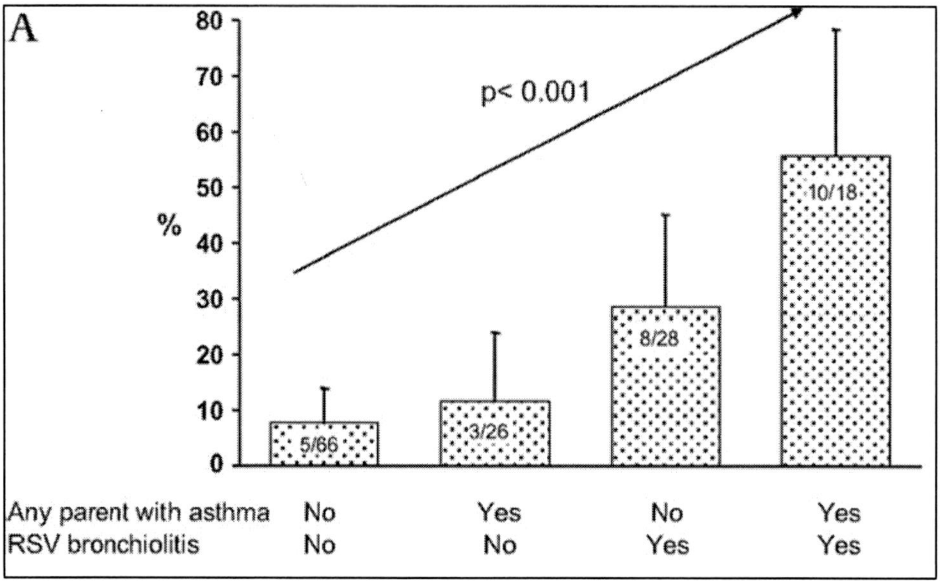

Adapted from Thorax 2010;65:1045-52.

Figure 8. Proportion (%) with current asthma/ recurrent wheeze in RSV and control cohorts with respect to heredity for asthma.

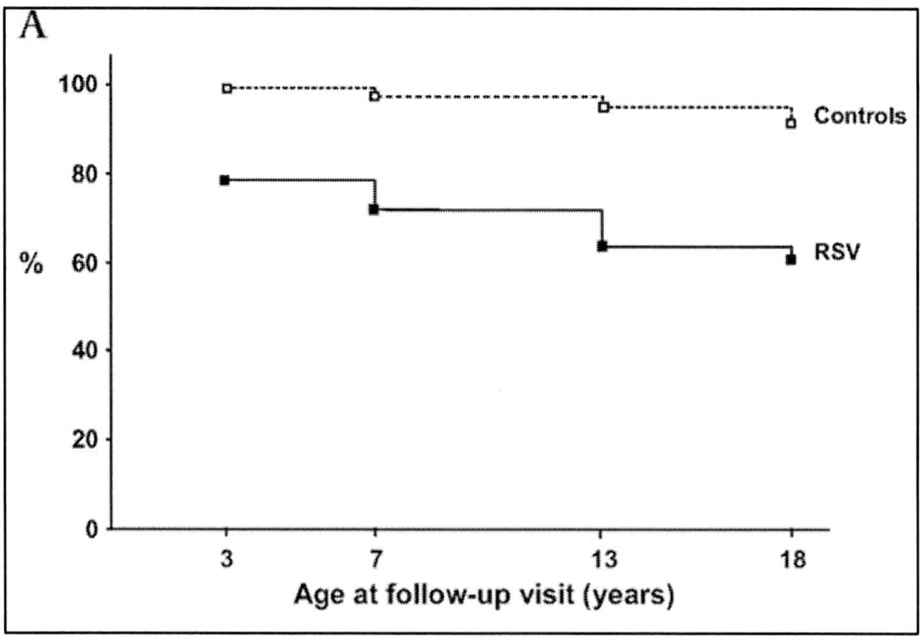

Adapted from Thorax 2010;65:1045-52.

Figure 9. Proportion (%) of subjects in the RSV and control cohorts who never had an asthma diagnosis at follow-up at ages 3, 7, 13 and 18 years.

This gene-environment idea is lent support by a large epidemiological study [109] done in Tennessee, USA, in which investigators noted that infants who were born roughly 120 days before the time of the year at which RSV prevalence was at its peak had the highest rate of admissions to hospital for wheezing illnesses. Follow-up revealed that the timing of birth with respect to the peak of the winter bronchiolitis season was also associated with a high risk for developing asthma. These findings suggest that infants who are at the highest risk for severe RSV bronchiolitis are also most likely to develop asthma.

Moreover, they suggest an association between wheezing illnesses due to RSV infection in early life and the subsequent expression of persistent wheezing and asthma when a child begins school. However, an association between RSV infection and asthma has not been seen in all investigators.

For example, longitudinal data from Tucson Children's Respiratory Study [110] indicate that RSV LRI before a child is 3 years of age are associated with subsequent wheezing and asthma in early childhood, but not beyond age 11 years. Furthermore, Thomsen et al., [111] assessed the association between admission to hospital due to RSV infection and development of asthma based on a twin registry in Denmark. They concluded that severe RSV infections do not cause asthma but, instead, that a genetic predisposition to both RSV bronchiolitis and asthma exists.

Distinguishing which bronchiolitis patients are at a particular risk for persistent wheezing and asthma in later life is essential for planning of an optimal treatment for early-life wheezers. [112]

3) Lung Function after RSV Infection

Longitudinal studies have revealed permanent loss of lung function after bronchiolitis. Later lung function abnormalities have been documented after severe bronchiolitis in infancy [107] and after mild early-life wheezing, [113] and even years after cessation of wheezing. [114] Subnormal findings in flow-volume spirometry were present at the age of 18-20 years in 30% and AHR in 41% of former bronchiolitis patients in the Finnish cohort study. [114] In non-atopic transient and persistent wheezers, lung function gradually improved, but on average, remained subnormal through childhood even after 5-10 symptom-free years. [113]

4) Recurrent Wheezing in Atopic Children after RSV Infection

Although RSV LRIs in early life are followed by later wheezing, it is unclear whether there is a causal relationship between this and an atopic tendency. Studies from Australia seem to suggest that early-life respiratory infections with RSV in conjunction with atopic sensitization may contribute to the risk for subsequent development of persistent asthma. [116] A prospective cohort of 263 children at high risk of atopy demonstrates significant associations between RSV-induced wheeze LRI in the first year of life and the subsequent development of persistent wheeze at 5 years. [116](Table 7)

This suggests viral infections interact with atopy in infancy to promote later asthma. Notably the occurrence of both of these events during this narrow developmental window is associated with maximal risk for subsequent asthma, which suggests a contribution from both classes of inflammatory insults to disease pathogenesis. Protection of high-risk children against the effects of severe respiratory infection during infancy may represent an effective strategy for primary asthma prevention. [116]

Table 7. Predictors of current wheeze at 5 years of age in relation to time of atopic sensitization

Type of ARI	Never atopic OR (95% CI) *P* value	Atopic by age of 2 years OR (95% CI) *P* value	Atopic after 2 years OR (95% CI) *P* value
Whole population regardless of ARI history	**0.4 (0.2-0.8) 0.006***	**3.1 (1.5-6.4) 0.05**	**2.9 (1.4-5.8) 0.05**
Any wheezy LRI in first year	1.4 (0.4-5.1) 0.6	**3.4 (1.2-9.7) 0.02**	0.5 (0.1-3.5) 0.5
No. of wheezy LRI *(linear model)*	1.1 (0.5-2.8) 0.8	**2.4 (1.2-4.7) 0.01**	0.9 (0.2-4.1)0.9
0	Comparison group	Comparison group	Comparison group
1	1.6 (0.4-6.9) 0.5	1.9 (0.7-5.5) 0.2	(≥1) 0.5 (0.1-3.4) 0.5
≥2	1.0 (0.1-9.1) 1.0	**7.1 (1.3-38.4) 0.02**	NA
Any febrile infections in first year	1.2 (0.4-3.8) 0.8	1.2 (0.8-1.8) 0.4	1.8 (0.3-9.6) 0.5
Any febrile URI	1.3 (0.4-4.1) 0.7	0.9 (0.5-1.5) 0.9	1.4 (0.3-7.1) 0.7
Any febrile LRI	1.0 (0.2-3.8) 1.0	**4.2 (1.5-11.8) 0.006**	1.3 (0.2-9.9) 0.8
Any wheezy or febrile LRI	1.0 (0.3-3.4) 1.0	**3.9 (1.4-10.5) 0.007**	0.7 (0.1-3.9) 0.7
Any wLRI associated with rhinovirus or RSV	0.8 (0.2-4.0) 0.8	**4.1 (1.3-12.6) 0.02**	0.9 (0.1-6.4) 0.9
Any wLRI associated with rhinovirus	1.6 (0.3-8.7) 0.6	**3.2 (1.1-9.5) 0.03**	2.1 (0.3-18.5) 0.5
Any wLRI associated with RSV	1.6 (0.3-8.7) 0.6	3.6 (1.0-13.3) 0.06	Insufficient number

NA, Not applicable.

*Data in boldface are statistically significant at the .05 level.

Adapted from J Allergy Clin Immunol 2007;119:1105-10.

5) Wheezing after RSV LRI in Preterm Infants

Studies have reported that acute RSV LRI in infancy may lead to long-term airway morbidity and gestational age may affect the development of airway reactivity, [117] and premature infants have been documented to be at high risk for serious or fatal RSV infection. [118] A previous study demonstrated that RSV LRI during early infancy of preterm infants was associated with an increased risk for early childhood wheezing by age 3 years. [119](Table 8)

Table 8. Rates of serious early childhood wheezing between ages 2 and 3 years stratified by other variables of interest

Variable	RSV Cohort, No. (%)	Control Cohort, No. (%)	*P*
Gestational age			
≤32 wk*	4/20 (20.0)	4/50 (8.0)	0.213
33-36 wk	22/118 (18.6)	12/158 (7.6)	0.009*
Parental atopy			
Yes*	16/107 (15.0)	9/111 (8.1)	0.113
No	40/218 (18.3)	32/392 (8.2)	<0.001
Parental asthma			
Yes*	4/34 (11.8)	3/34 (8.8)	1.000
No	52/291 (17.9)	38/469 (8.1)	<0.001

Adapted from Clin Ther 2010;32:2422-32.

6) Long-Term Outcome of Early Childhood Wheezing

Over half of the former bronchiolitis patients have suffered from recurrent wheezing episodes at 2-3 years of age, and 25-54% have been symptomatic at 4-6 years of age. [120] Although the tendency for wheezing decreases over time, still 15-30% have asthma during the early school years, [121] which is more than the 4-10% prevalence of asthma among school children observed in population-based studies in Scandinavian countries. [122]

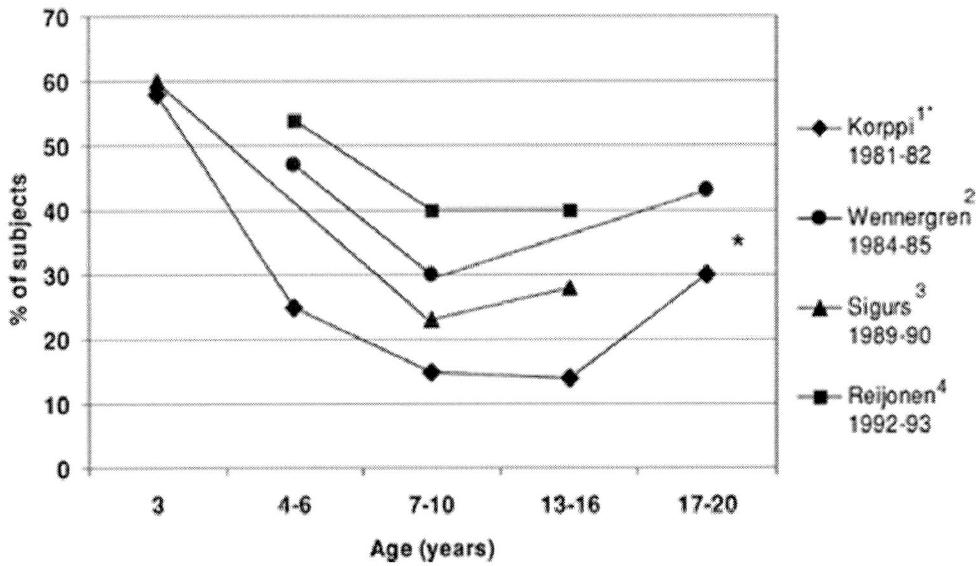

Adapted from Acta Paediatr 2008;97:5-11.

Figure 10. subsequent asthma until school age after hospitalization for bronchiolitis in early life.

Children with wheezing severe enough to need hospitalization at less than 24 months of age form a group at a particular risk for asthma and other respiratory disorders in later life. There are 4 prospective follow-up studies after hospitalization for bronchiolitis, two from Finland and two from Sweden, which have continued until more than 10 years of age. [112](Figure 10) As seen in Figure 10, 14-40% of former bronchiolitis patients had asthma in adolescence. [107, 123].

The prevalence of modest to severe asthma at 17-20 years of age was 16-30%, and the prevalence of all asthma cases was 41-43%. [115, 124].

7) Cellular and Molecular Linking RSV Infection to Asthma

RSV-induced LRI constitutes a proven risk factor for the development of childhood asthma. Cellular and molecular studies of RSV infection in human cell lines and neurologic evidence in animal models have demonstrated a possible causal relationship between RSV-induced LRI during infancy and asthma later in life [117].

Epithelial cells are the first line of defense of the airway, and their exposure to RSV causes signals the release of several chemokines and cytokines. These inflammatory mediators damage the epithelium and cause loss of epithelial cells, leading to increased airway permeability, mucous plugging, and decreased clearance. The degree of epithelial damage is correlated with the magnitude of inflammation and AHR. [117, 125] One of the earliest events in response to RSV infection is the initial innate cytokine response, with a time-dependent increase in expression. The early cytokines, including the Type 1 IFN-α/β, IL-12, and IL-18, have been detected in the respiratory secretions of infants with RSV infection. [126] As shown in Figure 11, RSV infection upregulates the expression of several cytokines and chemokines, such as IL-1β, IL-6, IL-8, TNF-α, MIP1α, RANTES, and the adhesion molecule ICAM-1, in cultured epithelial cells. [117, 127].

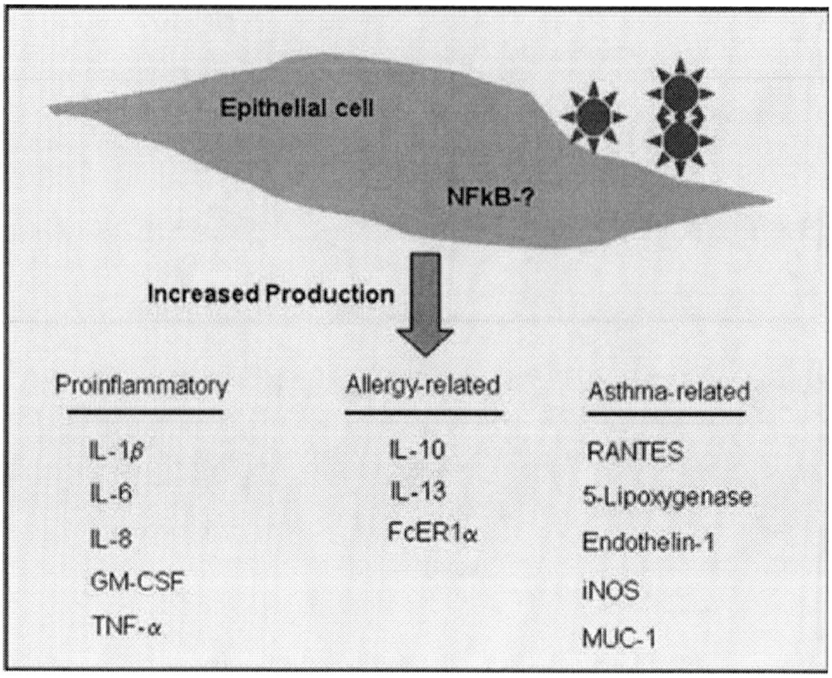

Adapted from Acta Paediatr 2008;97:5-11.

Figure 11. Epithelial cell as the target of RSV and possible role of NF- κ B in mediating RSV-induced activation of genes.

During the acute stage of infection, airway epithelial cells can initiate primary local inflammatory responses by directly responding with cytokine secretion to inflammatory stimuli or by amplifying an inflammatory event previously initiated by activated macrophages, eosinophils, or lymphocytes. [117](Table 9).

Table 9. Common inflammatory cells and mediators in the upper and lower airway in RSV infection

Immune response	Immune mechanism(s)
Inflammatory cells	Eosinophills Mast cells Basophills Dendritic cells Neutrophills Th2 lymphocytes
Mediators	Histamine Cysteinyl leukotrienes Prostaglandins Kinins Cytokines Chemokines

Adapted from Clin Microbiol Rev 2008;21:495-504.

These cell types may have important roles in controlling infection; however, inappropriate expression of inflammatory mediators may be linked to AHR and exacerbation of RSV-associated asthma. [128, 129] In addition to the impact on immunogenicity due to the actions of the cytokines and chemokines they produce, bronchial epithelial cells also express adhesion molecules, such as ICAM-1, and MHC class II molecules, which enable them to present antigens directly to T cells. [116] The relationships between atopy, RSV infection in early life, clinical bronchiolitis, and the development of asthma are rather complex. RSV infections may be related to asthma through an airway injury mechanism through a Th2 pathway. [130].

6. Treatment

Present treatment for infants hospitalized with RSV are primarily supportive and aimed at maintaining adequate oxygenation and ventilator support and hydration. [131] Initial assessment of respiratory status should include a measure of oxygenation and oxygen should be given when there is clinical evidence of respiratory distress even before full assessment is completed. [132] Fluid and nutritional status should also be assessed early and decisions made about use of intravenous fluids, nasogastric feeding, or maintenance of frequent oral feedings. After the use of oxygen therapy and attention of fluid and nutritional status, the evidence base for all other therapies drops sharply. [131]

1) Antiviral Therapy (Ribavirin)

1.1. Background

RSV spreads from respiratory secretions through close contact with infected persons or contact with contaminated surfaces, on which it survives for up to several hours. Despite this impressive burden of disease, the treatment of RSV today remains largely supportive and unchanged since the discovery of this virus in 1957. Only one drug (ribavirin) is currently licensed by the US FDA to treat RSV, and its use remains limited and controversial. Aerosolized ribavirin is not licensed for use in many countries due to its high cost and concern of potential harm to healthcare professionals. [133]

1.2. Pharmacology

Ribavirin is a synthetic nucleotide analog that is converted through cellular kinases into 5' triphosphate nucleotide. In this form it is thought to interfere with RNA metabolism and viral reproduction. [134] Its mechanisms of action are thought to include hypermutation and inhibition of RNA polymerases, but the exact mechanism of action is unknown. The primary serious adverse effect of ribavirin is hemolytic anemia through erythrocyte trapping and it is teratogenic in all non-primitive animal species on which it has been tested at higher levels than administered to people. [134]

1.3. Efficacy

Although aerosolized ribavirin has good antiviral in vitro activity against RSV, subsequent double-blind placebo-controlled studies in mechanically ventilated RSV patients have failed to show positive effects and even found prolongation of mechanical ventilation and the duration of hospital stays. [135] The AAP has recommended that ribavirin may be considered in high-risk children for serious RSV disease since 1996. [136] Early use has been shown to reduce the morbidity and mortality in high-risk patients such as adult and pediatric bone marrow transplantation patients.

1.4. Conclusion

When considering the lack of unequivocal evidence, the price of the product, the difficult administration of the product and the fear of adverse events, there is no place for the routine use of ribavirin in the treatment of either ventilated or non-ventilated patients with RSV LRI. The use of ribavirin in highest risk patients, such as bone marrow transplant recipients, remains controversial. [134]

2) Bronchodilator

2.1. Background

Airway obstruction secondary to inflammation and constriction of the smaller airways plays an important role in the pathogenesis of serious RSV infection. There is also a strong association with RSV and post-bronchiolitis wheezing and asthma. [104, 107] Considering the similarities between bronchiolitis, post-bronchiolitis wheezing and asthma, it is not surprising that research has focused on bronchodilator therapy in the treatment of RSV infection. [134]

2.2. Pharmacology

Bronchodilators or β2 mimetics act on the β2 receptors in bronchial smooth muscle and dilate the bronchi and bronchioles, hence increasing airflow. [134]

2.3. Efficacy

Short-acting β2 agonists such as albuterol/salbutamol and anticholinergics such as ipratropium bromide and theophylline have all been evaluated in the treatment of RSV LRI, but the results are conflicting. [134] Overall, in patients with RSV-induced respiratory failure, up to 50% will respond to inhaled β-agonists. [137] However, large meta-analyses have either shown no beneficial effects or only a modest short-term improvement in the overall average clinical scores when comparing bronchodilators to placebo in infants with mild-to-moderate disease. [138]

Another randomized double-blind controlled trial in infants admitted to hospital with bronchiolitis found no positive acute effects on respiratory effort and no reduction in the length of hospital stay with the use of nebulized adrenalin when compared to placebo. [139]

2.4. Conclusion

The routine use of nebulized bronchodilator therapy in children with RSV LRI is no longer recommended. [134]

3) Corticosteroids

3.1. Background

There is a large body of evidence in favor of the notion that RSV is an immune-mediated disease. [16, 75, 93] The peak of disease coincides with the development of specific T and B cell responses, rather than with the peak of viral replication. [140] The results with the association between RSV and post-bronchiolitis wheezing and asthma, suggest that not so much viral cytotoxicity but rather the immune response and excessive airway inflammation play an extensive role in the pathogenesis of serious RSV disease. [134] There is convincing evidence that Th1 and Th2 cytokine patterns determine the type of immune response to RSV infection and that the spectrum of cytokine expression affects the control mechanisms involved in the regulation of disease pathogenesis and chronicity. [141]

3.2. Pharmacology

Steroid hormones are synthesized from cholesterol in the adrenal cortex and produce an anti-inflammatory response through leukocyte adhesion and the production of prostaglandins and leukotrienes, hence potentially decreasing bronchiolar swelling and airway obstruction. [134]

3.3. Efficacy

A large meta-analysis showed a significant improvement in the clinical symptoms, length of stay and duration of symptoms. [142] However, later meta-analyses and systemic reviews found no evidence in favor of corticosteroids. [143] A recent systematic review evaluated the effect of inhaled corticosteroids, started during the acute phase of bronchiolitis, on the prevention of post-bronchiolitis wheezing. Due to the small number of patients included and the inability to pool all clinical outcomes, strong recommendations could not be made. [144]

3.4. Conclusion

The general consensus is that systemic corticosteroids are not indicated in therapy against RSV LRI. Because the disease process produced by RSV infection is primarily inflammatory, other therapeutic approaches that target this inflammatory process may be successful. [134]

4) Antibiotics

4.1. Background

Although RSV disease is of viral origin, nearly half of all hospitalized infants with RSV LRI are treated with antibiotics. [145] Although an apparent contradiction, antibiotics are often initiated upon initial presentation of a distressed infant, with consolidation on a chest radiograph or during the course of the disease when concurrent bacterial infection is suspected. [134]

4.2. Pharmacology

Macrolide, through their ability for preventing the production of pro-inflammatory mediators and cytokines, may exert therapeutic effects independently of their antibacterial activity. [134] Clarithromycin, one of the newer macrolides, suppresses cytokine production via inhibition of NF-κB inhibition. [146] Immunomodulation further results from inhibition of neutrophil migration, an increase in phagocytosis and NK cell activity and induction of eosinophil apaptosis. [147]

4.3. Efficacy

Pulmonary bacterial co-infection is common in children ventilated for severe RSV bronchiolitis. The rates of positive bacterial culture from bronchoalveolar lavage and endotracheal aspirates in infants admitted to the ICU with RSV infection vary from 33 to 44%. [148] In a double–blind randomized placebo-controlled trial, clarithromycin reduced the length of hospital stay, duration of need for supplemental oxygen and plasma cytokine levels and readmission rates to the hospital after discharge. [147] Another recent randomized controlled trial did not show a beneficial effect of azithromycin in children hospitalized for RSV LRI. [149]

4.4. Conclusion

Unjustified use of antibiotics must be avoided because of concern about the development of antimicrobial resistance. Although RSV LRI can mimic bacterial pneumonia, antibiotics should not be used in non-ventilated children with RSV unless concomitant bacterial infection is proven. Empirical antibiotics therapy may be justified in children admitted to the ICU with probable signs of bacterial co-infection, pending the results of definitive cultures. The regular use of macrolides in children with RSV LRI does not appear justified. [134] Antibiotics need to be used cautiously owing to the potential for side effects, cost to the patient and the community and increasing bacterial resistance to antibiotics. [150]

5) Surfactant Therapy

Surfactant is a potentially promising therapy and it may play a role in the host immunity. In the three RTC, use of surfactant was associated with a decrease in duration of mechanical ventilation and a decrease in ICU length of stay.

There was no mortality or adverse effects of surfactant administration reported among the patients in these trials. The administration of exogenous surfactant to mechanically ventilated infants and children with bronchiolitis appears to be reasonably safe. However, the limited available data and differences among the published trials make it difficult for the clinician to draw particularly strong inferences about its effects in this population. [151]

6) Ventilator Supportive Therapy

Current practice regarding ventilator support is largely based on clinical judgment and case reports. Strategies for the use of ventilation should be tailored to the underlying disease type. Infants with diffuse consolidation should be treated with PEEP or high volume strategy high frequency oscillation ventilation. Infants who are hyperinflated could achieve greater benefit from slow rates and long expiratory times. [152]

7) Palivizumab Therapy

Palivizumab has proven efficacy for prophylaxis of RSV in infants with prematurity or CHD. Despite a paucity of data, palivizumab is sometimes used to prevent progression when high-risk patients present with RSV URI, or as therapy when any patient presents with severe RSV LRI. [153]

According to a systematic review of the literature on the use of palivizumab as therapy for RSV, when used for prophylaxis, the drug was generally well tolerated however, RCTs with sufficient power are needed to assess the efficacy of palivizumab in preventing progression of RSV URI and in treating severe RSV infection. [153]

7. Prevention

Although RSV bronchiolitis has a self-limiting course in most children and can usually be managed conservatively at home, a number of cases require hospitalization because of marked hypoxia and the impossibility of maintaining adequate hydration and regular feeding. [154] Approximately 1% of hospitalized children with bronchiolitis require admission to an ICU, where mortality is less than 1% in otherwise healthy patients but can reach 3.5% in children at risk of cardiac disease or CLD. [154] RSV spreads readily in the community, particularly among children who have close contact with infected patients or contaminated surfaces or objects. [154]

Nosocomial infections are common in pediatric wards. However, universal prevention for RSV infection is still not possible. There is no vaccine against RSV, the use of passive immunization has disadvantages, intravenous RSV immunoglobulins are very expensive and show poor efficacy, and humanized monoclonal antibodies are also expensive.

1) RSV vaccine

1.1. Background: Challenges for Developing a RSV Vaccine

With lack of adequate treatment, research focused on vaccine development as early as the 1960s. The highest risk group for severe RSV infection is infants less than 6 months of age. Thus, an RSV vaccine would ideally be administered as soon as possible after birth. [155] In practice, an initial dose would likely be administered at or before age of 2 months. Full term infants acquire maternal antibodies during the latter half of gestation and antibody levels remain relatively high for 6 months after birth. [155] This would coincide with the time when an RSV vaccine would need to stimulate a protective immune response in the presence of maternal antibody. [155] Several studies indicate that infants under 8 months of age have a reduced serum antibody response to natural RSV infection compared with older children. This diminished immunity may be due to an immature immune system, but it may also be caused by suppression of the immune response by maternal antibodies. [155]

1.2. Pharmacology

In the mid-1960s, formalin-inactivated (FI)-RSV vaccine lot 100 was administered intramuscularly to infants and children, 2 months to 7 years old. [155] A vaccine is an antigenic preparation that is used for establishing immunity to a disease. After vaccination, the body recognizes the protein coat on the virus and responds by neutralizing the agent before it can enter cells and by destroying infected cells before they can multiply. A FI-RSV vaccine offered no protection against naturally acquired RSV, but rather led to enhanced disease and increased mortality when patients were subsequently infected with RSV in the next season. [155] Although FI-RSV was highly immunogenic and elicited high ELISA titers of RSV antibody, the elicited antibodies were non-neutralizing, did not inhibit virus fusion, and were not protective. [156] The mechanism responsible for this vaccine-associated enhanced disease was not completely understood until reactive carbonyl groups due to formalin inactivation of the virus were recently found to be responsible.

1.3. Efficacy

In view of the severity of disease in particular in neonates, elderly and immunocompromised individuals, these populations are the primary targets for vaccination. [58](Table 10)

Table 10. Primary target populations for RSV vaccination

Group	Age-related risk factors	Special risk factors	Potential sequelae of RSV infection
Newborns	Low lung elasticity Immaturity of immune system	Prematurity Congenital heart disease Congenital immunodeficiency	Bronchiolitis Recurrent wheezing, asthma Otitis media
Elderly	Reduced lung elasticity		Sudden infant death syndrome Pneumonia
Immuno compromised	Impaired immune system	Transplantation Chemotherapy Cystic fibrosis	Pneumonia

Adapted from Rev Med Virol 2007;17:5-34.

1.4. Conclusion

At present, no vaccine against RSV is available. Considering its history and the criteria that an RSV vaccine must meet, such as efficacy against antigenically divergent strains in a very young population, vaccine development against RSV is a challenging field. [155]

2) Immunoglobulins

2.1. Background

Due to the lack of a safe RSV vaccine, much research has focused on immunoglobulins in the prevention of RSV infection.

2.2. Pharmacology

Immunoglobulins are glycoproteins that bind to a specific antigen and neutralize it. RSV polyclonal hyperimmune globulin (RSV IG) was prepared from donors with high serum titers of RSV-neutralizing antibody. [134]

2.3. Efficacy

Standard intravenous immune globulin was neither protective nor therapeutic in patients with RSV bronchiolitis due to insufficient titers of antibodies. [157] RSV IG overcame this problem and was licenced and recommended by the AAP in 1996. [158] RSV IG given as treatment to infants with severe RSV has a positive effect on lowering viral titers, but this was not correlated with improved clinical outcomes. [159] Passive immunization with RSV IG is only effective as long as enough neutralizing antibody titer is achieved and monthly administration of this product is cumbersome. [134] RSV IG is no longer commercially available.

2.4. Conclusion

Immunoglobulins have no place in the treatment of RSV LRI.

3) Palivizumab

3.1. Palivizumab for RSV Prevention

Palivizumab, which is produced by recombinant DNA technology, is an IgG1 humanized monoclonal antibody against an epitope in the A antigenic site of the RSV F protein that neutralizes RSV and prevents viral binding to cells. [133]

When given intramuscularly, it carries no risk of viral transmission, will not interfere with routine vaccination schedules, and shortage is theoretically avoidable. Palivizumab was approved by the US FDA for prevention of RSV disease in high-risk infants in 1998, including premature infants and infants with BPD or hemodynamically significant CHD. [133] The Committee on Infectious Disease (COID) of the AAP has published guidelines for consideration of palivizumab use. [160] In their 2009 statement, the COID suggested further restrictions in these indications compared with those published in 2006 based on cost considerations. [133, 161](Table 11)

Table 11. Comparison of 2006 and 2009 Committee on Infectious Disease of the American Academy of Pediatrics guidelines for palivizumab

	2006 guidelines [1]	2009 guidelines [2]
Chronic lung disease of infancy	Consider ≤24 months of age; five doses	No change
Congenital heart disease	Consider ≤24 months of age; five doses	No change
≤28 weeks GA	During first RSV season (≤12 months of age)	No change
29–32 weeks GA	29 weeks, 0 days to 32 weeks, 0 days; up to 6 months of age at start of RSV season	29 weeks, 0 days through to **31 weeks, 6 days**; up to 6 months of age at start of RSV season
32–35 weeks GA	32 weeks, 1 day through 35 weeks, 0 days; ≤6 months at start of RSV season AND two of five risk factors (childcare attendance, school-aged siblings, exposure to environmental air pollutants, congenital airway abnormalities and severe neuromuscular disease)	32 weeks, 0 days through to **34 weeks 6 days**; **<3 months of age at start of RSV season; three doses maximum (stop dosing at ≥90 days of age); one of two risk factors (childcare attendance and sibling[s] <5 years of age)**

[†]2009 changes in bold.
GA: Gestational age; RSV: Respiratory syncytial virus.

Adapted from Expert Rev Anti Infect Ther 2011;9:27-32.

3.2. Palivizumab for Preterm Infants

According to a systematic review conducted for efficacy and safety of palivizumab in preterm infants and its cost effectiveness in the United Kingdom, palivizumab prophylaxis is safe and efficious, but cost effectiveness has yet to be demonstrated. Palivizumab passive RSV immunization for five months over the RSV season reduces the risk of developing RSV illness by approximately 50%. [162] Although monoclonal antibodies have proven to be effective in providing projection to high-risk infants, their introduction in resource poor settings might be limited by high cost associated with them. Candidate vaccines for active immunization of infants against RSV hold greatest promise. Introduction of a low cost vaccine against RSV would reduce the inequitable distribution of burden due to childhood LRI and will most likely have a high impact on morbidity and mortality due to severe LRI. [163]

4) Motavizumab

Motavizumab, an investigational monoclonal antibody developed by affinity maturation of palivizumab, has significantly higher affinity for RSV F protein than palivizumab. [164] Compared with palivizumab, motavizumab was up to 20-fold more potent in microneutralization studies and, in the cotton rat model, reduced nasal and lung RSV titers 25-and 100-fold, respectively. The phase 3, randomized, double-blind, palivizumab-controlled study revealed that motavizumab recipients experienced 50% fewer RSV LRI than palivizumab recipients. [165] Motavizumab may offer an improved alternative in prophylaxis for serious RSV disease in infants and children at high risk. [165] Motavizumab proved non-inferior to palivizumab in preventing hospitalizations related to RSV infection, and reduced the number of medically-attended outpatient visits for RSV LRI. [166]

5) Leukotriene (LT) Modifier

CysLT levels in children with RSV bronchiolitis were significantly higher than in control subjects. In a recent study, Han et al., suggested that cysLT may play a critical role during RSV infection. [167] They showed that LT modifier during primary infection attenuated the AHR and airway inflammation after reinfection with RSV in mice. [168] Also, LT modifier treatment recently demonstrated reduced eosinophil degranulation and a decrease in recurrent wheezing episodes in post-RSV bronchitis in infants. [169]

In conclusion, despite more than four decades of study, the treatment of RSV remains supportive. Bronchodilators, corticosteroids and antiviral have all failed to demonstrate significant efficacy in this disease.

The role of antiviral agents is limited at present, with no new agents near availability. Even with improved antibody prophylaxis or proper therapeutic agents for acute RSV disease, the long-term airway morbidity may not be diminished. Prevention should be the key road to follow. New insights into its pathogenesis and genetic predispositions should lead to the development of innovative vaccines and effective immunoglobulins, thereby enabling control of RSV disease worldwide.

REFERENCES

[1] Garcia-Garcia ML, Calvo C, Falcon A, Pozo F, Perez-Brena P, De Cea JM, et al. Role of emerging respiratory viruses in children with severe acute wheezing. *Pediatr. Pulmonol.* 2010;45:585-91.

[2] Paramore LC, Mahadevia PJ, Piedra PA. Outpatient RSV lower respiratory infections among high-risk infants and other pediatric populations. *Pediatr. Pulmonol.* 2010;45:578-84.

[3] Principi N, Esposito S. Antigen-based assays for the identification of influenza virus and respiratory syncytial virus: Why and how to use them in pediatric practice. *Clin. Lab. Med.* 2009;29:649-60.

[4] Nair H, Nokes DJ, Gessner BD, Dherani M, Madhi SA, Singleton RJ, et al. Global burden of acute lower respiratory infections due to respiratory syncytial virus in young children: a systematic review and meta-analysis. *Lancet* 2010;375:1545-55.

[5] Welliver RC, Checchia PA, Bauman JH, Fernandes AW, Mahadevia PJ, Hall CB. Fatality rates in published reports of RSV hospitalizations among high-risk and otherwise healthy children. *CMRO* 2010;26:2175-81.

[6] Garcia CG, Bhore R, Soriano-Fallas A, Trost M, Chason R, Ramilo O, et al. Risk factors in children hospitalized with RSV bronchiolitis versus non-RSV bronchiolitis. *Pediatrics* 2010;126:e1453-e60.

[7] Mcintosh K. Respiratory syncytial virus. In: Kliegman RM, Behrman RE, Jenson HB, Stanton BF, eds, *Nelson Textbook of Pediatrics.* 18th ed. Philadelphia: Saunders Elsevier 2007:1388-90.

[8] Yoo Y, Yu J, Kim DK, Choi SH, Kim CK, Koh YY. Methacholine and adenosine 5'-monophosphate challenges in children with post-infectious bronchiolitis obliterans. *Eur. Respir. J.* 2006;27:36-41.

[9] Lange W. Uber eine eigentumliche erkrankung der klemen: Branche and bronchiolen (Bronchitis rt bronchiolitis obliterans). *Dtsch Arch. Klin. Med.* 1901;70:342.

[10] Mauad T, Dolhnikoff M, The Sao Paulo Bronchiolitis Obliterans Study Group. Histology of childhood bronchiolitis obliterans. *Pediatr. Pulmonol.* 2002;33:466-74.

[11] Fischer GB, Teper A, Colom AJ. Acute viral bronchiolitis and its sequelae in developing countries. *Paediatr. Respir. Rev.* 2002;3:298-302.

[12] Chang AB, Masel JP, Masters B. Post-infectious bronchiolitis obliterans: clinical, radiological and pulmonary function sequelae. *Pediatr. Radiol.* 1998;28:23-9.

[13] Morichi S, Kawashima H, Ioi H, Yamanaka G, Kashiwagi Y, Hoshika A, et al. Classification of acute encephalopathy in respiratory syncytial virus infection. J Infect Chemother 2011 Jun 7. Epub ahead of print.

[14] Sweetman LL, Ng YT, Butler IJ, Bodensteiner JB. Neurologic complications associated with respiratory syncytial virus. *Pediatr. Neurol.* 2005;32:307-10.

[15] Mizuguchi M, Yamanouchi H, Ichiyama T, Shiomi M. Acute encephalopathy associated with influenza and other viral infections. *Acta Neurol. Scand.* 2007;115(Suppl 186):45-56.

[16] Durbin JE, Durbin RK. Respiratory syncytial virus-induced immunoprotection and immunopathology. *Viral Immunol.* 2004;17:370-80.

[17] Varga SM, Braciale TJ. RSV-induced immunopathology: Dynamic interplay between the virus and host immune response. *Virology* 2002;295:203-7.

[18] Wilkins C, Gale M Jr. Recognition of viruses by cytoplasmic sensors. Curr Opin Immunol 2010;22:41-7.

[19] Takeuchi O, Akira S. MDA5/RIG-1 and virus recognition. *Curr. Opin. Immunol.* 2008;20:17-22.

[20] Saito T, Hirai R, Loo YM, Owen D, Johnson CL, Sinha SC, et al. Regulation of innate antiviral defenses through a shared repressor domain in RIG-1 and LGP2. *Proc. Natl. Acad. Sci. USA* 2007;104:582-7.

[21] Kawai T, Takahashi K, Sato S, Coban C, Kumar H, Kato H, et al. IPS-1, an adaptor triggering RIG-1-and Mda5-mediated type 1 interferon induction. *Nat. Immunol.* 2005;6:981-8.

[22] Seth RB, Sun L, Ea CK, Chen ZJ. Identification and characterization of MAVS, a mitochondrial antiviral signaling protein that activates NF-κB and IRF 3. *Cell* 2005;122:669-82.

[23] Xu LG, Wang YY, Han KJ, Li LY, Zhai Z, Shu HB. VISA is an adaptor protein required for virus-triggered INF-ß signaling. *Mol. Cell* 2005;19:727-40.

[24] Meylan E, Curran J, Hofmann K, Moradpour D, Binder M, Bartenschlager R, et al. Cardif is an adaptor protein in the RIG-1 antiviral pathway and is targeted by hepatic C virus. *Nature* 2005;437:1167-72.

[25] Collins PL, Crowe JE, Jr. Respiratory syncytial virus and metapneumovirus. In: Knipe DM, Howley PM eds. *Fields Virology*, 5th edition. Philadelphia: Lippincott Williams and Wilkins, 2007, 1602-41.

[26] Zuppan C, Robinson C, Langston C. 1995. Viral pneumonia in infants and children, pp. 111-153. In: Askin F, langstin C, Berstein J, et al, eds. *Pulmonary Disease*, Vol 18, Karger, New York.

[27] Biron CA. Role of early cytokines, including alpha and beta interferons (IFN-α/ß), in innate and adaptive immune responses to viral infections. *Semin. Immunol.* 1998;10:383-90.

[28] Le Bon A, Tough DF. Links between innate and adaptive immunity via type 1 interferon. *Curr. Opin. Immunol.* 2002;14:432-6.

[29] Atreya PL, Kulkarni S. Respirarory syncytial virus strain A2 is resistant to the antiviral effects of Type 1 interferons and human MxA. *Virology* 1999;261:227-41.

[30] Goodbourn S, Didcock L, Randall RE. Interferons: cell signaling, immune modulation, antiviral responses and virus countermeasures. *J. Gen. Virol.* 2000;81:2341-64.

[31] Gotoh B, Komatsu T, Takeuchi K, Yokoo J. Paramyxovirus strategies for evading the interferon response. *Rev. Med. Virol.* 2002;12:337-57.

[32] He B, Paterson RG, Stock N, Durbin JE, Durbin RK, Goodboum S, et al. Recovery of paramyxovirus simian virus 5 with a V protein lacking the conserved cysteine-rich domain: the multifunctional V protein blocks both interferon-beta induction and interferon signaling. *Virology* 2002;303:15-32.

[33] Bossert B, Marozin S, Conzelmann KK. Nonstructural proteins NS1 and NS2 of bovine respiratory syncytial virus block activation of interferon regulatory factor 3. *J. Virol.* 2003;77:8661-8.

[34] Schlender J, Bossert B, Buchholz U, Conzelmann KKl. Bovine respiratory syncytial virus nonstructural proteins NS1 and NS2 cooperatively antagonize alpha/beta interferon-induced antiviral response. *J. Virol.* 2000;74:8234-42.

[35] Spann KM, Tran KC, Chi B, Rabin RL, Collins PL. Suppression of the induction of alpha, beta and lambda interferons by the NS1 and NS2 proteins of human respiratory syncytial virus in human epithelial cells and macrophages. *J. Virol.* 2004;78:4363-9.

[36] Kurt-Jones EA, Popova L, Kwinn L, Haynes LM, Jones LP, Tripp RA, et al. Pattern recognition receptors TLR4 and CD14 mediate response to respiratory syncytial virus. *Nat. Immunol.* 2000;1:398-401.

[37] Hatada EN, Krappmann D, Scheidereit C. NF-kappaB and the innate immune response. *Curr. Opin. Immunol.* 2000;12:52-8.

[38] Levine S, Klaiber-Franco R, Paradiso PR. Demonstration that glycoprotein G is the attachment protein of respiratory syncytial virus. *J. Gen. Virol.* 1987;68:2521-4.

[39] Techaarpornkul S, Barretto N, Peeples ME. Functional analysis of recombinant respiratory syncytial virus deletion mutants lacking the small hydrophobic and/or attachment glycoprotein gene. *J. Virol.* 2001;75:6825-34.

[40] Teng MN, Whitehead SS, Collins PL. Contribution of the respiratory syncytial virus G glycoprotein and its secreted and membrane-bound forms to virus replication in vitro and in vivo. *Virology* 2001;289:283-96.

[41] Barr F, Pedigo H, Johnson TR, Shepherd VL. Surfactant protein-A enhances uptake of respiratory syncytial virus by monocytes and U937 macrophages. *Am. J. Respir. Cell Mol. Biol.* 2000;23:586-92.

[42] Ghildyal R, Hartley C, Varrasso A, Meanger J, Voelker DR, Anders EM, et al. Surfactant protein A binds to the fusion glycoprotein of respiratory syncytial virus and neutralizes virion infectivity. *J. Infect Dis.* 1999;180:2009-13.

[43] Hickling TP, Bright H, Wing K, Gower D, Martin SL, Sim RB, et al. A recombinant trimeric surfactant protein D carbohydrate recognition domain inhibits respiratory syncytial virus infection in vitro and in vivo. *Eur. J. Immunol.* 1999;29:3478-84.

[44] LeVine AM, Elliot J, Whitsett JA, Srikiatkhachom A, crouch E, DeSilva N, et al. Surfactant protein-d enhances phagocytosis and pulmonary clearance of respiratory syncytial virus. *Am. J. Respir. Cell Mol. Biol.* 2004;31:193-9.

[45] LeVine AM, Gwozdz J, Stark J, Bruno M, Whitsett J, Korfhagen T. Surfactant protein-A enhances respiratory syncytial virus clearance in vivo. *J. Clin. Invest* 1999;103:1015-21.

[46] Cannon MJ, Openshaw PJ, Askonas BA. Cytotoxic T cells clear virus but augment lung pathology in mice infected with respiratory syncytial virus. *J. Exp. Med.* 1998;168:1163-8.

[47] Graham BS, Bunton LA, Rowland J, Wright PF, Karzon DT. Respiratory syncytial virus infection in anti-mu-treated mice. *J. Virol.* 1991;65:4936-42.

[48] Graham BS, Bunton LA, Wright PF, Karzon DT. Role of T lymphocytes subsets in the pathogenesis of primary infection and rechallenge with respiratory syncytial virus in mice. *J. Clin. Invest* 1991;88:1026-33.

[49] Durbin JE, Johnson TR, Durbin RK, Mertz SE, Morotti RA, Peebles RS, et al. The role of IFN in respiratory syncytial virus pathogenesis. *J. Immunol.* 2002;168:2944-52.

[50] Byeon JH, Lee JC, Choi IS, Yoo Y, Park SH, Choung JT. Comparison of cytokine responses in nasopharyngeal aspirates from children with viral lower respiratory tract infections. *Acta Paediatr* 2009;98:725-30.

[51] Alwan WH, Openshaw PJ. Distinct patterns of T- and B-cell immunity to respiratory syncytial virus induced by individual viral proteins. *Vaccine* 1993;11:431-7.

[52] Alwan WH, Record FM, Openshaw PJ. CD4+ T cells clear virus but augment disease in mice infected with respiratory syncytial virus. Comparison with the effects of CD8+ T cells. *Clin. Exp. Immunol.* 1992;88:527-36.

[53] Alwan WH, Kozlowska WJ, Openshaw PJ. Distinct types of lung disease caused by functional subsets of antiviral T cells. *J. Exp. Med.* 1994;179:81-9.

[54] Openshaw PJ, Clarke SL, Record FM. Pulmonary eosinophilic response to respiratory syncytial virus infection in mice sensitized to the major surface glycoprotein G. *Int. Immunol.* 1992;4:493-500.

[55] Srikiatkhachorn A, Braciale TJ. Virus-specific CD8+ T lymphocytes downregulate T helper cell type 2 cytokine secretion and pulmonary eosinophilia during experimental murine respiratory syncytial virus infection. *J. Exp. Med.* 1997;186:421-32.

[56] Srikiatkhachorn A, Braciale TJ. Virus-specific memory and effector T lymphocytes exhibit different cytokine responses to antigens during experimental murine respiratory syncytial virus infection. *J. Virol.* 1997;71:678-85.

[57] Srikiatkhachorn A, Chang W, Braciale TJ. Induction of Th-1 and Th-2 responses by respiratory syncytial virus attachment glycoprotein is epitope and major histocompatibility complex independent. *J. Virol.* 1999;73:6590-7.

[58] van Drunen Littel-van den Hurk S, Mapletoft JW, Arsic N, Kovacs-Nolan J. Immunopathology of RSV infection: prospects for developing vaccines without this complication. *Rev. Med. Virol.* 2007;17:5-34.

[59] Altman JD, Moss PA, Goulder PJ, Barouch DH, McHeyzer-Williams MG, Bell JI, et al. Phenotypic analysis of antigen-specific T lymphocytes. *Science* 1996;274.94-6.

[60] Openshaw PJ, Anderson K, Wertz GW, Askonas BA. The 22,000-kilodalton protein of respiratory syncytial virus is a major target for K^d-restricted cytotoxic T lymphocytes from mice primed by infection. *J. Virol* 1990;64:1683-9.

[61] Chang J, Braciale TJ. Respiratory syncytial virus infection suppresses lung CD8+ T-cell effector activity and peripheral CD8+ T-cell memory in the respiratory tract. *Nat. Med.* 2002;8:54-60.

[62] Wagner D, Muelenaer P, Henderson FW, Snyder MH, Reimer CB, Walsh EE, et al. Serum immunoglobulin G antibody subclass response to respiratory syncytial virus F and G glycoproteins after first, second, and third infections. *J. Clin. Microbiol.* 1989;27:589-92.

[63] Welliver RC, Kaul TN, Putnam TI, Sun M, Riddlesberger K, Ogra PL. The antibody response to primary and secondary infection with respiratory syncytial virus: kinetics of class-specific responses. *J. Pediatr.* 1980;98:808-13.

[64] Falsey AR, Walsh EE. Relationship of serum antibody to risk of respiratory syncytial virus infection in elderly adults. *J. Infect Dis.* 1998;177:463-6.

[65] Piedra PA Jewell AM, Cron SG, atmar RL, Glezen WP. Correlates of immunity to respiratory syncytial virus (RSV) associated-hospitalization: establishment of minimum protective threshold levels of serum neutralizing antibodies. *Vaccine* 2003;21:3479-82.

[66] Atkins JT, Karimi P, Morris BH, McDavid G, Shim S. Prophylaxis for respiratory syncytial virus with respiratory syncytial virus-immunoglobulin intravenous among preterm infants of thirty-two weeks gestation and less: reduction in incidence, severity of illness and cost. *Pediatr. Infect. Dis. J.* 2000;19:138-43.

[67] Le Bon A, Schiavoni G, D'Agostino G, Gresser I, Belardelli F, Tough DF. Type 1 interferons potently enhance humoral immunity and can promote isotype switching by stimulating dendritic cells in vivo. *Immunity* 2001;14:461-70.

[68] Palucka K, Banchereau J. How dendritic cells and microbes interact to elicit or subvert protective immune responses. *Curr. Opin. Immunol.* 2002;14:420-31.

[69] Openshaw PJ, Dean GS, Culley FJ. Links between respiratory syncytial virus bronchiolitis and childhood asthma: clinical and research approaches. *Pediatr. Infect. Dis. J.* 2003;22:S58-S64.

[70] Jafri HS, Chavez-Bueno S, Mejias A, Gomez AM, Rios AM, Nassi SS, et al. Respiratory syncytial virus induces pneumonia, cytokine response, airway obstruction, and chronic inflammatory infiltrates associated with long-term airway hyperrepsponsiveness in mice. *J. Infect Dis.* 2004;189:1856-65.

[71] Schwarze J, Ciesiewicz G, Hamelmann E, Joetham A, Shultz LD, Lamers MC, et al. IL-5 and eosinophilis are essential for the development of airway hyperresponsiveness following acute respiratory syncytial virus infection. *J. Immunol.* 1999;162:2997-3004.

[72] Tekkanat KK, Maassab H, Miller A, Berlin AA, Kunkel SL, Lukacs NW. RANTES (CCL5) production during primary respiratory syncytial virus infection exacerbates airway disease. *Eur. J. Immunol* 2002;32:3276-84.

[73] Mukherjee S, Lindell DM, Berlin AA, Morris SB, Shanley TP, Hershenson MB, et al. IL-17-induced pulmonary pathogenesis during respiratory viral infection and exacerbation of allergic disease. *Am. J. Pathol.* 2011;179:248-58.

[74] Hall CB, Walsh EE, Long CE, Schnabel KC. Immunity to and frequency of reinfection with respiratory syncytial virus. *J. Infect. Dis.* 1991;163:693-8.

[75] Kruijsen D, Bakkers MJ, van Uden NO, Viveen MC, van der Sluis TC, Kimpen JL, et al. Serum antibodies critically affect virus-specific CD4+/CD8+ T cell balance during respiratory syncytial virus infections. J Immunol 2010;185:6489-98.

[76] Lamprecht CL, Krause HE, Mufson MA. Role of maternal antibody in pneumonia and bronchiolitis due to respiratory syncytial virus. *J. Infect. Dis.* 1976;134:211-7.

[77] Bruhn FW, Yeager AS. Respiratory syncytial virus in early infancy. Circulating antibody and the severity of infection. *Am. J. Dis. Child* 1977;131:145-8.

[78] Polack FP, Teng MN, Collins PL, Prince GA, Exner M, Regele H, et al. A role for immune complexes in enhanced respiratory syncytial virus disease. *J. Exp. Med.* 2002;196:859-65.

[79] de Jong JM, Schuurhuis DH, Ioan-Facsinay A, Welling MM, Camps MG, van der Voort EI, et al. Dendritic cells, but not macrophages or B cells, activate major histocompatibility complex class II-restricted CD4+ T cells upon immune-complex uptake in vivo. *Immunology* 2006;119:499-506.

[80] Hamano Y, Arase H, Saisho H, Saito T. Immune complex and Fc receptor-mediated augmentation of antigen presentation for in vivo Th cell responses. *J. Immunol.* 2000;164:6113-9.

[81] Schuurhuis DH, Ioan-Facsinay A, Nagelkerken B, van Schip JJ, Sedlik C, Melief CJ, et al. Antigen-antibody immune complexes empower dendritic cells to efficiently prime specific CD8+ CTL responses in vivo. *J. Immunol.* 2002;168:2240-6.

[82] van Montfoort N, de Jong JM, Schuurhuis DH, van der Voort EI, Camps MG, Huizinga TW, et al. A novel role of complement factor C1q in augmenting the presentation of antigen captured in immune complexes to CD8+ T lymphocytes. *J. Immunol.* 2007;178:7581-6.

[83] Hashimoto K, Durbin JE, Zhou W, Collins RD, Ho SB, Kolls JK, et al. Respiratory syncytial virus infection in the absence of STAT 1 results in airway dysfunction, airway mucus, and augmented IL-17 levels. *J. Allergy Clin. Immunol.* 2005;116:550-7.

[84] Hashimoto K, Graham BS, Ho SB, Adler KB, Collins RD, Olson SJ, et al. Respiratory syncytial virus in allergic lung inflammation increases Muc5ac and gob-5. *Am. J. Respir. Crit. Care Med.* 2004;170:306-12.

[85] Ye P, Rodriguez FH, Kanaly S, Stocking KL, Schurr J, Schwarzenberger P, et al. Requirement of interleukin 17 receptor signaling for lung CXC chemokine and granulocyte colony-stimulating factor expression, neutrophil recruitment, and host defense. *J. Exp. Med.* 2001;194:519-27.

[86] Osorio F, LeibundGut-Landmann S, Lochner M, Lahl K, Sparwasser T, Eberl G, et al. DC activated via dectin-1 convert Treg into IL-17 producers. *Eur. J. Immunol.* 2008;38:3274-81.

[87] Chintakuntlawar AV, Chodosh J. Chemokine CXCL1/KC and its receptor CXCR2 are responsible for neutrophil chemotaxis in adenoviral keratitis. *J. Interferon Cytokine Res.* 2009;29:657-66.

[88] Vieira SM, Lemos HP, Grespan R, Napimoga MH, Dal-Secco D, Freitas A, et al. A crucial role for TNF-alpha in mediating neutrophil influx induced by endogenously generated or exogenous chemokines. KC/CXCL1 and LIX/CXCL5. *Br. J. Pharmacol.* 2009;158:779-89.

[89] Crowe CR, Chen K, Pociask DA, Alcorn JF, Krivich C, Enelow RI, et al. Critical role of IL-17RA in immunopathology of influenza infection. *J. Immunol.* 2009;183:5301-10.

[90] Larranaga CL, Ampuero SL, Luchsinger VF, Carrion FA, Aguilar NV, Morales PR, et al. Impaired immune response in severe human lower tract respiratory infection by respiratory syncytial virus. *Pediatr Infect Dis. J.* 2009;28:867-73.

[91] Welliver TP, Garofalo RP, Hosakote Y, Hintz KH, Avendano L, Sanchez K, et al. Severe human lower respiratory tract illness caused by respiratory syncytial virus and influenza virus is characterized by the absence of pulmonary cytotoxic lymphocyte responses. *J. Infect. Dis.* 2007;195:1126-36.

[92] Reed JL, Brewah YA, Delaney T, Welliver T, Burwell T, Benjamin E, et al. Macrophage impairment underlies airway occlusion in primary respiratory syncytial virus bronchiolitis. *J. Infect. Dis.* 2008;198:1783-93.

[93] Braciale TJ. Respiratory syncytial virus and T cells: Interplay between the virus and the host adaptive immune system. *Proc. Am. Thorac. Soc.* 2005;2:141-6.

[94] Henrickson KJ, Hall CB. Diagnostic assays for respiratory syncytial virus disease. *Pediatr .Infect. Dis.* J. 2007;26:S36-S40.

[95] Hall CB, Powell KR, MacDonald NE, Gala CL, Menegus ME, Suffin SC, et al. Respiratory syncytial viral infection in children with compromised immune function. *N. Engl. J. Med.* 1986;315:77-81.

[96] Chandwani S, Borkowsky W, Krasinski K, Lawrence R, Welliver R. Respiratory syncytial virus infection in human immunodeficiency virus-infected children. *J. Pediatr.* 1990;117:251-4.

[97] Dowell SF, Anderson LJ, Gary HE Jr, Erdman DD, Plouffe JF, File TM Jr, et al. Respiratory syncytial virus is an important cause of community-acquired lower respiratory infection among hospitalized adults. *J. Infect. Dis.* 1996;174:456-62.

[98] Henrickson KJ. Advances in the laboratory diagnosis of viral respiratory disease. *Pediatr. Infect. Dis. J.* 2004;23:S6-S10.

[99] Subbarao EK, Dietrich MC, De Sierra TM, Black CJ, Super DM, Thomas F, et al. Rapid detection of respiratory syncytial virus by a biotin-enhanced immunoassay: test performance by laboratory technologists and housestaff. *Pediatr. Infect. Dis. J.* 1989;8:865-9.

[100] Henrickson KJ. Cost-effective use of rapid diagnostic techniques in the treatment and prevention of viral respiratory infections. *Pediatr. Ann.* 2005;34:24-31.

[101] Pavia AT. Viral infections of the lower respiratory tract: Old viruses, new viruses, and the role of diagnosis. *CID* 2011;52:S284-S289.

[102] Roh KH, Kim J, Nam MH, Yoon S, Lee CK, Lee K, et al. Comparison of the Seeplex reverse transcription PCR assay with the R-mix viral culture and immunofluorescence techniques for detection of eight respiratory viruses. *Ann. Clin. Lab. Sci.* 2008;38:41-6.

[103] American Academy of Pediatrics Subcommittee on Diagnosis and Management of Bronchiolitis. Diagnosis and management of bronchiolitis. *Pediatrics* 2006;118:1774-93.

[104] Busse WW, Lemanske RF Jr, Gern JE. Role of viral respiratory infections in asthma and asthma exacerbations. *Lancet* 2010;376:826-34.

[105] Martinez FD, Wright AL, Taussig LM, Holberg CJ, Halonen M, Morgan WJ. Asthma and wheezing in the first six years of life. The Group Health Meedical Associates. *N. Engl. J. Med.* 1995;332:133-8.

[106] Perez-Yarza EG, Moreno A, Lazaro P, Mejias A, Ramilo O. The association between respiratory syncytial virus infection and the development of childhood asthma. *Pediatr. Infect. Dis. J.* 2007;26:733-9.

[107] Sigurs N, Gustaffson PM, Bjarnason R, Lundberg F, Schmidt S, Sigurbergsson F, et al. Severe respiratory syncytial virus bronchiolitis in infancy and asthma and allergy at age 13. *Am. J. Respir. Crit. Care Med.* 2005;171:137-41.

[108] Sigurs N, Aljassim F, Kjellman B, Robinson PD, Sigurbergsson F, Bjarnason R, et al. Asthma and allergy patterns over 18 years after severe RSV bronchiolitis in the first year of life. *Thorax* 2010;65:1045-52.

[109] Wu P, Dupont WD, Griffin MR, Carroll KN, Mitchel EF, Gebretsadik T, et al. Evidence of a causal role of winter virus infection during infancy in early childhood asthma. *Am. J. Respir. Crit. Care Med.* 2008;178:1123-9.

[110] Stein RT, Sherrill D, Morgan WJ, Holberg CJ, Halonen M, Taussig LM, et al. Respiratory syncytial virus in early life and risk of wheeze and allergy by age 13 years. *Lancet* 1999;354:541-5.

[111] Thomsen SF, van der Sluis S, Stensballe LG, Posthuma D, Skytthe A, Kyvik KO, et al. Exploring the association between severe respiratory syncytial virus infection and asthma: a registry-based twin study. *Am. J. Respir. Crit. Care Med.* 2009;179:1091-7.

[112] Piippo-Savolainen E, Korppi M. Wheezy babies-wheezy adults? Review on long-term outcome until adulthood after early childhood wheezing. *Acta Paediatr.* 2008;97:5-11.

[113] Turner SW, Young S, Landau LI, Le Souef PN. Reduced lung function both before bronchiolitis and at 11 years. *Arch. Dis. Child* 2002;87:417-20.

[114] Taussig LM, Wright AL, Holberg CJ, Halonen M, Morgan WJ, Martinez FD. Tucson children's respiratory study: 1980 to present. *J. Allergy Clin. Immunol.* 2003;111:661-75.

[115] Piippo-Savolainen E, Remes S, Kannisto S, Korhonen K, Korppi M. Asthma and lung function 20 years after wheezing in infancy: results from a prospective follow-up study. *Arch. Pediatr. Adolesc. Med.* 2004;158:1070-6.

[116] Kusel MM, de Klerk NH, Kebadze T, Vohma V, Holt PG, Johnston SL, et al. Early-life respiratory viral infections, atopic sensitization, and risk of subsequent development of persistent asthma. *J. Allergy Clin. Immunol.* 2007;119:1105-10.

[117] Mohapatra SS, Boyapalle S. Epidemiologic, experimental, and clinical links between respiratory syncytial virus infection and asthma. *Clin. Microbiol. Rev.* 2008;21:495-504.

[118] Respiratory syncytial virus. In: Pickering LK, Baker CJ, Long SS, McMillan JA, eds. Red Book: 2006 Report of the Committee on Infectious Diseases. 27th ed. *Elk Grove Village*, Ⅲ: American Academy of Pediatrics; 2006;560-6.

[119] Romero JR, Stewart DL, Buysman EK, Fernandes AW, Jafri HS, Mahadevia PJ. Serious early childhood wheezing after respiratory syncytial virus lower respiratory tract illness in preterm infants. *Clin. Ther.* 2010;32:2422-32.

[120] Kuikka L, Reijonen T, Remes K, Korppi M. Bronchial asthma after early childhood wheezing: a follow-up until 4.5-6 years of age. *Acta Paediatr.* 1994;83:744-8.

[121] Sigurs N, Bjarnason R, Sigurbergsson F, Kjellman B. Respiratory syncytial virus bronchiolitis in infancy is an important risk factor for asthma and allergy at age 7. *Am. J. Respir Crit. Care Med.* 2000;161:1501-7.

[122] Forsberg B, Pekkanen J, Clench-Aas J, Martensson MB, Stjemberg N, Bartonova P, et al. Childhood asthma in four regions in Scandinavia: risk factors and avoidance effects. *Int. J. Epidemiol.* 1997;26:610-9.

[123] Hyvarinen M, Piippo-Savolainen E, Korhonen K, Korppi M. Teenage asthma after severe infantile bronchiolitis or pneumonia. *Acta Paediatr* 2005;94:1378-83.

[124] Goksor E, Amark M, Alm B, Gustafsson PM, Wennergren G. Asthma symptoms in early childhood-what happens then? *Acta Paediatr* 2006;95:471-8.

[125] Matsuse H, Behera AK, Kumar M, Rabb H, Lockey RF, Mahapatra SS. Recurrent respiratory syncytial virus infections in allergen-sensitized mice lead to persistent airway inflammation and hyperresponsiveness. *J. Immunol.* 2000;164:6583-92.

[126] Garofalo RP, Hintz KH, Hill V, Ogra PL, Welliver RC. Production of interferon gamma in respiratory syncytial virus infection of humans is not associated with interleukins 12 and 18. *J. Med. Virol.* 2004;73:289-94.

[127] Thomas LH, Friedland JS, Sharland M, Becker S. Respiratory syncytial virus-induced RANTES production from human bronchial epithelial cells is dependent on nuclear

factor–kappa B nuclear binding and is inhibited by adenovirus-mediated expression of inhibitor of kappa B alpha. *J. Immunol.* 1998;161:1007-16.

[128] Ehlenfield DR, Cameron K, Welliver RC. Eosinophilia at the time of respiratory syncytial virus bronchiolitis predicts childhood reactive airway disease. *Pediatrics* 2000;105:79-83.

[129] Schwarze J, Hamelmann E, Bradley KL, Takeda K, Gelfand EW. Respiratory syncytial virus infection results in airway hyperresponsiveness and enhanced airway sensitization to allergen. *J. Clin. Invest* 1997;100:226-33.

[130] Stein RT. Long-term airway morbidity following viral LRTI in early infancy: recurrent wheezing or asthma? *Pediatr. Respir. Rev.* 2009;10(Suppl 1):29-31.

[131] Mitchell I. Treatment of RSV bronchiolitis: drugs, antibiotics. *Paediatr Respir. Rev.* 2006;10(Suppl 1) 14-15.

[132] Unger S, Cunningham S. Effect of oxygen supplementation on length of stay for infants hospitalized with acute viral bronchiolitis. *Pediatrics* 2008;121:470-5.

[133] Krilov LR. Respiratory syncytial virus disease: update on treatment and prevention. *Expert Rev. Anti Infect Ther.* 2011;9:27-32.

[134] Faber TE, Kimpen JL, Bont LJ. Respiratory syncytial virus bronchiolitis: prevention and treatment. *Expert Opin. Pharmacother* 2008;9:2451-8.

[135] Guerguerian AM, Gauthier M, Label MH, Farrell CA, Lacroix J. Ribavirin in ventilated respiratory syncytial virus bronchiolitis. A randomized, placebo-controlled trial. *Am. J. Respir. Crit. Care Med.* 1999;160:829-34.

[136] American Academy of Pediatrics, Committee on Infectious Diseases. Reassessment of indications for ribavirin therapy in respiratory syncytial virus infections. *Pediatrics* 1996;97:137-40.

[137] Hammer J, Numa A, Newth CJ. Albuterol responsiveness in infants with respiratory failure caused by respiratory syncytial virus infection. *J. Pediatr.* 1995;127:485-90.

[138] Gadomski AM, Bhasale AL. Bronchodialtors for bronchiolitis. *Cochrane Database Syst. Rev.* 2006;3:CD001266.

[139] Wainwright C, Altamirano L, Cheney J, Barber S, Price D, Moloney S, et al. A multicenter, randomized, double-blind, controlled trial of nebulized epinephrine in infants with acute bronchiolitis. *N. Engl. J. Med.* 2003;349:27-35.

[140] Openshaw PJ. Antiviral immune responses and lung inflammation after respiratory syncytial virus infection. *Proc. Am. Thorac. Soc.* 2005;2:121-5.

[141] Tripp RA, Oshansky C, Alvarez R. Cytokines and respiratory syncytial virus infection. *Proc. Am. Thorac. Soc.* 2005;2:147-9.

[142] Garrison MM, Christakis DA, Harvey E, Cummings P, Davis RL. Systemic corticosteroids in infant bronchiolitis: A meta-analysis. *Pediatrics* 2000;105:E44

[143] Patel H, Platt R, Lozano JM, Wang EE. Glucocorticoids for acute viral bronchiolitis in infants and young children. *Cochrane Database Syst. Rev.* 2004;3:CD004878.

[144] Blom D, Ermers M, Bont L, van Aalderen WM, van Woensel JB. Inhaled corticosteroids during acute bronchiolitis in the prevention of post-bronchiolitis wheezing. *Cochrane Database Syst. Rev.* 2007;1:CD004881.

[145] Behrendt CE, Decker MD, Burch DJ, Watson PH. International variation in the management of infants hospitalized with respiratory syncytial virus. International RSV Study Group. *Eur. J. Pediatr.* 1998;157:215-20.

[146] Ichiyama T, Nishikawa M, Yoshitomi T, Hasegawa S, Matsubara T, Hayashi T, et al. Clarithromycin inhibits NF-kappaB activation in human peripheral blood mononuclear cells and pulmonary epithelial cells. *Antimicrob. Agents Chemother.* 2001;45:44-7.

[147] Tahan F, Ozcan A, Koc N. Clarithromycin in the treatment of RSV bronchiolitis: a double-blind, randomised, placebo-controlled trial. *Eur. Respir. J.* 2007;29:91-7.

[148] Thornburn K, Harigopal S, Reddy V, Taylor N, van Saene HK. High incidence of pulmonary bacterial co-infection in children with severe respiratory syncytial virus (RSV) bronchiolitis. *Thorax* 2006;61:611-5.

[149] Kneyber MC, van Woensel JB, Uijtendaal E, Uiterwaal CS, Kimpen JL: Dutch Antibiotics in RSV Trial (DART) Research Group. Azithromycin does not improve disease course in hospitalized infants with respiratory syncytial virus (RSV) lower respiratory tract disease: a randomized equivalence trial. *Pediatr. Pulmonol.* 2008;43:142-9.

[150] Spurling GK, Doust J, Del Mar CB, Ericksson L. Antibiotics for bronchiolitis in children. *Cochrane Database Syst. Rev.* 2011;6:CD005189.

[151] Ventre K, Haroon M, Davison C. Surfactant therapy for bronchiolitis in critically ill infants. *Cochrane Database Syst. Rev.* 2006;3:CD005150.

[152] Greenough A. Role of ventilation in RSV disease: CPAP, ventilation, HFO, ECMO. *Pediatr. Respir. Rev.* 2009;10(Suppl 1):26-8.

[153] Hu J, Robinson JL. Treatment of respiratory syncytial virus with palivizumab: a systematic review. World J Pediatr 2010;6:296-300.

[154] American Academy of Pediatrics. Subcommittee on Diagnosis and Management of Bronchiolitis. Diagnosis and management of bronchiolitis. *Pediatrics* 2006;118:1774-93.

[155] Schickli JH, Dubovsky F, Tang RS. Challenges in developing a pediatric RSV vaccine. *Human vaccines* 2009;5:582-91.

[156] Prince GA, Jenson AB, Hemming VG, Murphy BR, Walsh EE, Horswood RL, et al. Enhancement of respiratory syncytial virus pulmonary pathology in cotton rats by prior intramuscular inoculation of formalin-inactivated virus. *J. Virol.* 1986;57:721-8.

[157] Meissner HC, Fulton DR, Groothuis JR, Geggel RL, Marx GR, Hemming VG, et al. Controlled trial to evaluate protection of high-risk infants against respiratory syncytial virus disease by using standard intravenous immune globulin. *Antimicrob. Agents Chemother* 1993;37:1655-8.

[158] American Academy of Pediatrics, Committee on Infectious Diseases and Committee on Fetus and Newborn. Respiratory syncytial virus immune globulin intravenous: Indications for use. *Pediatrics* 1997;99:645-50.

[159] Fuller H, Del Mar C. Immunoglobulin treatment for respiratory syncytial virus infection. *Cochrane Database Syst. Rev.* 2006;18:CD004883.

[160] American Academy of Pediatrics. Respiratory syncytial virus. In: Red Book; 2006 Report of the Committee on Infectious Diseases. 27th edition. Pickering LK, Baker CJ, Long SS, McMillan JA, eds. *American Academy of pediatrics.* Elk Grove Village, IL, USA, 2006;560-6.

[161] American Academy of Pediatrics. Respiratory syncytial virus. In: Red Book; 2009 Report of the Committee on Infectious Diseases. 28th edition. Pickering LK, Baker CJ, Kimberlin DW, Long SS, eds. American Academy of Pediatrics. *Elk Grove Village*, IL, USA, 2009;560-9.

[162] Fitzgerald DA. Preventing RSV bronchiolitis in vulnerable infants: The role of palivizumab. *Pediatr. Respir Rev.* 2009;10:143-7.

[163] Nair H, Verma VR, Theodoratou E, Zgaga L, Huda T, Simoes EA, et al. An evaluation of the emerging interventions against respiratory syncytial virus (RSV)-associated acute lower respiratory infections in children. *BMC Publlic Health* 2011;11(Suppl 3):S30.

[164] Wu H, Pfarr DS, Tang Y, An LL, Patel NK, Watkins JD, et al. Ultra-potent antibodies against respiratory syncytial virus: effects of binding kinetics and binding valence on viral neutralization. *J. Mol. Biol.* 2005;350:126-44.

[165] Carbonell-Estrany X, Simões EA, Dagan R, Hall CB, Harris B, Hultquist M, et al. Motavizumab for prophylaxis of respiratory syncytial virus in high-risk children: A noninferiority trial. *Peidatrics* 2010;125:e35.

[166] Welliver RC. Pharmacotherapy of respiratory syncytial virus infection. *Curr. Opin. Pharmacol.* 2010;10:289-93.

[167] Kim CK, Koh JY, Han TH, Kim DK, Kim BI, Koh YY. Increased levels of BAL cystcinyl leukotrienes in acute RSV bronchiolitis. *Acta Paediatr.* 2006;95:479-85.

[168] Han J, Jia Y, Takeda K, Shiraishi Y, Okamoto M, Dakhama A, et al. Montelukast during primary infection prevents airway hyperresponsiveness and inflammation after reinfection with respiratory syncytial virus. *Am. J. Respir. Crit. Care Med.* 2010;182:455-63.

[169] Kim CK, Choi J, Kim HB, Callaway Z, Shin BM, Kim JT, et al. A randomized intervention of montelukast for post-bronchiolitis: Effect on eosinophil degranulation. *J. Pediatr.* 2010;156:749-54.

In: Respiratory Syncytial Virus ISBN 978-1-62100-835-4
Editors: Haneul Nam and Gippeum Kun, pp. 123-147

Chapter 3

RESPIRATORY SYNCYTIAL VIRUS INFECTION: PREVENTION, DIAGNOSIS, AND TREATMENT

Beatriz Gómez**[*]**

Facultad de Medicina, Universidad Nacional Autónoma de México,
Ciudad Universitaria, México D.F., México

ABSTRACT

Estimates from the World Health Organization indicate that, worldwide, respiratory syncytial virus (RSV) is responsible for 64 million infections and 160,000 deaths per annum. Both short- and long-term morbidity and mortality are particularly significant for infants. RSV accounts for more than 60% of acute lung respiratory tract infection in children and more than 80%, in infants less than a year of age. RSV is recognized as a significant cause of disease in the elderly population, with an average incidence of 5.5%, about twice that of influenza. Outbreaks occur yearly during the winter season and the infection recurs naturally throughout life.

One diagnostic challenge is that respiratory infections, which can be caused by several viral pathogens in addition to RSV, usually present with signs and symptoms that are nearly indistinguishable by clinical diagnosis. The rapid and accurate detection of RSV provides pathogen-specific diagnosis, allows implementation of appropriate measures to control infection, and improves the management of patients.

Current treatment strategies (*e.g.*, ribavirin) for these patients are limited, but several new drug interventions (*e.g.*, MBX300, RSV604, ALN-RSV01) are under investigation. Several other preventive agents and strategies have been developed (*e.g.*, RSV-IGIV, palivizumab) others are in the pipeline (*e.g.*, motavizumab) or are under development. Although RSV was discovered 40 years ago and despite the importance of RSV as a pathogen, there are as yet no safe and effective vaccines. This is due to a number of factors that complicate the development of such a vaccine, with the basic difficulty being that natural infection imparts only transient and partial immunity to re-infection. At present, prophylaxis with passive antibody therapy is the only specific treatment; thus, patient care remains largely supportive.

[*] Email: begomez@unam.mx

However, there are good reasons to think that the scene may soon change. As the pace of development of antiviral drugs and vaccines accelerates, novel therapies are set to make a major impact in the management of this very common infection. Although their use and effect are difficult to anticipate, such interventions could ultimately lead to the interruption of transmission of RSV, thereby resulting in profound changes in the impact of RSV on human health. Thus, it is possible that, in the foreseeable future, such therapeutic tools may have a major impact not only on the management of this infection, but also on prevention of the disease.

In this chapter, we review the clinical condition of individuals infected with RSV, with a focus on the populations at highest risk and the squeal to the infection. In addition, we review the prevention and treatment strategies that were used in the past and those currently in use for these high-risk patients, as well as possible future strategies for the development of vaccines and antiviral drugs. This review should provide a single, valuable source of information to clinicians and to investigators.

1. Introduction

1.1. Virus: Characteristics, Genomic Organization, and Proteins

Respiratory syncytial virus (RSV) is an enveloped, non-segmented, single-stranded, negative-sense RNA virus of order Mononegavirales, family Paramyxoviridae, subfamily Pneumovirinae. The virions are pleomorphic, consisting of a nucleocapsid contained within a bilayer formed from the host-cell plasma membrane (1). RSV particles enter host cells by membrane fusion with the target cells, a process that is mediated by the viral fusion (F) protein. Fusion of infected cells with their neighbors produces multinucleated cells (synycytia) (2, 3). Gene expression and genome replication take place in the cytoplasm; progeny virions bud through the plasma membrane into the surrounding milieu (4, 5).

The nucleocapsid contains the RNA genome (15,222 nucleotides) consisting of ten genes that encode 11 proteins (*vide infra*), of which eight are structural and two are not packed in the virion. The ten viral genes (*N1*, *N2*, *N*, *P*, *M*, *SH*, *G*, *F*, *M2*, and *L*) are arranged sequentially and each is flanked with conserved gene start and gene end transcription signals. Viral proteins are synthesized by an RSV-specific, RNA-dependent, RNA-polymerase complex that is composed of viral components—genomic RNA and the L, N, P, and M2–1 proteins (5); RNA polymerase attaches to the only promoter at the 3′ leader end; mRNA is synthesized in a polar gradient (4-6).

Individual gene is transcribed into a separate, capped, polyadenylated mRNA that encodes a single viral protein, with the exception of the M2 mRNA, which contains two overlapping, open-reading frames that, by means of a ribosomal stop-restart mechanism, are expressed as two distinct proteins, M2-1 and M2-2, which are factors involved in transcription and in modulating the balance between transcription and RNA replication, respectively. In the genome, the leader (Le) sequence at the 3′ end and the trailer (Tr) sequence at the 5′ end are important for the initiation of transcription and replication, respectively (4, 5, 7).

RNA replication involves the synthesis of the full-length, positive-sense intermediate, and the antigenome, which is copied into progeny genomes. As they are synthesized, the

RNAs of both the antigenome and genome become encapsidated with nucleocapsid (N) protein. The N protein encapsidates the genomic RNA as its positive-sense antigenome. The large (L) protein is the major polymerase subunit and contains the catalytic domains. The phosphoprotein (P) is an essential cofactor in RNA synthesis; it is thought to associate with free N and L proteins. The two non-structural viral products (NS1 and NS2) accumulate in infected cells, but are present in only trace amounts in mature virions (6). NS1 and NS2 antagonize the interferon (IFN) response (8, 9).

Four viral proteins are associated with the lipid bilayer: the matrix (M) protein, which lines the inner-envelope surface, is required for viral assembly (5); the heavily glycosylated (G), fusion (F), and small hydrophobic (SH) proteins are transmembrane, surface glycoproteins. The SH protein is not required for viral replication or syncytia formation. G and F proteins play an important role in infectivity and pathogenesis, as they are the only neutralizing and the major protecting virus antigen (5, 10, 11). The G protein is responsible for attachment of virus particles to the host cell (12, 13), but the F protein can also provide this function The genome RNA is encapsidated by the nucleocapsid protein (N) which, together with the P and L proteins form the RNA replication unit (5) nucleocapsid.

1.2. Clinical Manifestations: Infection, Recurrent Infections, Chronic Sequelae, and Risk Factors for Severe Disease

Clinical Manifestations. Infection. RSV is a prevalent and highly infectious virus, more so than any other respiratory virus. Worldwide, it is a very important pathogen, causing acute upper- and lower-respiratory-tract infections (URT and LRT), respectively, especially in infants and young children (14-20). It is considered to be the most frequent cause of pneumonia and bronchiolitis, which bronchiolitis is the single most common cause for the hospitalization of infants (20-23). Recently estimates made by the World Health Organization (WHO) indicate that worldwide, RSV causes 64 million cases of morbidity and 160,000 deaths each year and accounts for more than 60% of acute LRTI in children and more than 80%, in infants (5, 14). In the United States of America (USA), RSV infection accounts for 23.0–39.5% of the hospitalizations of children for any respiratory-tract illness and results in 120,000 childhood hospitalizations and up to 500 deaths annually (15, 24, 27). For children younger than one year of age, RSV is responsible for 19-fold more deaths than is influenza (15, 24-28).

RSV is also an important cause of morbidity and mortality in the elderly and the immunocompromised (29-31). In the elderly, is the second leading cause of viral death, with a reported 5.5% annual incidence; in high-risk adult population, the incidence rises to 10%. In the wintertime, RSV accounts for up to 25% of the mortality attributed to influenza (29). In elderly persons, RSV causes pneumonia and exacerbations of chronic obstructive pulmonary disease (COPD) (31), thus contributing substantially to the number of deaths in the elderly population during the winter season (32). In the USA, there are an estimated 14,000–60,000 RSV-related hospitalizations and 1,500–7,000 deaths in people >65 years due to RSV infection each year (15, 24, 28, 33).

Infection by virus starts in the nose and/or the eyes by the introduction of viral particles in an aerosol or by direct contact with fluids containing the virus (34, 35). Once the virus has penetrated the cells of the epithelium, replication of the virus takes place in the nasopharynx;

the incubation period is 4–5 days, although in some cases it is longer (36, 37). Normally, infection is confined to the superficial cells of the respiratory epithelium and is restricted to the respiratory epithelium (14, 34). Virus can be spread to the lower respiratory tract (LRT), probably through aspiration of secretions, although the possibility of transmission by cell-to-cell fusion cannot be discarded (38). The inflammatory response associated with this infection is extremely complex (39) and involves the release of multiple cytokines and chemokines from epithelium cells and from infiltrating immunocytes, local neuro-immune interactions, and mast-cell degranulation with variable release of leukotrines (40-43).

In adults, symptoms of viral infection usually manifest as rhinorrhea, cough, and low-grade fever; however, in premature infants, the elderly, and imunosuppressed patients, bronchiolitis and pneumonia are frequent (14, 29, 44), in older children, RSV is likely to be a contributor to otitis media (45). Clinical signs of bronchiolitis include increased airway resistance, air trapping, and wheezing (21, 46-48).

The pathologies caused by human RSV include bronchitis, bronchiolar epithelial necrosis, bronchiolar occlusion, parenchyma inflammation, and alveolar exudation (49). Disease caused by RSV is especially severe in children between 1–3 months old, even though maternal antibodies are usually present (50).

Recurrent infections. RSV is a respiratory pathogen that has the ability to re-infect symptomatically throughout the lifespan, even within a short interval after the previous infection (11, 51, 52); re-infection is not related to different virus serotypes (53, 54). Children who suffer from severe RSV infections in infancy are prone to recurrent episodes of wheezing and asthma in later childhood (43, 55-58), prevention of RSV infection in the first year of life may possibly reduce the frequency of post-viral wheezing in later life.

RSV presents a single serotype with two antigenic subgroups (59). Virus antigenic dimorphism was established with monoclonal antibodies which identified extensive differences in the G protein and few in protein F (60-62) RSV strains vary genetically and antigenically and have been classified into two broad groups, A and B with additional variability detected within the groups, A virus are more virulent than subgroup B and replicate to higher titers in the respiratory tract (5, 63).

Re-infection can occur during the same RSV season and across all age groups. Moreover, re-infection can occur even in the presence of high serum antibody titers, although the course of the disease is attenuated. Re-infection is favored by exposure to a heavy virus load (48, 63).

Re-Infections may occur by repeated exposure to the same viral isolate, so that antigenic variation is not strictly required for re-infections to occur (11, 27, 47, 51, 64).

Immunity to RSV, which is induced by natural infection, is permanent but not protective (5). The first two episodes of infection typically occur during the first two years of life, and these episodes tend to be the most severe (65). Most subsequent infections run a milder course, frequently being localized in the upper respiratory tract (URT): however, the illness can progress to an LRTI having more severe symptoms (47, 52).

Antigenic variability may contribute to the capacity of the virus to establish re-infections and may pose a challenge to the design of a vaccine (5) . The most extensive genetic and antigenic diversity is found in the attachment glycoprotein G, restriction fragment analysis of the cDNA of G protein revealed 12 restriction patterns for group A and seven for group B (59, 62). During individual epidemic periods, viruses of both antigenic groups may co-circulate, although the viruses of one group may predominate (66). When there are epidemics in which the same group predominates in consecutive years, the dominant viruses are genetically different from year to year (5). It remains unclear to what extent frequent re-infection by RSV reflects inadequate or inappropriate responses by the host (67).

Chronic Sequelae. The link between RSV infection and the development of sequelae (wheezing, asthma, or apnea) has long been a matter of debate (68). The association between RSV infection and subsequent wheezing is sustained by epidemiological studies and is reinforced by reports that documented that more than 50% of infants who had severe RSV infection in early life presented subsequent episodes of wheezing, which in some cases persisted until 11 years of age or older (56, 57, 69). RSV bronquiolitis in infancy has been reported to be an important risk factor for subsequent asthma and allergy (57, 69). It is possible that wheezing and asthma could be explained either by pre-existing genetic susceptibility factors that contribute to the risk of RSV bronchiolitis and the subsequent wheezing episodes (49); by the RSV infection causing an alteration of the airway structure and/or inducing an aberrant immune response, by the persistence of RSV in the host cells (68-70).

Apnea is a well-known complication of RSV infection in infants; on occasion, the apnea may be so severe as to cause death (71). As early as 1956, the virus was isolated in infants under six months of age, who had required hospitalization for RSV infection (72). The highest incidence of apnea occurs in premature infants and in infants less than one month of age. In most cases, however, apnea is self-limited and does not recur in subsequent RSV infections. An interesting observation is that apnea is frequently the first clinical manifestation of RSV infection and may occur regardless of the severity of other RSV-related symptoms (73).

Risk. The risk of severe RSV disease is increased by factors related to the ability of the host to control and withstand a respiratory tract infection. Significant risk factors are young age (<6 months), premature birth (≤35 weeks of gestation), bronchopulmonary dysplasia, congenital heart disease, immunodeficiency or immunosuppression, male gender, exposure to smoking, crowded day care, the first or second RSV infection in life, unusually narrow airways, low birth weight (5, 44, 48), a low titer of RSV-specific serum antibodies, and old age (44).

Environmental factors such as the ones that affect lung function (*e.g.*, household tobacco use) or that increase exposure to infection (*e.g.*, day care, multiple siblings, hospitalization) have been reported as playing an important role (33, 74). The participation of a genetic predisposition in severe RSV disease has been observed 1) through association of susceptibility with a family history of asthma or severe infant LRT disease and 2) through differences in susceptibility between ethnic, racial, and gender groups (65, 75). Recent studies have shown an association between an increased incidence of severe pediatric RSV disease and genetic polymorphisms in genes that code for cytokines and chemokines (76). It should be noted that these studies are preliminary and are at times inconsistent.

There is also evidence that RSV may cause persistent infection. Persistence of RSV has been demonstrated in guinea pigs (77) in cows, (78), and mice (79). The year-round persistence of RSV in patients with COPD has been detected and is associated with airway inflammation and accelerated decline in forced expiratory volume (FEV1) (31, 80).

1.3. Epidemiology: Geographic and age Distribution, Seasonality, and Transmission

Geographic Distribution and Seasonality. LRTI caused by RSV occurs epidemically, and the appearance of epidemics seems to vary with latitude, altitude, and climate, with the epidemic pattern tending to appear in clusters. The season in which RSV epidemics occur depends on geographic location and altitude. Though it varies from one continent to another, outbreaks usually begin in costal areas. Seasonal RSV outbreaks occur each year throughout the world; however, the peak and duration of the seasonal outbreak vary from one year to the next. Outbreaks occur during the winter months: in the northern hemisphere, the annual epidemics normally start in November, peak in January and February, and end in May; in the southern hemisphere, the epidemic season run from May through September. In the tropics, epidemics peak during the rainy season (5, 48).

Age distribution. By the age of two, almost all children have been infected with RSV and a high percentage (80%) have experienced at least two infections (5, 14, 21, 46), with most of the children suffering only mild symptoms, such as rhinorrhea, cough, fever, and sometimes wheezing, the infection generally resolving in less than two weeks (47, 53). However, 25–40% of these children develop lower respiratory signs indicative of viral bronchiolitis or pneumonia (15, 51, 72).

Transmission. RSV transmission is principally done by direct contact with respiratory secretions with the subsequent inoculation of nasopharyngeal or conjunctiva mucus membranes, or by entry of large respiratory droplets into the nose or eyes (34). The stability of RSV in aerosol particles is related to humidity and temperature: the virus is stable in >90% humidity and at 4°C, and remains viable on hard surfaces for up to six hours, on rubber gloves for 90 minutes, and on skin for 20 minutes (14).

The prolonged survival of RSV highlights the need for the washing of hands and for taking precautions when in contact with others in order to limit the spread of RSV (14, 81). The incubation period ranges from 2–8 days; on average, the period in which individuals shed virus is limited to about eight days (63, 75). Rarely, immunocompetent individuals can shed for up to three weeks; however, in immunocompromised individuals, viral shedding is prolonged significantly and can continue for several months (5, 44).

RSV is an important cause of nosocomial infections, which appears to be spread by contact or by aerosols (82). Hospital staff appears to play a major role in viral spread and have infection rates of 25–50% during RSV epidemics. The probability that an infant or child will acquire the infection in a hospital ward increases with the duration of stay and the number of patients in the room (21, 83).

1.4 Section Summary

RSV is a negative, single-stranded RNA virus of the Paramyxoviridae family. Its genome includes ten genes and code for 11 proteins, three of which, F, G and SH, are transmembrane glycoproteins. G protein mediates RSV attachment to the host cell and the F protein promotes the entry of the virus into the host cell through fusion of viral and host membranes. F and G proteins are the most important antigens of RSV. Through antigen-neutralization assays, two RSV groups, A and B, were differentiated; within these groups, there is further variability.

Both antigenic variants are usually present during seasonal outbreaks, although the one that prevails may vary from year to year.

Prevalent around the world, RSV is the most important cause of LRTI in infants and young children. The WHO estimates that, worldwide, RSV accounts for 64 million infections and 160,000 deaths per annum, and for more than 60% of acute LRTI in children 80% in infants less than a year of age. Moreover, RSV is an important cause of disease in the elderly population, with an average incidence about twice that of influenza. Almost all children have been infected with RSV at least once by the time they are two years of age, resulting in approximately 24 hospitalizations per 1,000 infants and up to one million deaths worldwide each year.

RSV clinical disease varies from rhinitis and otitis media to bronchiolitis and pneumonia, which are associated with considerable morbidity and mortality. Because prior infection does not confer persistent protective immunity, re-infections are common throughout life, although the severity decreases. Factors that favor respiratory tract infections increase the risk of severe RSV disease. Transmission occurs through inoculation of the nasopharyngeal or conjunctiva mucosa with respiratory secretions from infected individuals. Viral shedding persists for approximately one week, but can be significantly prolonged in immunocompromised individuals.

2. Prevention

2.1. Active Immunization: Vaccine

Despite the importance of RSV as a pathogen and the more than 50 years of RSV research, the immunopathologic features and the incomplete immunity associated with RSV disease in infants remain difficulties for the development of effective vaccines and treatments. To date, there is no licensed vaccine for prophylaxis of RSV infection. This is due to a number of factors that complicate the development of an effective and safe vaccine (84-86).

First, because the most serious RSV disease occurs between 2–7 months of age, vaccination should be done the first few weeks after birth; however, the presence of maternal antibodies might interfere immune responses due to the administered vaccines, especially in the first few weeks of life (87). Full-term infants acquire maternal antibodies during the latter half of gestation and antibody levels remain relatively high for six months post partum. This would coincide with the time when an RSV vaccine would be administered. Therefore, an ideal RSV vaccine would need to stimulate a protective immune response in the infant, even though maternal antibodies are present (85, 87, 88).

Second. Although RSV infections induce both B-cell (antibody) and T-cell responses, these immune responses to natural infection do not prevent frequent re-infections, whether by the identical or closely related RSV. Re-infections occur in all age groups. This inability to prevent infection may be the consequence of a highly prevalent or contagious virus. Other possible explanations are that the initial RSV infection permanently alters the characteristics of adaptive immune effectors (or memory), or that RSV persists in the host a possibility that cannot be discarded (5) .

Finally, unintended consequences can result. An example is the experience of enhanced disease that resulted after vaccination with a formalin-inactivated vaccine. In the 1960s, a study was carried out to evaluate a formalin-inactivated RSV vaccine mixed with alum adjuvant (FI-RSV) that was administered to children by intramuscular injection. During the next winter season, 80% of the vaccinated children required hospitalization and some died, whereas in the control group, only 2.5% of the children were hospitalized. The clinical disease in vaccinated infants was indistinguishable from typical RSV (89, 90). The FI-RSV resulted in a predisposition for exacerbated pulmonary disease in infants, which was attributed to an imbalance in the Th1/Th2 immune response, although the exact cause has not been elucidated (90-93). Such untoward results make it difficult to proceed with vaccine testing in infants. It is likely that an effective and safe vaccine needs to elicit a balanced immune response, including RSV-specific neutralizing antibodies, CD8 T-cells, Th1/Th2 CD4 T-cells, and preferably secretory IgA (87, 91).

Various strategies have been employed to develop a safe and effective RSV vaccine (84). One of the major current approaches to developing such a vaccine is through the use of live-attenuated RSV strains for intranasal administration. This strategy accomplishes several goals: it induces local mucosal and systemic immunity; the intranasal route partially escapes the interference effects of maternal serum antibodies; compared with inactivated vaccines, live attenuated intranasal vaccines are more immunogenic and provide broader protection; and live, attenuated vaccines are not associated with enhanced disease (91, 94, 95). It is unlikely that a single vaccination will impart complete protection against RSV disease, as evidenced by natural re-infection occurring throughout life (5, 52, 96).

Several candidates for live-attenuated RSV vaccine have been developed by conventional cold passage and/or chemical mutagenesis and have been evaluated in a clinical setting. Second generation live-attenuated RSV also has been generated by reverse genetics and tested in RSV-naïve, 1–2 month-old infants (97). Results from that study showed that protective immunity could be achieved in a majority of the recipients. However, for this live-attenuated RSV approach, it is quite challenging to determine whether or not the balance between over attenuation and under attenuation is most appropriate for a safe and effective vaccine (98).

2.2. Passive Immunization: Antibodies, Human Immunoglobulin and Humanized Monoclonal Antibodies

Because antibodies interfere with pathogen binding and facilitate the opsonization, neutralization, and clearance of viruses, they are attractive therapeutic agents. Currently, only two antibodies have been approved for the treatment of RSV. A polyclonal antibody, human immunoglobulin, a hyper-immune polyclonal globulin (99), and a humanized monoclonal antibody, palivizumab (64, 100-102).

Human Immunoglobulin. Respiratory syncytial virus immunoglobulin intravenous (RSV-IVIG) is a pooled, polyclonal human immunoglobulin that has been purified from donors with high-RSV-neutralizing antibody titers, which is meant to be administered by monthly intravenous infusion during the RSV season. A significant decrease in RSV-related hospitalizations was seen when RSV-IVIG was administered to high-risk infants who were premature or who had chronic lung disease. RSV-IVIG has drawbacks in that it can interfere with the immune response to live virus vaccines and it requires delaying of immunization with the measles/mumps/rubella (MMR). The major disadvantages of RSV-IVIG are the following: 1) the need for repeated venous access and a long intravenous infusion (4–6 h), with the consequent need of medical supervision in a hospital setting; 2) the recommended dose of 15 ml/ kg presents a significant risk of fluid overload to sensitive infants, thus necessitating frequent diuretic therapy; and the combined costs of acquisition and of supervised administration of the immunoglobulin are high (99, 103).

Monoclonal Antibodies. There are several advantages to the use of monoclonal antibodies: they are less likely to exert an immunosuppressive effect in children; they carry essentially no risk of transmitting blood-borne infections or other plasma-associated adverse effects; they contain higher titers of neutralizing antibody, and therefore can be prepared in smaller volumes suitable for intramuscular administration in either outpatient or home setting; and they obviate the risk of fluid overload and need for diuretic rescue.

Monoclonal anti-RSV antibodies target a single viral epitope. Palivizumab is a humanized, monoclonal IgG1 antibody produced by recombinant DNA technology (64, 101). The only mAb approved by the United States Food and Drug Administration (FDA) for RSV, palivizumab targets the highly conserved F glycoprotein of RSV, thereby inhibiting viral entry into host cells (27, 101). Because palivizumab has not been demonstrated to provide a clinical benefit for the treatment of RSV disease, it is indicated only for use in RSV prevention (104). The most commonly reported adverse events are URTI, otitis media, fever, rhinitis, rash, diarrhea, cough, vomiting, gastroenteritis, and wheezing. Severe hypersensitivity can occur, but the incidence is rare, with less than one case of anaphylaxis per 100,000 patients (101, 103, 104). Motavizumab (MEDI-524) is a second-generation, humanized IgG1 monoclonal antibody, developed from palivizumab, with ~70-fold higher affinity for the RSV F glycoprotein and 20-fold greater neutralizing capacity however, it has not as yet been approved by FDA (105).

2.3. Pharmacological Agents: Nucleoside Analogues and Pharmacological Drugs

Nucleoside Analogue. Antiviral therapy for RSV is limited. Ribavirin, a synthetic nucleoside analog with broad virustatic activity *in vitro*, is the only licensed antiviral approved for treatment of severe RSV disease (106). Ribavirin has broad antiviral activity and inhibits viral multiplication by several mechanisms, *i.e.*, inhibition of viral polymerase (107). However, its clinical benefits are small and occur only in a fraction of RSV-infected patients; thus, its use is now limited mainly to immune severe RSV patients (108). Ribavirin has been administered by aerosol to infants with severe RSV bronchiolitis and to RSV-infected, immunocompromised patients; however, it showed little efficacy (46, 108-111).

Although ribavirin effectively inhibits RSV replication in vitro (107), its lack of efficacy in vivo is not surprising because the first clinical symptoms usually appear towards the end of the exponential viral replication in the lungs, which is followed by rapid decline of virus titers (5). Thus, by the time the classical signs of bronchiolitis are diagnosed, little virus remains in the lungs, while the immune inflammatory response of the host dominates the pathophysiology. Hence, the therapeutic use of a virustatic agent like ribavirin requires immediate intervention at clinical onset, which is, logistically, nearly impossible to achieve (112-114).

Pharmacological Agents. Two different approaches are used to design antiviral drugs: to interfere with the life cycle of the virus or to target the host response to RSV infection. The latter approach is in the early stage of investigation.

Six different drugs are currently in pre-clinical and clinical trials; their targets are RSV proteins G, F, N, or L. These drug candidates and their mechanisms are the following: 1) MBX300 inhibits viral attachment by acting against G protein (115); 2) VP-14637 interferes with F protein activity, thereby inhibiting fusion with, and entry into, the host by the virion; (116) 3) ALN-RSV01 and RSV604 work against the N protein, through siRNA or protein inhibitor, respectively (117) 4) YM53403 and AUG-2PPMO derivatives of Benzappein and peptide conjugate phosphorodiamidate morpholino oligomers (PMO), respectively, are inhibitors of L protein (118).

Attachment inhibitor. MBX-300 (Microbiotix) targets the RSV attachment (G) protein; it has been in development for the oral treatment of RSV infection. Given either before or several hours after infection, it reduces the number of replicating virus, suggesting that the antiviral effect is achieved by inhibition of the protein. Phase I trials showed that the drug was well absorbed in humans and that a single daily dose was sufficient to achieve efficacious antiviral levels (107, 115, 119). Clinical trials are underway (120).

Fusion inhibitors. RSV infects target cells by fusing the lipid viral membrane with the lipid membrane of the host, thus inhibition of this process reduces viral load and syncytia formation (5). During membrane fusion, F protein undergoes a conformational change that exposes hydrophobic epitopes (116, 121). Several compounds have been developed which bind to these epitopes (122), but these attempts frequently have failed. To date, VP-14637 (ViroPharma) N is the only candidate for licensing. VP-14637 is a small molecule that inhibits RSV entry into host cells and can be delivered directly to the infection site. The technology is suited for use in infants and was under development by ViroPharma. The drug, which interacts directly with the F protein, was tested in an inhaled formulation in Phase I trials to evaluate the safety and pharmacokinetic profile (123).

Short Interfering RNAs. RNA interference (RNAi) is a natural process that occurs in the cytoplasm and leads to degradation of mRNA. Inside a cell, viral RNA can be targeted by small interfering RNAs (siRNAs) that are synthesized to target any endogenous mRNA sequence in a cell or an exogenous sequence carried by a virus. The antisense strand of the siRNA binds in a sequence-specific manner to existing mRNAs in the cytoplasm, which leads to cleavage and subsequent release of the inactivated fragments of the complementary mRNA. This process interrupts the synthesis of the corresponding protein (124)

N protein inhibitors. ALN-RSV01 (Alnylam Pharmaceuticals) inhibits the replication of RSV by interrupting the synthesis of the viral N protein. In mice, ALN-RSV01 (2 mg/kg, single dose) can protect against RSV infection, and the results of placebo-controlled, healthy-volunteer studies have demonstrated that the drug is active after nasal delivery (125, 126). Phase II trials with an inhaled formulation are continuing (120).

RSV-604 is an oral benzodiazepine under development by Arrow Therapeutics (Novartis) that targets the N protein. Like that for YM-53403 (Yamanouchi Pharmceutical), its probable mechanism of anti-RSV activity is inhibition of viral RNA polymerase. It has a broad activity spectrum against many clinical isolates of RSV antigenic subgroups A and B. In contrast to most fusion inhibitors, RSV604 was shown to be active when administered after infection

(117). Phase I trials showed that the drug was well absorbed in humans, and that a single daily dose was sufficient to achieve antiviral levels. Clinical trials are continuing (120).

L protein inhibitors. YM-53403 (Yamanouchi Pharmaceutical) is a novel compound that targets the L protein. Its activity against both subgroups A and B has been demonstrated, presumably YM-53403 acts by interfering with RNA synthesis; it has a higher potency than ribavirin (118). Preclinical studies are ongoing for YM-53403 and AUG-2 PPMO (Avi Bio Pharma (120).

Morpholino oligomers are synthetic molecules consisting of approximately 25 nucleic acid bases chosen to bind to and block specific RNA molecules, thus preventing transcription of gene products. Two antisense PMOs targeting the sequence of RSV L protein mRNA has been tested for anti-RSV activity in cells and in mice. In infected cells in tissue culture, these PMOs reduced viral titers by >100-fold, with minimal toxicity. Intranasal administration of PMOs to BALB/c mice before RSV inoculation reduced viral titers by 1.2 $\log_{10}$ on Day 5 after infection, and attenuated pulmonary inflammation at Day 7 (127).

2.4 Section Summary

Despite the importance of RSV to health, there is as yet no licensed vaccine. This situation is due to different factors, in that viral immunity is partially protective; newborn infants are the primary targeted population, yet the presence of maternal antibodies might interfere with the vaccine and the experience with a vaccine in the 1960s, in which pulmonary disease, probably due to unbalanced Th2 immune response, resulted. Of the various candidates for a vaccine, the live-attenuated vaccine presents advantages, in that it induces a balanced immune response, can be delivered through the mucosa, and is efficacious in infants, in whom maternal antibodies are present.

At present, two antibodies are indicated for RSV prevention: a highly concentrated polyclonal antibody, obtained from the plasma of healthy individuals, and the monoclonal antibody, palivizumab, that targets the F protein. Both are administered prophylactically to patients (infants) at-risk. The RSV-IGIV became the first FDA-approved agent for RSV prevention, but has been replaced by palivizumab. Motavizumab, a next-generation, humanized, monoclonal antibody, with improved activity against RSV *in vitro*, is currently undergoing FDA evaluation for licensing in the USA.

Ribavirin, the only antiviral drug approved for RSV treatment, inhibits viral multiplication because its clinical benefits are limited, its use is now restricted mainly to immunocompromised patients or to the early treatment of severe RSV. Ribavirin spray can reduce the severity of the disease and the amount of virus load, but does not reduce the duration of hospitalization.

Currently, six different drugs are in pre-clinical and clinical trials; their targets are the RSV proteins G, F, N or L. Their mechanisms are based on inhibiting viral attachment, fusion, and interference with the N and L proteins that are involved in intracellular replication.

It should be noted that some of the most effective means of reducing the spread of RSV infection are physical ones: efficient hand washing and care when in contact with others.

3. Diagnosis

Clinical signs and symptoms can make presumptive diagnosis of RSV infection in infants, by chest radiographs showing hyperinflation, or by the rapid detection of antigen by using an immunofluorescence technique with monoclonal antibodies. In a presumptive diagnosis is important to consider the season of the year and whether other members of the family have respiratory illness either concurrent with, or just prior to, the patient's episode of RSV infection (14). Clinical signs and symptoms of viral respiratory tract illness generally are not helpful in differentiating RSV-related from non–RSV-related LRTI (21).

Reliable diagnosis depends on the laboratory assays; rapid antigen-detection tests may be helpful in diagnosing RSV as the cause of LRT disease (bronchiolitis) among children (21). It is advisable to carry out such tests, because when information is received in a timely manner, necessary precautions may be taken to reduce the risk of nosocomial and/or nursing homes infection (14). In addition, the rapid identification of the virus causing of the infection can reduce the use of antibiotics, which in most cases of RSV LTRI should be avoided (128).

A variety of laboratory methods, which detect the presence of RSV in respiratory secretions, are available to aid in the diagnosis of RSV infection in children and adults (100, 129). In general, children have several logs higher concentrations of RSV in their secretions than do adults immunocompromised individuals and the elderly often have lower concentration (44).

3.1 Sample Collection and Transport

Specimens are obtained by aspiration or by nasal or nasopharyngeal secretion, or by nasal swab. As the virus is easily inactivated, the samples should be kept cold (4 °C) and, as quickly as possible, be inoculated into a monolayer of cells sensitive to RSV. Usually human heteroploid cell lines (HEp-2, HeLa, or A549) are used for primary isolation; presence of the virus is confirmed by the cytopathic effect that appears after 3–7 days of incubation (37 °C). Frequently, false-negative results are due to poor quality samples (130).

Currently available methods for diagnosis of RSV infections include cell culture (CC), serology, or direct examination of respiratory secretions by various techniques. These include direct and indirect tests that use electron microscopy, indirect and direct immunofluorescent antibody (IFA) tests, enzyme-linked immunoassays (EIAs), and nucleic acid amplification, *e.g*, polymerase chain reaction (PCR) (129, 131).

3. 2 Direct and Indirect Techniques

For many years cell culture (CC) was considered the gold standard for diagnosing respiratory viral infections; an advantage of CC is its ability to detect viral co-infections. In addition, the isolated virus can be stored for future epidemiological and diagnostic studies. However, CC has disadvantages, in that it requires special specimen-handling procedures to maintain viral viability; requires a long assay time, (average, 2–5 days); is expensive due to the cost of reagents and labor per test, and has low-to-poor sensitivity compared to tests that use nucleic acid amplification. Thus, in many settings, CC is being replaced by nucleic acid amplification assays that have greater sensitivity and provide more rapid results (129, 132, 133).

Antigen-based assay. The direct detection of viral antigen is a common assay that is used in most clinical laboratories to diagnose RSV infection. Several tests are available that provide clinicians with the means for rapid diagnosis, with information being obtained in few hours, Another advantage of these tests is that they do not require virus viability; this is especially important when the transportation time is prolonged. Antigen-based assays include indirect and direct IFA tests, EIA, and mmunoassays. Of the commercially available, rapid, diagnostic assays, EIAs usually have the best combination of sensitivity, specificity, and ease of use. Although the specificity is low, EIA has sufficient sensitivity and specificity to provide reliable results. Antigen-based methods are frequently used because they are inexpensive, easy to perform, and easy to interpret; however, antigen detection methods are often thousands of times less sensitive than are molecular assays. Because of the small amount of viral antigen that is usually present in the nasopharyngeal aspirates collected from RSV-infected adults, current antigen-detection assays may lack the sensitivity to detect RSV antigen in such cases. RT-PCR may be required to detect and diagnose RSV in adults(134, 135).

Molecular Assays. Molecular assays have become the new gold standard for respiratory virus detection because they are significantly more sensitive and specific than are either CC or antigen assays: an increase in sensitivity between 12–50% is frequently obtained when positive controls are included. The nucleic acid techniques detect specific nucleic acid sequences; PCR is the prototype of this technique. PCR amplifies a DNA segment of 100–1,000 base pairs by using short oligonucleotide primers and a thermostable Taq polymerase; the assay sensitivity can be as low as 1–10 copies of the target DNA. For the detection of RNA sequences, it is necessary to obtain, prior to the assay, the complementary DNA by reverse transcriptase. Amplified DNA can be detected by gel analyses and real-time determinations can be obtained by using probes conjugated to fluorescein. It is important that each laboratory establish the sensitivity and specificity of the assay, as well as the predictive value of a positive or negative result. The great sensitivity of RT-PCR assays extends the time during which the virus may be detected in specimens, as compared to that of other methods (44, 130, 136).

Serology. Serology usually is not helpful for diagnosis of acute respiratory virus infections because 10–30% of patients with documented respiratory viral infections will remain serologically negative (17).

3. 3 Section Summary

During the RSV season, the use of rapid laboratory tests to detect the virus may be helpful in diagnosing RSV as the cause of LRT disease, primarily bronchiolitis, in children. RSV is identified by four principal techniques: virus in cell culture, serology, immunofluorescence assays that detect antigen, and nucleic acid/PCR-based tests. The new gold standards for RSV detection are antigen detection by molecular assays, EIA and PCR, as these methods are highly specific and sensitive compared with CC or other immunoassays.

4. TREATMENT

4.1 Support Care

The majority of RSV infections are confined to the URT and lead to symptoms of the common cold, coryza, cough, and hoarseness; such mild, self-limited illnesses are treated in an outpatient setting. Only infants having respiratory distress or difficulty in feeding or those requiring supplemental oxygen are taken to the hospital. Due to the lack of cffective medications, current treatment relies on supportive care, which basically is directed to ensuring adequate oxygenation, improving respiration, and taking care that the infant is adequately hydrated and has its nutritional needs met. Infants hospitalized with RSV bronchiolitis often have decreased nutritional intake due to respiratory distress and tachypnea and, therefore, need nutritional support.

RSV URTI in infants is often accompanied by fever and may lead to lethargy and poor feeding. Although specific treatment is usually not required, in some cases, analgesics/antipyretics and nasal decongestants may be helpful in reducing discomfort and symptoms, thus making feeding easier and allowing an adequate supply of oral fluids, such that the majority of infants hospitalized with RSV infection may be discharged within 72 hours (21).

4.2 Pharmacological Interventions

Existing treatment. Because there are no effective drugs to treat RSV patients with severe LTRI, medical treatment is focused on drugs designed to overcome airway obstruction and the resulting respiratory distress. The therapeutic agents commonly used in the settings of RSV infection are bronchodilators, β2-agonists, nebulized epinephrine, and antimuscarinics, such as ipratropium bromide; however, in general, results of these interventions have been disappointing (128, 137).

Bronchodilators are frequently used for infants with wheezing due to RSV LRTI. Studies assessing the effects of these bronchodilators on lung function and clinical outcome yielded conflicting results and concluded that bronchodilator treatment can improve clinical symptom scores in the short term in viral LRTI cases, but that such treatment does not reduce the duration of hospitalization and increases treatment cost. (128, 137).

The use of epinephrine, B-agonists and albuterol in the treatment of RSV bronchiolitis was evaluated in the Cochrane Reviews published between 1998 and 2003. The authors concluded that the available data do not support the use of epinephrine in an in-patient setting, but that for outpatients, epinephrine may produce a modest short-term improvement and, therefore, would be preferable to albuterol in the treatment of bronchiolitis. In summary, epinephrine, b-agonists, and albuterol have not been shown to have consistent benefits in the treatment of RSV bronchiolitis (137, 138).

Another widely used approach was (and often still is) the use of corticosteroids in order to control inflammation in the airway and the subsequent respiratory symptoms. Studies that used low-dose or high-dose inhaled corticosteroids, as well as systemic application, yielded conflicting results. The majority of those studies failed to demonstrate relevant reductions in LRTI symptoms, length of hospital stay, or need for mechanical ventilation. An analysis of studies comparing systemic glucocorticoid treatment to placebo did not find any between-group difference in the length of hospital stay or in the clinical score for infants and young children with LRTI (139).

For infants with LRTI who required mechanical ventilation, surfactant has been used. A Cochrane meta-analysis, which included three studies that showed some reduction in the duration of mechanical ventilation and in the length of stay in intensive care, concluded that there were no sufficiently powered data to provide reliable estimates of surfactant effects on ventilated infants with LRTI (137, 140).

A promising new development is the inhalation of hypertonic saline. A recent trial of this treatment reported a 26% reduction in the length of hospitalization for infants with acute viral bronchiolitis (141). This treatment could become a new, useful tool for the management of viral LRTI. To confirm whether inhalation of hypertonic saline has a beneficial effect, future studies focus on children under six months of age; and exclude non-effective therapies.

4.3 Section Summary

Current treatment for severe viral LRTI in infants relies on supportive measures only. These measures include supplementation of oxygen, monitoring of apnea, feeding by nasal/gastric tube or intravenous fluids, and, if required, respiratory support with nasal, bi-level, positive-airway pressure (BiPAP), or intubation and mechanical ventilation.

Supportive care is the mainstay of therapy for RSV disease and is directed toward ensuring adequate oxygenation, improving pulmonary hygiene, and meeting fluid and nutrition requirements. Severe respiratory failure requires mechanical ventilatory support. A variety of anti-inflammatory compounds have been, or now are, in clinical trials to treat bronchiolitis, as well as the reactive airway disease developing after bronchiolitis, although these compounds often have failed to demonstrate significant effects. These therapies principally target the hyper-inflammatory response and not the agent inducing this response.

Consistent benefit in the treatment of RSV disease has not been obtained with administered or inhaled corticosteroids; therefore, their use is not recommended. For routine treatment, ribavirin is not recommended, but may be considered in immunocompromised individuals. Nebulized treatments with hypertonic saline may be an option to improve mucociliary clearance. Antibiotics are recommended only when evidence has confirmed the presence of a coexistent bacterial infection.

Conclusion

RSV is a prevalent and highly infectious virus, more so than other respiratory viruses. Worldwide, it is the most frequent cause of bronchiolitis and pneumonia in infants and young children; it is also a significant agent of morbidity and mortality in adults and in immunocompromised patients. Infections occur every year during the late fall, winter, or early spring. Almost every child has been infected with this virus at least once by the time they are two years of age. Transmission occurs through inoculation of the nasopharyngeal or conjunctiva mucosa with respiratory secretions from infected individuals or through inhalation of viral particles. Viral shedding persists for approximately one week, but can be significantly prolonged in immunocompromised individuals. Hand washing, and isolation are highly effective in preventing the spread of RSV infection.

RSV, an RNA virus of the Paramyxoviridae family, has two surface proteins, F and G, which are the major antigens and are critical for virulence. Previous infections do not result in persistent immunity, and re-infections are frequent. There is no licensed vaccine, though inactivated vaccines are being evaluated. The best, safest, and most effective option for passive prophylaxis is use of the humanized monoclonal antibody, palivizumab, the use of which is currently limited to infants at high risk for severe respiratory disease. Of the many candidates for RSV treatment being evaluated, six are currently in pre-clinical or clinical trials; they target four RSV proteins, F, G, N, and L. Presumptive diagnosis of RSV infection should be confirmed by detection of the RSV antigen or genome. Despite many attempts to develop vaccines and anti-viral drugs for RSV infection, supportive care remains the most effective therapy.

Acknowledgment

The author thanks Veronica Yakoleff for editing the manuscript and for helpful comments. Work from the authors laboratory was supported by grants from Consejo Nacional de Ciencia y Tecnología, Dirección General de Asuntos del Personal Académico and Facultad de Medicina, Universidad Nacional Autónoma de México, México.

References

[1] Norrby E, Marusyk H, Orvell C. *Morphogenesis of respiratory syncytial virus in a green monkey kidney cell line (Vero).* J Virol. 1970 Aug;6(2):237-42.

[2] Hallak LK, Spillmann D, Collins PL, Peeples ME. *Glycosaminoglycan sulfation requirements for respiratory syncytial virus infection.* J Virol. 2000 Nov;74(22):10508-13.

[3] Smith BJ, Lawrence MC, Colman PM. *Modelling the structure of the fusion protein from human respiratory syncytial virus.* Protein Eng. 2002 May;15(5):365-71.

[4] Cowton VM, McGivern DR, Fearns R. *Unravelling the complexities of respiratory syncytial virus RNA synthesis.* J Gen Virol. 2006 Jul;87(Pt 7):1805-21.

[5] Collins PL, Crowe JEJ. *Respiratory Syncytial Virus and Metapneumovirus.* In: Knipe DM, Howler PM, editors. Fields Virology. Philadelphia, P. A.: Lippincott Williams & Wilkins; 2007. p. 1601-46.

[6] Huang YT, Collins PL, Wertz GW. *Characterization of the 10 proteins of human respiratory syncytial virus: identification of a fourth envelope-associated protein.* Virus Res. 1985 Mar;2(2):157-73.

[7] Barik S. *The structure of the 5' terminal cap of the respiratory syncytial virus mRNA.* J Gen Virol. 1993 Mar;74 (Pt 3):485-90.

[8] Lo MS, Brazas RM, Holtzman MJ. *Respiratory syncytial virus nonstructural proteins NS1 and NS2 mediate inhibition of Stat2 expression and alpha/beta interferon responsiveness.* J Virol. 2005 Jul;79(14):9315-9.

[9] Spann KM, Tran KC, Collins PL. *Effects of nonstructural proteins NS1 and NS2 of human respiratory syncytial virus on interferon regulatory factor 3, NF-kappaB, and proinflammatory cytokines.* J Virol. 2005 May;79(9):5353-62.

[10] Bukreyev A, Yang L, Fricke J, Cheng L, Ward JM, Murphy BR, et al. *The secreted form of respiratory syncytial virus G glycoprotein helps the virus evade antibody-mediated restriction of replication by acting as an antigen decoy and through effects on Fc receptor-bearing leukocytes.* J Virol. 2008 Dec;82(24):12191-204.

[11] Walsh EE, Peterson DR, Falsey AR. *Risk factors for severe respiratory syncytial virus infection in elderly persons.* J Infect Dis. 2004 Jan 15;189(2):233-8.

[12] Levine S, Klaiber-Franco R, Paradiso PR. *Demonstration that glycoprotein G is the attachment protein of respiratory syncytial virus.* J Gen Virol. 1987 Sep;68 (Pt 9):2521-4.

[13] Teng MN, Whitehead SS, Collins PL. *Contribution of the respiratory syncytial virus G glycoprotein and its secreted and membrane-bound forms to virus replication in vitro and in vivo.* Virology. 2001 Oct 25;289(2):283-96.

[14] Hall CB, Douglas RG, Jr., Geiman JM. *Respiratory syncytial virus infections in infants: quantitation and duration of shedding.* J Pediatr. 1976 Jul;89(1):11-5.

[15] Shay DK, Holman RC, Roosevelt GE, Clarke MJ, Anderson LJ. *Bronchiolitis-associated mortality and estimates of respiratory syncytial virus-associated deaths among US children, 1979-1997.* J Infect Dis. 2001 Jan 1;183(1):16-22.

[16] Kim HW, Canchola JG, Brandt CD, Pyles G, Chanock RM, Jensen K, et al. *Respiratory syncytial virus disease in infants despite prior administration of antigenic inactivated vaccine.* Am J Epidemiol. 1969 Apr;89(4):422-34.

[17] Dowell SF, Anderson LJ, Gary HE, Jr., Erdman DD, Plouffe JF, File TM, Jr., et al. *Respiratory syncytial virus is an important cause of community-acquired lower respiratory infection among hospitalized adults.* J Infect Dis. 1996 Sep;174(3):456-62.

[18] Tregoning JS, Schwarze J. *Respiratory viral infections in infants: causes, clinical symptoms, virology, and immunology.* Clin Microbiol Rev. Jan;23(1):74-98.

[19] Paramore LC, Ciuryla V, Ciesla G, Liu L. *Economic impact of respiratory syncytial virus-related illness in the US: an analysis of national databases.* Pharmacoeconomics. 2004;22(5):275-84.

[20] Monto AS, Ullman BM. *Acute respiratory illness in an American community.* The Tecumseh study. JAMA. 1974 Jan 14;227(2):164-9.

[21] Hall CB, Weinberg GA, Iwane MK, Blumkin AK, Edwards KM, Staat MA, et al. *The burden of respiratory syncytial virus infection in young children.* N Engl J Med. 2009 Feb 5;360(6):588-98.

[22] Stott EJ, Taylor G. *Respiratory syncytial virus.* Brief review. Arch Virol. 1985;84(1-2):1-52.

[23] Wright PF, Gruber WC, Peters M, Reed G, Zhu Y, Robinson F, et al. *Illness severity, viral shedding, and antibody responses in infants hospitalized with bronchiolitis caused by respiratory syncytial virus.* J Infect Dis. 2002 Apr 15;185(8):1011-8.

[24] Leader S, Kohlhase K. *Respiratory syncytial virus-coded pediatric hospitalizations, 1997 to 1999.* Pediatr Infect Dis J. 2002 Jul;21(7):629-32.

[25] Greenough A. *Respiratory syncytial virus infection: clinical features, management, and prophylaxis.* Curr Opin Pulm Med. 2002 May;8(3):214-7.

[26] Meissner HC, Rennels MB, Pickering LK, Hall CB. *Risk of severe respiratory syncytial virus disease, identification of high risk infants and recommendations for prophylaxis with palivizumab.* Pediatr Infect Dis J. 2004 Mar;23(3):284-5.

[27] Simoes EA, Carbonell-Estrany X. *Impact of severe disease caused by respiratory syncytial virus in children living in developed countries.* Pediatr Infect Dis J. 2003 Feb;22(2 Suppl):S13-8; discussion S8-20.

[28] Thompson WW, Shay DK, Weintraub E, Brammer L, Cox N, Anderson LJ, et al. *Mortality associated with influenza and respiratory syncytial virus in the United States.* JAMA. 2003 Jan 8;289(2):179-86.

[29] Falsey AR, Walsh EE. *Respiratory syncytial virus infection in adults.* Clin Microbiol Rev. 2000 Jul;13(3):371-84.

[30] Falsey AR. *Respiratory syncytial virus infection in elderly and high-risk adults.* Exp Lung Res. 2005 Sep;31 Suppl 1:77.

[31] Falsey AR, Formica MA, Hennessey PA, Criddle MM, Sullender WM, Walsh EE. *Detection of respiratory syncytial virus in adults with chronic obstructive pulmonary disease.* Am J Respir Crit Care Med. 2006 Mar 15;173(6):639-43.

[32] Iwane MK, Edwards KM, Szilagyi PG, Walker FJ, Griffin MR, Weinberg GA, et al. *Population-based surveillance for hospitalizations associated with respiratory syncytial virus, influenza virus, and parainfluenza viruses among young children.* Pediatrics. 2004 Jun;113(6):1758-64.

[33] Howard TS, Hoffman LH, Stang PE, Simoes EA. *Respiratory syncytial virus pneumonia in the hospital setting: length of stay, charges, and mortality.* J Pediatr. 2000 Aug;137(2):227-32.

[34] Hall CB, Douglas RG, Jr., Schnabel KC, Geiman JM. *Infectivity of respiratory syncytial virus by various routes of inoculation.* Infect Immun. 1981 Sep;33(3):779-83.

[35] Kim HW, Arrobio JO, Brandt CD, Jeffries BC, Pyles G, Reid JL, et al. *Epidemiology of respiratory syncytial virus infection in Washington, D.C. I. Importance of the virus in different respiratory tract disease syndromes and temporal distribution of infection.* Am J Epidemiol. 1973 Sep;98(3):216-25.

[36] Aujard Y, Fauroux B. *Risk factors for severe respiratory syncytial virus infection in infants.* Respir Med. 2002 Apr;96 Suppl B:S9-14.

[37] Finger R, Anderson LJ, Dicker RC, Harrison B, Doan R, Downing A, et al. *Epidemic infections caused by respiratory syncytial virus in institutionalized young adults.* J Infect Dis. 1987 Jun;155(6):1335-9.

[38] McNamara PS, Smyth RL. *The pathogenesis of respiratory syncytial virus disease in childhood.* Br Med Bull. 2002;61:13-28.

[39] Openshaw PJ, Tregoning JS. *Immune responses and disease enhancement during respiratory syncytial virus infection.* Clin Microbiol Rev. 2005 Jul;18(3):541-55.

[40] van Schaik SM, Tristram DA, Nagpal IS, Hintz KM, Welliver RC, 2nd, Welliver RC. *Increased production of IFN-gamma and cysteinyl leukotrienes in virus-induced wheezing.* J Allergy Clin Immunol. 1999 Apr;103(4):630-6.

[41] Piedimonte G, Renzetti G, Auais A, Di Marco A, Tripodi S, Colistro F, et al. *Leukotriene synthesis during respiratory syncytial virus bronchiolitis: influence of age and atopy.* Pediatr Pulmonol. 2005 Oct;40(4):285-91.

[42] Volovitz B, Welliver RC, De Castro G, Krystofik DA, Ogra PL. *The release of leukotrienes in the respiratory tract during infection with respiratory syncytial virus: role in obstructive airway disease.* Pediatr Res. 1988 Oct;24(4):504-7.

[43] Zeng R, Li C, Li N, Wei L, Cui Y. *The role of cytokines and chemokines in severe respiratory syncytial virus infection and subsequent asthma.* Cytokine. Jan;53(1):1-7.

[44] Hall CB, Powell KR, MacDonald NE, Gala CL, Menegus ME, Suffin SC, et al. *Respiratory syncytial viral infection in children with compromised immune function.* N Engl J Med. 1986 Jul 10;315(2):77-81.

[45] Chonmaitree T, Revai K, Grady JJ, Clos A, Patel JA, Nair S, et al. *Viral upper respiratory tract infection and otitis media complication in young children.* Clin Infect Dis. 2008 Mar 15;46(6):815-23.

[46] Hall CB. *Respiratory syncytial virus.* Isr J Med Sci. 1983 Oct;19(10):889-91.

[47] Henderson FW, Collier AM, Clyde WA, Jr., Denny FW. *Respiratory-syncytial-virus infections, reinfections and immunity. A prospective, longitudinal study in young children.* N Engl J Med. 1979 Mar 8;300(10):530-4.

[48] Welliver RC. *Review of epidemiology and clinical risk factors for severe respiratory syncytial virus (RSV) infection.* J Pediatr. 2003 Nov;143(5 Suppl):S112-7.

[49] Smyth RL, Openshaw PJ. *Bronchiolitis.* Lancet. 2006 Jul 22;368(9532):312-22.

[50] Aherne W, Bird T, Court SD, Gardner PS, McQuillin J. *Pathological changes in virus infections of the lower respiratory tract in children.* J Clin Pathol. 1970 Feb;23(1):7-18.

[51] Hall CB, Walsh EE, Long CE, Schnabel KC. *Immunity to and frequency of reinfection with respiratory syncytial virus.* J Infect Dis. 1991 Apr;163(4):693-8.

[52] Hall CB, Long CE, Schnabel KC. *Respiratory syncytial virus infections in previously healthy working adults.* Clin Infect Dis. 2001 Sep 15;33(6):792-6.

[53] Glezen WP, Taber LH, Frank AL, Kasel JA. *Risk of primary infection and reinfection with respiratory syncytial virus.* Am J Dis Child. 1986 Jun;140(6):543-6.

[54] Walsh EE, Hall CB, Briselli M, Brandriss MW, Schlesinger JJ. *Immunization with glycoprotein subunits of respiratory syncytial virus to protect cotton rats against viral infection.* J Infect Dis. 1987 Jun;155(6):1198-204.

[55] Fjaerli HO, Farstad T, Rod G, Ufert GK, Gulbrandsen P, Nakstad B. *Acute bronchiolitis in infancy as risk factor for wheezing and reduced pulmonary function by seven years in Akershus County, Norway.* BMC Pediatr. 2005;5:31.

[56] Pullan CR, Hey EN. *Wheezing, asthma, and pulmonary dysfunction 10 years after infection with respiratory syncytial virus in infancy.* Br Med J (Clin Res Ed). 1982 Jun 5;284(6330):1665-9.

[57] Sigurs N, Gustafsson PM, Bjarnason R, Lundberg F, Schmidt S, Sigurbergsson F, et al. *Severe respiratory syncytial virus bronchiolitis in infancy and asthma and allergy at age 13.* Am J Respir Crit Care Med. 2005 Jan 15;171(2):137-41.

[58] Welliver RC, Wong DT, Sun M, Middleton E, Jr., Vaughan RS, Ogra PL. *The development of respiratory syncytial virus-specific IgE and the release of histamine in nasopharyngeal secretions after infection.* N Engl J Med. 1981 Oct 8;305(15):841-6.

[59] Zlateva KT, Lemey P, Moes E, Vandamme AM, Van Ranst M. *Genetic variability and molecular evolution of the human respiratory syncytial virus subgroup B attachment G protein.* J Virol. 2005 Jul;79(14):9157-67.

[60] Sullender WM, Mufson MA, Anderson LJ, Wertz GW. *Genetic diversity of the attachment protein of subgroup B respiratory syncytial viruses.* J Virol. 1991 Oct;65(10):5425-34.

[61] Anderson LJ, Hierholzer JC, Tsou C, Hendry RM, Fernie BF, Stone Y, et al. *Antigenic characterization of respiratory syncytial virus strains with monoclonal antibodies.* J Infect Dis. 1985 Apr;151(4):626-33.

[62] Johnson PR, Spriggs MK, Olmsted RA, Collins PL. *The G glycoprotein of human respiratory syncytial viruses of subgroups A and B: extensive sequence divergence between antigenically related proteins.* Proc Natl Acad Sci U S A. 1987 Aug;84(16):5625-9.

[63] Fodha I, Vabret A, Ghedira L, Seboui H, Chouchane S, Dewar J, et al. *Respiratory syncytial virus infections in hospitalized infants: association between viral load, virus subgroup, and disease severity.* J Med Virol. 2007 Dec;79(12):1951-8.

[64] Simoes EA, Groothuis JR, Carbonell-Estrany X, Rieger CH, Mitchell I, Fredrick LM, et al. *Palivizumab prophylaxis, respiratory syncytial virus, and subsequent recurrent wheezing.* J Pediatr. 2007 Jul;151(1):34-42, e1.

[65] Holberg CJ, Wright AL, Martinez FD, Ray CG, Taussig LM, Lebowitz MD. *Risk factors for respiratory syncytial virus-associated lower respiratory illnesses in the first year of life.* Am J Epidemiol. 1991 Jun 1;133(11):1135-51.

[66] Zlateva KT, Vijgen L, Dekeersmaeker N, Naranjo C, Van Ranst M. *Subgroup prevalence and genotype circulation patterns of human respiratory syncytial virus in Belgium during ten successive epidemic seasons.* J Clin Microbiol. 2007 Sep;45(9):3022-30.

[67] White LJ, Waris M, Cane PA, Nokes DJ, Medley GF. *The transmission dynamics of groups A and B human respiratory syncytial virus (hRSV) in England & Wales and Finland: seasonality and cross-protection.* Epidemiol Infect. 2005 Apr;133(2):279-89.

[68] Korppi M, Hyvarinen M, Piippo-Savolainen E. *Asthma after early RSV infection--how to control?* Pediatr Infect Dis J. 2008 Feb;27(2):191-2; author reply 2.

[69] Stein RT, Sherrill D, Morgan WJ, Holberg CJ, Halonen M, Taussig LM, et al. *Respiratory syncytial virus in early life and risk of wheeze and allergy by age 13 years.* Lancet. 1999 Aug 14;354(9178):541-5.

[70] Sikkel MB, Quint JK, Mallia P, Wedzicha JA, Johnston SL. *Respiratory syncytial virus persistence in chronic obstructive pulmonary disease.* Pediatr Infect Dis J. 2008 Oct;27(10 Suppl):S63-70.

[71] Bruhn FW, Mokrohisky ST, McIntosh K. *Apnea associated with respiratory syncytial virus infection in young infants.* J Pediatr. 1977 Mar;90(3):382-6.

[72] Chanock RM, Kim HW, Vargosko AJ, Deleva A, Johnson KM, Cumming C, et al. *Respiratory syncytial virus. I. Virus recovery and other observations during 1960 outbreak of bronchiolitis, pneumonia, and minor respiratory diseases in children.* JAMA. 1961 May 27;176:647-53.

[73] Church NR, Anas NG, Hall CB, Brooks JG. *Respiratory syncytial virus-related apnea in infants. Demographics and outcome.* Am J Dis Child. 1984 Mar;138(3):247-50.

[74] Hall CB, Douglas RG, Jr., Geiman JM, Messner MK. N*osocomial respiratory syncytial virus infections.* N Engl J Med. 1975 Dec 25;293(26):1343-6.

[75] Boyce TG, Mellen BG, Mitchel EF, Jr., Wright PF, Griffin MR. *Rates of hospitalization for respiratory syncytial virus infection among children in medicaid.* J Pediatr. 2000 Dec;137(6):865-70.

[76] Hoebee B, Bont L, Rietveld E, van Oosten M, Hodemaekers HM, Nagelkerke NJ, et al. *Influence of promoter variants of interleukin-10, interleukin-9, and tumor necrosis factor-alpha genes on respiratory syncytial virus bronchiolitis.* J Infect Dis. 2004 Jan 15;189(2):239-47.

[77] Hegele RG, Hayashi S, Bramley AM, Hogg JC. *Persistence of respiratory syncytial virus genome and protein after acute bronchiolitis in guinea pigs.* Chest. 1994 Jun;105(6):1848-54.

[78] Valarcher JF, Bourhy H, Lavenu A, Bourges-Abella N, Roth M, Andreoletti O, et al. *Persistent infection of B lymphocytes by bovine respiratory syncytial virus.* Virology. 2001 Dec 5;291(1):55-67.

[79] Mejias A, Chavez-Bueno S, Gomez AM, Somers C, Estripeaut D, Torres JP, et al. *Respiratory syncytial virus persistence: evidence in the mouse model.* Pediatr Infect Dis J. 2008 Oct;27(10 Suppl):S60-2.

[80] Wilkinson TM, Donaldson GC, Johnston SL, Openshaw PJ, Wedzicha JA. *Respiratory syncytial virus, airway inflammation, and FEV1 decline in patients with chronic obstructive pulmonary disease.* Am J Respir Crit Care Med. 2006 Apr 15;173(8):871-6.

[81] Halasa NB, Williams JV, Wilson GJ, Walsh WF, Schaffner W, Wright PF. *Medical and economic impact of a respiratory syncytial virus outbreak in a neonatal intensive care unit.* Pediatr Infect Dis J. 2005 Dec;24(12):1040-4.

[82] Hall CB, Douglas RG, Jr. *Clinically useful method for the isolation of respiratory syncytial virus.* J Infect Dis. 1975 Jan;131(1):1-5.

[83] Hall CB. *Respiratory syncytial virus: its transmission in the hospital environment.* Yale J Biol Med. 1982 May-Aug;55(3-4):219-23.

[84] Dudas RA, Karron RA. *Respiratory syncytial virus vaccines.* Clin Microbiol Rev. 1998 Jul;11(3):430-9.

[85] Lee MS, Walker RE, Mendelman PM. *Medical burden of respiratory syncytial virus and parainfluenza virus type 3 infection among US children. Implications for design of vaccine trials.* Hum Vaccin. 2005 Jan-Feb;1(1):6-11.

[86] Yamazaki H, Tsutsumi H, Matsuda K, Nagai K, Ogra PL, Chiba S. *Effect of maternal antibody on IgA antibody response in nasopharyngeal secretion in infants and children during primary respiratory syncytial virus infection.* J Gen Virol. 1994 Aug;75 (Pt 8):2115-9.

[87] Kovarik J, Siegrist CA. *Immunity in early life.* Immunol Today. 1998 Apr;19(4):150-2.

[88] Osborn JJ, Dancis J, Rosenberg BV. *Studies of the immunology of the newborn infant. III. Permeability of the placenta to maternal antibody during fetal life.* Pediatrics. 1952 Oct;10(4):450-6.

[89] Kapikian AZ, Mitchell RH, Chanock RM, Shvedoff RA, Stewart CE. *An epidemiologic study of altered clinical reactivity to respiratory syncytial (RS) virus infection in children previously vaccinated with an inactivated RS virus vaccine.* Am J Epidemiol. 1969 Apr;89(4):405-21.

[90] Murphy BR, Walsh EE. *Formalin-inactivated respiratory syncytial virus vaccine induces antibodies to the fusion glycoprotein that are deficient in fusion-inhibiting activity.* J Clin Microbiol. 1988 Aug;26(8):1595-7.

[91] Polack FP, Teng MN, Collins PL, Prince GA, Exner M, Regele H, et al. *A role for immune complexes in enhanced respiratory syncytial virus disease.* J Exp Med. 2002 Sep 16;196(6):859-65.

[92] Prince GA, Curtis SJ, Yim KC, Porter DD. *Vaccine-enhanced respiratory syncytial virus disease in cotton rats following immunization with Lot 100 or a newly prepared reference vaccine.* J Gen Virol. 2001 Dec;82(Pt 12):2881-8.

[93] Waris ME, Tsou C, Erdman DD, Day DB, Anderson LJ. *Priming with live respiratory syncytial virus (RSV) prevents the enhanced pulmonary inflammatory response seen after RSV challenge in BALB/c mice immunized with formalin-inactivated RSV.* J Virol. 1997 Sep;71(9):6935-9.

[94] Karron RA, Wright PF, Crowe JE, Jr., Clements-Mann ML, Thompson J, Makhene M, et al. *Evaluation of two live, cold-passaged, temperature-sensitive respiratory syncytial virus vaccines in chimpanzees and in human adults, infants, and children.* J Infect Dis. 1997 Dec;176(6):1428-36.

[95] Wright PF, Karron RA, Belshe RB, Thompson J, Crowe JE, Jr., Boyce TG, et al. *Evaluation of a live, cold-passaged, temperature-sensitive, respiratory syncytial virus vaccine candidate in infancy.* J Infect Dis. 2000 Nov;182(5):1331-42.

[96] Parrott RH, Kim HW, Arrobio JO, Hodes DS, Murphy BR, Brandt CD, et al. *Epidemiology of respiratory syncytial virus infection in Washington, D.C. II. Infection and disease with respect to age, immunologic status, race and sex.* Am J Epidemiol. 1973 Oct;98(4):289-300.

[97] Collins PL, Murphy BR. *New generation live vaccines against human respiratory syncytial virus designed by reverse genetics.* Proc Am Thorac Soc. 2005;2(2):166-73.

[98] Schickli JH, Dubovsky F, Tang RS. *Challenges in developing a pediatric RSV vaccine.* Hum Vaccin. 2009 Sep;5(9):582-91.

[99] O'Shea TM, Sevick MA, Givner LB. *Costs and benefits of respiratory syncytial virus immunoglobulin to prevent hospitalization for lower respiratory tract illness in very low birth weight infants.* Pediatr Infect Dis J. 1998 Jul;17(7):587-93.

[100] Johnston SL, Siegel CS. *Evaluation of direct immunofluorescence, enzyme immunoassay, centrifugation culture, and conventional culture for the detection of respiratory syncytial virus.* J Clin Microbiol. 1990 Nov;28(11):2394-7.

[101] Johnson S, Oliver C, Prince GA, Hemming VG, Pfarr DS, Wang SC, et al. *Development of a humanized monoclonal antibody (MEDI-493) with potent in vitro and in vivo activity against respiratory syncytial virus.* J Infect Dis. 1997 Nov;176(5):1215-24.

[102] Groothuis JR, Simoes EA, Levin MJ, Hall CB, Long CE, Rodriguez WJ, et al. *Prophylactic administration of respiratory syncytial virus immune globulin to high-risk infants and young children.* The Respiratory Syncytial Virus Immune Globulin Study Group. N Engl J Med. 1993 Nov 18;329(21):1524-30.

[103] Groothuis JR. *Safety of palivizumab in preterm infants 29 to 32 weeks' gestational age without chronic lung disease to prevent serious respiratory syncytial virus infection.* Eur J Clin Microbiol Infect Dis. 2003 Jul;22(7):414-7.

[104] Subramanian KN, Weisman LE, Rhodes T, Ariagno R, Sanchez PJ, Steichen J, et al. *Safety, tolerance and pharmacokinetics of a humanized monoclonal antibody to respiratory syncytial virus in premature infants and infants with bronchopulmonary dysplasia.* MEDI-493 Study Group. Pediatr Infect Dis J. 1998 Feb;17(2):110-5.

[105] Abarca K, Jung E, Fernandez P, Zhao L, Harris B, Connor EM, et al. *Safety, tolerability, pharmacokinetics, and immunogenicity of motavizumab, a humanized, enhanced-potency monoclonal antibody for the prevention of respiratory syncytial virus infection in at-risk children.* Pediatr Infect Dis J. 2009 Apr;28(4):267-72.

[106] Sidwell RW, Huffman JH, Khare GP, Allen LB, Witkowski JT, Robins RK. *Broad-spectrum antiviral activity of Virazole: 1-beta-D-ribofuranosyl-1,2,4-triazole-3-carboxamide.* Science. 1972 Aug 25;177(50):705-6.

[107] Sidwell RW, Barnard DL. *Respiratory syncytial virus infections: recent prospects for control.* Antiviral Res. 2006 Sep;71(2-3):379-90.

[108] Barry W, Cockburn F, Cornall R, Price JF, Sutherland G, Vardag A. *Ribavirin aerosol for acute bronchiolitis.* Arch Dis Child. 1986 Jun;61(6):593-7.

[109] Hall CB, McBride JT, Walsh EE, Bell DM, Gala CL, Hildreth S, et al. *Aerosolized ribavirin treatment of infants with respiratory syncytial viral infection. A randomized double-blind study.* N Engl J Med. 1983 Jun 16;308(24):1443-7.

[110] Rodrigucz WJ, Parrott RH. *Ribavirin aerosol treatment of serious respiratory syncytial virus infection in infants.* Infect Dis Clin North Am. 1987 Jun;1(2):425-39.

[111] Smith DW, Frankel LR, Mathers LH, Tang AT, Ariagno RL, Prober CG. *A controlled trial of aerosolized ribavirin in infants receiving mechanical ventilation for severe respiratory syncytial virus infection.* N Engl J Med. 1991 Jul 4;325(1):24-9.

[112] Everard ML, Swarbrick A, Rigby AS, Milner AD. T*he effect of ribavirin to treat previously healthy infants admitted with acute bronchiolitis on acute and chronic respiratory morbidity.* Respir Med. 2001 Apr;95(4):275-80.

[113] Guerguerian AM, Gauthier M, Lebel MH, Farrell CA, Lacroix J. *Ribavirin in ventilated respiratory syncytial virus bronchiolitis. A randomized, placebo-controlled trial.* Am J Respir Crit Care Med. 1999 Sep;160(3):829-34.

[114] Ventre K, Randolph AG. *Ribavirin for respiratory syncytial virus infection of the lower respiratory tract in infants and young children.* Cochrane Database Syst Rev. 2007(1):CD000181.

[115] Kimura K, Mori S, Tomita K, Ohno K, Takahashi K, Shigeta S, et al. *Antiviral activity of NMSO3 against respiratory syncytial virus infection in vitro and in vivo.* Antiviral Res. 2000 Jul;47(1):41-51.

[116] Lawless-Delmedico MK, Sista P, Sen R, Moore NC, Antczak JB, White JM, et al. *Heptad-repeat regions of respiratory syncytial virus F1 protein form a six-membered coiled-coil complex.* Biochemistry. 2000 Sep 26;39(38):11684-95.

[117] Chapman J, Abbott E, Alber DG, Baxter RC, Bithell SK, Henderson EA, et al. *RSV604, a novel inhibitor of respiratory syncytial virus replication.* Antimicrob Agents Chemother. 2007 Sep;51(9):3346-53.

[118] Sudo K, Miyazaki Y, Kojima N, Kobayashi M, Suzuki H, Shintani M, et al. *YM-53403, a unique anti-respiratory syncytial virus agent with a novel mechanism of action.* Antiviral Res. 2005 Feb;65(2):125-31.

[119] Douglas JL. *In search of a small-molecule inhibitor for respiratory syncytial virus.* Expert Rev Anti Infect Ther. 2004 Aug;2(4):625-39.

[120] Empey KM, Peebles RS, Jr., Kolls JK. *Pharmacologic advances in the treatment and prevention of respiratory syncytial virus.* Clin Infect Dis. 2010 May 1;50(9):1258-67.

[121] Zhao X, Singh M, Malashkevich VN, Kim PS. *Structural characterization of the human respiratory syncytial virus fusion protein core*. Proc Natl Acad Sci U S A. 2000 Dec 19;97(26):14172-7.

[122] Bonfanti JF, Roymans D. *Prospects for the development of fusion inhibitors to treat human respiratory syncytial virus infection*. Curr Opin Drug Discov Devel. 2009 Jul;12(4):479-87.

[123] Wyde PR, Laquerre S, Chetty SN, Gilbert BE, Nitz TJ, Pevear DC. *Antiviral efficacy of VP14637 against respiratory syncytial virus in vitro and in cotton rats following delivery by small droplet aerosol*. Antiviral Res. 2005 Oct;68(1):18-26.

[124] Barik S. *Silence of the transcripts: RNA interference in medicine*. J Mol Med. 2005 Oct;83(10):764-73.

[125] Alvarez R, Elbashir S, Borland T, Toudjarska I, Hadwiger P, John M, et al. *RNA interference-mediated silencing of the respiratory syncytial virus nucleocapsid defines a potent antiviral strategy*. Antimicrob Agents Chemother. 2009 Sep;53(9):3952-62.

[126] DeVincenzo J, Cehelsky JE, Alvarez R, Elbashir S, Harborth J, Toudjarska I, et al. *Evaluation of the safety, tolerability and pharmacokinetics of ALN-RSV01, a novel RNAi antiviral therapeutic directed against respiratory syncytial virus (RSV)*. Antiviral Res. 2008 Mar;77(3):225-31.

[127] Lai SH, Stein DA, Guerrero-Plata A, Liao SL, Ivanciuc T, Hong C, et al. *Inhibition of respiratory syncytial virus infections with morpholino oligomers in cell cultures and in mice*. Mol Ther. 2008 Jun;16(6):1120-8.

[128] Weisman LE. *Respiratory syncytial virus (RSV) prevention and treatment: past, present, and future*. Cardiovasc Hematol Agents Med Chem. 2009 Jul;7(3):223-33.

[129] Henrickson KJ. *Advances in the laboratory diagnosis of viral respiratory disease*. Pediatr Infect Dis J. 2004 Jan;23(1 Suppl):S6-10.

[130] Henrickson KJ, Hall CB. *Diagnostic assays for respiratory syncytial virus disease*. Pediatr Infect Dis J. 2007 Nov;26(11 Suppl):S36-40.

[131] Henrickson KJ. *Cost-effective use of rapid diagnostic techniques in the treatment and prevention of viral respiratory infections*. Pediatr Ann. 2005 Jan;34(1):24-31.

[132] Barenfanger J, Drake C, Mueller T, Troutt T, O'Brien J, Guttman K. *R-Mix cells are faster, at least as sensitive and marginally more costly than conventional cell lines for the detection of respiratory viruses*. J Clin Virol. 2001 Aug;22(1):101-10.

[133] Kuypers J, Wright N, Ferrenberg J, Huang ML, Cent A, Corey L, et al. *Comparison of real-time PCR assays with fluorescent-antibody assays for diagnosis of respiratory virus infections in children*. J Clin Microbiol. 2006 Jul;44(7):2382-8.

[134] Erdman DD, Weinberg GA, Edwards KM, Walker FJ, Anderson BC, Winter J, et al. *GeneScan reverse transcription-PCR assay for detection of six common respiratory viruses in young children hospitalized with acute respiratory illness*. J Clin Microbiol. 2003 Sep;41(9):4298-303.

[135] Fan J, Henrickson KJ, Savatski LL. *Rapid simultaneous diagnosis of infections with respiratory syncytial viruses A and B, influenza viruses A and B, and human parainfluenza virus types 1, 2, and 3 by multiplex quantitative reverse transcription-polymerase chain reaction-enzyme hybridization assay (Hexaplex)*. Clin Infect Dis. 1998 Jun;26(6):1397-402.

[136] Mahony JB. *Detection of respiratory viruses by molecular methods*. Clin Microbiol Rev. 2008 Oct;21(4):716-47.

[137] Gadomski AM, Bhasale AL. *Bronchodilators for bronchiolitis.* Cochrane Database Syst Rev. 2006;3:CD001266.

[138] Flores G, Horwitz RI. *Efficacy of beta2-agonists in bronchiolitis: a reappraisal and meta-analysis.* Pediatrics. 1997 Aug;100(2 Pt 1):233-9.

[139] Patel H, Platt R, Lozano JM, Wang EE. *Glucocorticoids for acute viral bronchiolitis in infants and young children.* Cochrane Database Syst Rev. 2004(3):CD004878.

[140] Liet JM, Millotte B, Tucci M, Laflammme S, Hutchison J, Creery D, et al. *Noninvasive therapy with helium-oxygen for severe bronchiolitis.* J Pediatr. 2005 Dec;147(6):812-7.

[141] Zhang L, Mendoza-Sassi RA, Wainwright C, Klassen TP. *Nebulized hypertonic saline solution for acute bronchiolitis in infants.* Cochrane Database Syst Rev. 2008(4):CD006458.

In: Respiratory Syncytial Virus ISBN 978-1-62100-835-4
Editors: Haneul Nam and Gippeum Kun, pp. 149-164

Chapter 4

Cellular Immunity and Immunoproteomics of HLA Class I Ligands in HRSV Infection

Daniel López
Centro Nacional de Microbiología,
Instituto de Salud "Carlos III" Spain

Abstract

Human respiratory syncytial virus (HRSV) is the single most important cause of serious airway illnesses such as bronchiolitis and pneumonia in infants and young children that require hospitalization with an attendant economic burden. Slight infections of this virus are reported in healthy adults while HRSV poses a severe health risk in immunocompromised individuals and in the elderly. Although multiple immune mechanisms are involved in HRSV disease and protection, the $CD8^+$ T lymphocytes are required to clear virus-infected cells. In last decades, several HRSV epitopes restricted by different major histocompatibility complex class I molecules of the mouse (H-2) or human (HLA) have been identified using murine models or cytolytic T lymphocytes of seropositive individuals respectively. In recent years, using high resolution mass spectrometry analysis of complex HLA-bound peptide pools, physiologically processed HLA ligands from HRSV have been identified. This knowledge could be used in the polyepitope vaccine development.

Introduction

Human respiratory syncytial virus (HRSV) [1], a *Pneumovirus* of the *Paramyxoviridae* family is an enveloped virus containing a negative-sense, single-stranded RNA of 15.2 kilobases. The HRSV genome is transcribed into 10mRNAs encoding 11 proteins since two overlapping open reading frames of M2 mRNA encode the M2-1 and M2-2 proteins respectively. The components of the polymerase complex are the nucleocapsid (N) protein, the catalytic subunit of the RNA-dependent RNA polymerase (L), the transcription factor (M2-1) and the phosphoprotein (P). M is the matrix protein whereas M2-2 is a regulatory factor in RNA synthesis. In addition, the non structural proteins NS1 and NS2 are antagonists of host type I interferons (IFN). Lastly, the viral envelope bears three transmembrane proteins (F, G and SH).

HRSV is the single most important cause of serious lower respiratory tract illnesses such as bronchiolitis and pneumonia in infants and young children [2-4]. In these acute lower respiratory infections due to HRSV, the case fatality ratio in children younger than 1 year of developing or industrialised countries is the 2.1% and 0.7% respectively [5]. Annually, the worldwide mortality from infection of this virus has been estimated in 66,000 to 199,000 deaths in young children and infants [5].

Although HRSV infections occur in people of all ages, usually mild infections are reported in healthy adults. In contrast this virus poses a serious health risk in immunocompromised individuals [6, 7] and in the elderly [8, 9]. Only in the United States, HRSV is estimated to cause approximately 13,000 annual deaths among adults who are elderly or have underlying cardiopulmonary and/or immunosuppressive conditions [9].

HRSV exists as a single serotype, but has two antigenic subgroups, A and B [10, 11]. The major source of antigenic differences between the two HRSV subgroups is the attachment G protein, a type II transmembrane glycoprotein with little homology to any other known viral protein. Between A and B subgroups A, the G protein varies by ~50% in amino acid sequence [12]. The nature of differences in this G protein indicates that both subgroups represent two lines of divergent evolution, rather than variants that differ only at a few major antigenic sites.

Although the airway epithelial cells are the primary site of HRSV replication *in vivo* (reviewed in [1]), this virus can infect both murine and human immune system cells, largely professional antigen-presenting cells (APCs). This infection induces maturation in murine and human macrophages and monocytes [13-16]. Also human plasmacytoid but not myeloid dendritic cells are activated by HRSV [17]. In addition, HRSV infection of mouse spleen B cells induces upregulation of typical activation markers such as CD86 and MHC class II [18, 19].

Innate and Humoral Response

The HRSV infection, as any other pathogenic illness, is controlled by the concerted action of different mechanisms and cells from host immune system. In the first phase, the cells of innate immune system as neutrophils infiltrate intensely the airways of ventilated HRSV-infected infants as shown their high presence in broncho-alveolar lavage samples of hospitalized infants [20]. In addition, abundant alveolar macrophages were detected in the lower respiratory tract in HRSV infection [21]. Moreover, the depletion of macrophages increases virus titers in the HRSV-infected lung by noteworthy inhibition of early inflammatory cytokines release [22].

Although the humoral response is not relevant in the course of the primary HRSV infection, the protection from following viral infections is mediated strongly through antibodies (Abs). In mice model, the depletion of B lymphocytes does not alter the rate of viral clearance in the primary infection but the clearance of virus after secondary infection was significantly diminished [23]. This decreased protection from secondary infection is associated with low titers of HRSV-specific Abs in the serum of infected patients [24].

Moreover, high titers of maternal acquired Abs inversely correlate with severe bronchiolitis in newborn infants [25]. Lastly, the passive immunization with HRSV-specific Abs reduces hospitalization from HRSV infection in high-risk infants [26].

Vaccination studies using HRSV F, G, M2 and P proteins have shown presence of specific Abs in blood serum, although this protection was associated only to the two major envelope glycoproteins (F and G proteins) [27]. Two different structures of the HRSV F protein: an immature folded form, and other mature cleaved form found in virions have been described [28, 29]. Although some neutralizing epitopes of the mature form are not found in the immature F protein, both forms induce similar humoral responses [30]. Among different virus isolates, the G protein with only a 50% identity is the less conserved protein. In contrast F protein shows a 90% identity between the two antigenic subgroups of HRSV [1]. Therefore, the majority of F-specific but few G-specific monoclonal Abs are cross-reactive [1] and thus, very few individual monoclonal Abs for G protein efficiently neutralize HRSV infectivity.

Both immunoglobulin A and G play are important in protection from HRSV infection. IgA is mainly associated with mucosal immunity. As HRSV initially replicates in apical respiratory epithelial cells from the lung airways thus, this IG subclass must be an essential factor in protection from initial HRSV infection. Fast and specific IgA Ab secretion in the upper airways of primary HRSV-infected mice could be detected [31]. Decreased HRSV-specific IgA titers in nasal wash correlated with increased infection in human adults [32]. Also, the intranasal administration of HRSV-specific IgA prior to HRSV infection enhances the antiviral protection in the mouse model [33], although this treatment is not as efficient as administration of HRSV-specific IgG to reduce overall pulmonary viral titers in these animals [34]. Also, reduced incidence of severe disease associated with lower-airway infection was found in both young individuals and elderly with high HRSV-neutralizing IgG Ab titers [32, 35].

Cellular Response

Multiple studies both animal models and infected infants or exposed adults indicate the key role of cellular immunity in the control of infection and the virus-induced inflammatory processes and airway damage by HRSV. This cellular response includes both secretion of chemokines and cytokines and $CD4^+$ or $CD8^+$ responses.

Chemokines and Cytokines

In the primary HRSV infection, both ciliated cells of the respiratory epithelium and lung-resident leukocytes release cytokines and chemokines quickly. These cell-signaling proteins recruit circulating leukocytes to the infected lung and thus, these immune cells release new cytokines mediating proinflammatory functions. Some of these cytokines and chemokines activate and recruit immune cells, but others suppress or regulate the proinflammatory state associated to HRSV infection. In summary, this intricate group of cytokines, chemokines, and multiple immune cells are all implicated in HRSV illness in humans. Even, differences in immunologic responses at birth may be determinant factor of the risk of RSV disease. The analysis of cytokines release from cord blood samples after stimulation with lipopolysaccharide either HRSV-hospitalized young subjects or healthy control children, low IL-1β, IL-2, IL-4, IL-5, and IL-10 but high IL-6 and IL-8 levels were found in hospitalized infants with HRSV disease [36]. In other studies, elevated IL-4 response [37] and decreased phytohemagglutinin-induced IL-13 secretion [38] were detected in umbilical cord blood cells of young children with risk of severe HRSV infection and asthma. Also, increased production of some Th2 cytokines such as IL-4, IL-5, and IL-13 has been associated with severe HRSV airway-disease in infants [38]. High IL-4 concentration was also observed in nasopharyngeal secretions of HRSV-infected children compared to control infants [39]. These results indicate that a Th2 polarization can enhance HRSV-associated disease. In addition, in other study an increased release of IL-17 associated to Th17 cells was detected in moderately HRSV cases as compared with severe sick patients but the mechanism was not elucidated [40]. In addition, a role of HRSV NS1 protein in the suppression of Th17 response with subsequent reduced protective adaptive response had been proposed [41].

IFNs are proteins secreted by host cells in response to the presence of intracellular pathogens including viruses. The genome of different viruses encodes IFN-suppressive proteins. Both HRSV nonstructural proteins NS1 and NS2 cooperatively antagonize the α/β IFN-induced response interfering with the host antiviral cytokine response in infected airway cells as well as suppressing plasmacytoid dendritic cell maturation [42].

Although the immune mechanism involved in HRSV illness and protection is not well characterized, humoral and cellular responses appear to play different roles in the antiviral protection as well as disease pathogenesis of HRSV infection. The specific antibody response prevents and limits the severity of HRSV infection but are not required for clearing primary infection [23]. However, T cell-mediated responses are required to abolish viral replication once HRSV infection is established as well as for the clearance of virus-infected cells in primary infection [43].

Studies in mouse model have shown that F and G glycoproteins prime different subsets of $CD4^+$ T cells. In these animals, G protein primes only $CD4^+$ T cells towards a Th2-type biased cytokine response [44] while F protein primes both $CD4^+$ and $CD8^+$ T cells toward a directed Th1-type cytokine response [45]. In contrast, G protein primes both Th1 and Th2 $CD4^+$ T cell response in humans [46].

Studies with HRSV-infected mice in which the $CD4^+$ and $CD8^+$ T-lymphocyte subpopulations were depleted individually or together by injections of specific Abs shown that both $CD4^+$ and $CD8^+$ lymphocyte subsets are important in clearing a primary infection [47]. Also, $CD4^+$ T cell responses are involved in pulmonary pathology during infection. Then, while IFN-γ secreting $CD4^+$ T cells (Th1-type cytokine response) clear virus in low lung pathology, the HRSV clearance by IL-4 secreting $CD4^+$ cells (Th2-type cytokine response) is strongly associated with important pulmonary damages, including eosinophilic infiltration [48, 49].

Several studies demonstrate the existence of HRSV-specific cytolytic T lymphocytes in peripheral blood mononuclear cells from young children with bronchiolitis [50, 51]. These $CD8^+$ T cells with an activated effector cell phenotype could be isolated from bronchoalveolar lavage samples and blood of infants with a severe primary respiratory HRSV infection [52]. Although also, the HRSV infection suppresses these lung effector activity by blocking IFN-γ secretion by the HRSV-specific T cells [53]. In addition in this study, fault the pulmonary CD8+ T-cell memory development by interfering with TCR-mediated signaling was also described [53]. Surprisingly, this alteration in effector function was only identified in $CD8^+$ T lymphocytes from HRSV-infected lung. Furthermore, the effector $CD8^+$ T cells that had migrated from the draining lymph nodes to other secondary lymphoid organs had no deficiency in their effector function. Moreover, the viral load after primary HRSV infection was significantly higher in the lungs of IFN-γ knockout mice than wild type animals [54]. Thus, during primary HRSV infection the IFN-γ production play a key role to the development of protection against HRSV-associated illness. The poor IFN-γ secretion mediated by HRSV maybe may contribute to its low immunogenicity and could explain the frequent reinfection observed in the human population. Moreover, the analysis of immune responses in several mouse strains with different major histocompatibility complex (MHC) haplotypes demonstrated that susceptibility to aftereffects in childhood HRSV infection was predominantly inherited [55]. Thus, MHC haplotype and its effect on $CD8^+$ T cell lymphocyte immune response play a central role in HRSV infection. In summary, all these results demonstrate a critical role of $CD8^+$ immune response in virus clearance.

Human cytotoxic T cells from normal healthy adults recognize almost six different HRSV proteins: F, N, M, M2-1, NS2, and SH but modest or no recognition of G, NS1 or P proteins was described [56]. Only the $CD8^+$ recognition of F and M2 proteins were associated with a recent infection and thus, these data shows the existence of a long term $CD8^+$ response against this virus [56]. Furthermore, induction of specific cytolytic T responses from HRSV F, N, and M2 proteins was found in the mouse model [57-60].

MHC Class I Epitopes

In cellular immunity, the recognition and killing of infected cells by $CD8^+$ cytolytic T lymphocytes (CTLs) first requires proteolytic degradation of newly synthesized viral proteins in the cytosol by the combined action of proteasomes and degradative peptidases [61]. This antigen processing generates short peptides of 8 to 12 residues that are translocated to the endoplasmic reticulum lumen by transporter associated with antigen processing (TAP), and subsequent N-terminal trimming by the metallo-aminoproteases ERAP1 and 2 is frequently required [62, 63]. Peptide binding to newly synthesized β2-microglobulin and MHC class I heavy chain generates stable peptide/MHC complexes. Usually, this interaction is made possible by two major anchor residues at position 2 and the C-terminus of the antigenic peptide [64, 65] that are deeply accommodated into specific pockets of the antigen recognition site of the MHC class I molecule [66, 67]. Finally, the stable trimolecular peptide-MHC-β_2-microglobulin complexes are transported to the cell membrane and presented for CTL recognition [68].

Different studies using CTL from seropositive individuals or murine models described several HRSV epitopes restricted by different MHC class I molecules of human (HLA) or mouse (H-2) respectively.

MURINE MHC CLASS I EPITOPES

Twenty years ago, Kulkarni et al. showed that the cytolytic activity of lung $CD8^+$ lymphocytes correlated with a protective cellular immune response in BALB/c mice vaccinated with a recombinant virus expressing the M2 protein of HRSV [69]. This HRSV protein induced resistance to virus infection in these $H\text{-}2^d$ mice (BALB/c) but not in $H\text{-}2^b$ or $H\text{-}2^k$ mouse strains [69]. The sequence SYIGSINNI, which spans residues 82-90 of the HRSV M2 protein and is conserved between subgroup A and B HRSV strains, was identified as the immunodominant K^d-restricted CTL epitope in $H\text{-}2^d$ mice. In this study, other two different M2 peptides were also identified as revevant epitopes (the different H-2 class I epitopes of HRSV identified are summarized in Table 1)[57]. Later, a new $H\text{-}2K^d$-restricted subdominant epitope with the amino acid sequence VYNTVISYI, spanning residues 127-135 of the same M2 protein, was also described [70]. In the same study, the frequency of specific T cells responding to both $M2_{82\text{-}90}$ (dominant) and $M2_{127\text{-}135}$ (subdominant) $H\text{-}2K^d$-restricted epitopes from HRSV M2 protein for both lymphoid and nonlymphoid tissues was studied in HRSV-infected mice. Following HRSV infection, the ratios of specific T lymphocytes for dominant and subdominant epitopes were either 3:1 in the spleen or 10:1 in the lung in primary response, secondary infection, and memory response [70].

Table 1. Summary of murine MHC class I epitopes of HRSV

Strain	H-2	Sequence [a]	Protein	Position	Reference
BALB/c	K^d	SY*I*GSINN*I*	Matrix 2	82-90	[57]
BALB/c	K^d	EY*A*LGVVG*V*	Matrix 2	71-79	[57]
BALB/c	K^d	NY*F*EWPPH*A*	Matrix 2	26-34	[57]
BALB/c	K^d	VY*N*TVISY*I*	Matrix 2	127-135	[70]
BALB/c	K^d	KY*K*NAVTE*L*	Fusion	85-93	[71]
BALB/c	K^d	ELQLLMQSTPPTNNR	Fusion	92-106	[72]
BALB/c	K^d	TY*M*LTNSE*L*	Fusion	249-257	[73]
BALB/c	K^d	TY*M*LTNSEL*L*	Fusion	249-258	[73]
C57Bl/6	D^b	NAIT*N*AKI*I*	Matrix	187-195	[75]

[a] The $H\text{-}2K^d$ or D^b anchor motifs are italicised.

To identify the epitope(s) involved in the protective HRSV F protein $CD8^+$ T response in BALB/c strain [59], a set of overlapping synthetic peptides corresponding to the complete HRSV F protein sequence of A2 strain was used [71]. The peptide spanning residues 85-93 was identified as the immunodominant $H\text{-}2K^d$-restricted epitope recognized by F-specific $CD8^+$ T lymphocytes from BALB/c mice. In contrast, no HRSV F-specific $CD8^+$ response was found to $H\text{-}2D^d$ or $H\text{-}2L^d$ class I alleles [71]. Following primary HRSV infection, the F-specific CTL response was 10-fold lower than the dominant M2-specific response previously described. With similar strategy of screening of overlapping synthetic peptides, a second $H\text{-}2K^d$-restricted epitope for HRSV F-specific $CD8^+$ CTL response was described [72]. An unusual long 15-mer peptide from the F protein (92–106 residues), which in contrast to other murine HRSV epitopes not contain the known allele-specific motif for $H\text{-}2K^d$ binding: Tyr at position 2 (P2) and aliphatic C-terminal residues (Table 1 and SYFPEITHI database: http://www.syfpeithi.de [65]) was identified. All residues of this atypical epitope appear to be required for efficient presentation to $CD8^+$ T lymphocytes [72]. As the interaction of this 15-mer epitope with the presenting H-$2K^d$ class I molecule was not studied, future studies are needed to clarify this unexpected protein structure.

With a different experimental strategy, the use of web software tools for predictive H-2^d binding analysis enabled the identification of other epitope in the F glycoprotein of the Long strain, F249–258. This epitope could be presented by K^d class I molecules either a 9-mer (TYMLTNSEL) or a 10-mer (TYMLTNSELL) peptide [73]. No hierarchy in CTL responses to F85–93 and F249–258 epitopes was found *in vivo* during a primary response, but F249–258 was found subdominant with respect to F85–93 in secondary responses and *in vivo* memory [73].

The BALB/c mice are among the most permissive mice but others murine strains are also susceptible to HRSV infection [74]. Thus, the overlapping synthetic peptide strategy, spanning the F, G, and M proteins of HRSV was used to identify the HRSV epitopes in H-2^b mice [75]. An H-$2D^b$-restricted CTL epitope from the RSV M protein NAITNAKII, corresponding to residues 187–195 was identified [75]. In these C57Bl/6 mice, the specific CTLs for M187–195 epitope were activated with comparable kinetics to the immunodominant epitope M2 82–90 in BALB/c mice.

HUMAN MHC CLASS I EPITOPES

Using a panel of overlapping peptides spanning the complete HRSV nucleoprotein the peptide ^{308}NPKASLLSL^{316} was the first human HRSV-specific CTL epitope identified from healthy volunteers [76]. Afterward with identical experimental approach, other four viral nucleoprotein epitopes were identified in association to HLA-A2 [77] or –B8 [78] positive donors (Table 2).

Also, overlapping peptide strategy with the HRSV fusion protein shown the existence of two HLA-B57 and –Cw12-restricted CTL epitopes from young children who had just recovered from severe HRSV infection [79] (Table 2). Identically, HLA-A1-restricted CTL specific for the peptide ^{109}RELPRFMNYT^{118} of fusion protein, was isolated in peripheral blood mononuclear cells from three healthy adult volunteers [80] (Table 2).

In other study, five epitopes derived from NS2, matrix, and matrix 2 proteins of HRSV and restricted by four different HLA class I alleles (HLA-A1, -A3, -B44 and -B51) were identified selecting peptides with suitable binding motifs using the SYFPEITHI prediction software [65] from healthy donors (Table 2). All these epitopes were detected in 4-5 different donors suggesting that each dominant epitope was specifically presented by the respective HLA class I allele [81].

Thus, thirteen different HRSV $CD8^+$ epitopes have been identified either ill infants or healthy adult donors (Table 2). These human epitopes were presented by three HLA-A, five –B, and one –C class I molecules indicating wide cellular immune control against this virus. All $CD8^+$ epitopes were peptides with canonical interactions for each presenting molecule. The only exception was the absence of anchor motif for HLA-A1 class I molecule (Asp or Glu at position 3 and aromatic C-terminal residue) in the ligand ^{109}RELPRFMNYT^{118} of the fusion protein [80]. This datum indicates the complexity and plasticity of interactions in HLA-peptide complexes.

In summary, different CTL epitopes have been identified in five of six HRSV proteins previously described as recognized by human CD8^{+} T cells [56] , thus only the identification of CTL epitopes from SH protein remains open and future studies are needed.

Table 2. Summary of human MHC class I epitopes of HRSV

HLA	Sequence[a]	Protein	Position	Reference
A2	Q*L*LSSSKY*T*	Nucleoprotein	16-24	[77]
A2	K*M*LKEMGE*V*	Nucleoprotein	137-145	[77]
B8	VML*R*WGVL*A*	Nucleoprotein	258-266	[78]
A2	I*L*NNPKAS*L*	Nucleoprotein	303-311	[77]
B7	N*P*KASLLS*L*	Nucleoprotein	308-316	[76]
A1	RELPRFMNYT	Fusion	109-118	[80]
B57	R*A*RRELPR*F*	Fusion	118-126	[79]
Cw12 [b]	IAVGLLLYC	Fusion	551-559	[79]
B51	I*P*YSGLLL*V*	Matrix	195-203	[81]
A1	YL*E*KESIY*Y*	Matrix	229-237	[81]
B44	A*E*LDRTEE*Y*	Matrix 2	64-72	[81]
A3	R*L*PADVLK*K*	Matrix 2	151-159	[81]
B51	L*A*KAVIHT*I*	NS2	41-49	[81]

[a] The HLA anchor motifs are italicised.

[b] No data of HLA-Cw12 anchor motif.

Human MHC Class I Ligands Identified by Mass Spectrometry

Usually, the endogenously sintetized MHC class I ligand is assumed to be the one that has the adequate anchor motifs, the minimal length, and the optimal antigenicity when tested as a synthetic peptide. In contrast, different evidences indicate that the simple extrapolation of either MHC binding strength or antigenicity is not sufficient to identify natural viral MHC class I ligands [82, 83]. All previous studies identifying several HRSV epitopes either mice or human were performed with synthetic peptides and no formal identification of natural epitopes was performed. Thus, the high-performance liquid chromatography (HPLC) coupled to high sensitivity mass spectrometry could be a useful technology to identify the endogenously processed HLA ligands derived from HRSV in infected cells.

The strategy of this experimental approach could be summarized as follows. First, the isolation of HLA-bound peptide repertoires from cells either not infected or infected with HRSV was done. Next, both HLA/peptide pools are fractionated by HPLC in consecutive runs and under same conditions to reduce alterations in the peptide elution patterns. Later, every HPLC fraction from each peptide pool is analyzed by MALDI-TOF mass spectrometry. Each spectrum of each single HPLC fraction of HRSV-infected cells is compared with the equivalent fraction of the uninfected cells. This comparison allows the selection of peptides found only in the HRSV-infected cells. Next, the corresponding MS/MS spectrum of each differential peptide is obtained by ion-trap mass spectrometry and its amino acid sequence is assigned with bioinformatics software. In addition, the sequences are validated by comparison with the MS/MS spectrum of the corresponding synthetic peptide. With this experimental strategy, the viral amino acid sequence ^{188}AITNAKII^{195}, of the HRSV matrix protein was identified as endogenously processed and presented in infected human cells [84]. This natural ligand uses alternative interactions to the anchor motifs previously described for its presenting HLA-Cw4 class I molecule (Table 3).

Previously, the ^{187}NAITNAKII^{195} nonamer has been described as a canonical H-2D^b-restricted CTL epitope [75] in C57Bl/6 mice (Table 1) with the anchor motifs for D^b molecules: Asn at position 5 and aliphatic C-terminal residue [85]. Therefore, two viral peptide species of different lengths but sharing identical antigenic core that differ only in the respective N-terminal residue were bound to either HLA-Cw4 or H-2D^b presenting class I molecules in the respective human or mouse infected cells. Surprisingly, both the human octamer and the mouse nonamer bound efficiently to HLA-Cw4 molecules, in spite of the lack of canonical anchors for interaction with the presenting molecule.

Tagging HRSV-infected cells with stable isotope-labeled amino acids expected to be anchor residues for two different HLA class I molecules (HLA-A2, and –B7) and then performing immunoprecipitation of HLA molecules and two-dimensional HPLC-mass spectrometry analysis, two different HRSV ligands were identified [86] (Table 3). The peptide ^{33}KLIHLTNAL^{41} of the NS1 protein was an HLA-A2-restricted ligand whereas the peptide ^{551}KARSTPVTL^{559} of the fusion protein was endogenously presented by HLA-B7 in human infected cells (Table 3).

Table 3. Summary of natural HLA class I ligands of HRSV identified by mass spectrometry

HLA	Sequence[a]	Protein	Position	Reference
Cw4	AITNAKII	Matrix	188-195	[84]
A2	K*L*IHLTNA*L*	NS1	33-41	[86]
B7	KARSTPVTL	Fusion	551-559	[86]
B27	H*R*QDINGKE*M*	Nucleoprotein	100-109	[87]
B27	R*R*ANNVLKNE*M*	Nucleoprotein	184-194	[87]
B27	K*R*YKGLLPKD*I*	Nucleoprotein	195-205	[87]
B27	S*R*SALLAQ*M*	Matrix	76-84	[87]
B27	V*R*NKDLNT*L*	Matrix	169-177	[87]
B27	K*R*LPADVLK*K*	Matrix 2	150-159	[87]
B27	G*R*NEVFSN*K*	Polymerase	2089-2097	[87]
B27	L*R*NEESEKMA*K*	Phosphoprotein	198-208	[87]
B27	H*R*FIYLIN*H*	NS2	37-45	[87]

[a] The HLA anchor motifs are italicised.

Then, in all previous studies single HRSV ligand presented by each HLA molecule was exposed on the cell membrane surface. Thus, this is the rule? Or conversely, could a particular HLA molecule present different ligands of this small virus simultaneously? To answer this question, HLA-B27 ligands isolated from large amounts of human healthy or

HRSV-infected cells were analyzed using ion trap mass spectrometry. With this analysis nine naturally presented HLA-B27 ligands from six different HRSV proteins in the same infected cells were found [87] (Table 3). These the nine HLA-B27 ligands represent 2% of the HRSV proteome, which is monitored by a single HLA class I allele. The extrapolation of these data for all HLA class I molecules suggest that the cellular immune response would monitor ~ 12% of the proteome of this small virus in heterozygous HLA-A, -B and -C infected individuals. In summary, these data suggest that the cellular immune pressure could be high in some small viruses as HRSV.

Perspectives of Polyepitope Vaccine Development against HRSV

HRSV lacks effective approved vaccine or antiviral therapy. Worldwide, this virus remains one of the pathogens deemed most important for vaccine development [88]. By means of different experimental approaches, potential HRSV vaccine candidates have been developed in the last years (reviewed in [89]), including inactivated or live attenuated virus strains, vector-based, and viral protein subunit/DNA-based candidates. On the other hand, against pathogens under cellular immune control as HRSV, the polyepitope vaccine strategy could be valuable. This vaccine includes a recombinant DNA construct inserted into a viral genome (generally adenovirus or vaccinia virus) encoding a chimerical protein where different HLA class I-presented epitopes from one or various pathogens are expressed. At present, multiepitope vaccine to costimulate multiple CTL responses targeted towards various antigens are being used against different pathogens including arenavirus, Epstein Barr virus, HIV, malaria and even several cancers (reviewed in [90]) but not with HRSV. These polyepitope vaccines are safe, easy to manufacture, thermostable, and cost effective. In this context, the high resolution mass spectrometry could be a useful and practical technology to identify naturally processed pathogen-derived peptides presented by HLA class I molecules. Later, these ligands could be included in multiepitope vaccine therapeutic approach that enhances cellular immune responses [91]. To conclude, as mutations that enable escape from host cellular immunity against HRSV do not appear to accumulate with time [1], thus this virus could be a candidate particularly adequate to the polyepitope vaccine development.

Conclusion

Recent studies using high-resolution mass spectrometry and associated technologies (immunoproteomics) have allowed the identification of different endogenously processed and presented HRSV ligands. These studies open up new perspectives in HLA-ligand-based vaccine development against this virus.

Acknowledgment

This work was supported by grants provided by the FIPSE Foundation.

REFERENCES

[1] Collins,P.L., Chanock,R.M., & Murphy,B.R. (2007). *Respiratory Syncytial Virus.* In Fields Virology, Lippincott Williams & Wilkins, ed., pp. 1443-1486.

[2] Hall,C.B. (2001). Respiratory syncytial virus and parainfluenza virus. N. Engl. *J. Med. 344*, 1917-1928.

[3] Shay,D.K. et al. (2001). Bronchiolitis-associated mortality and estimates of respiratory syncytial virus-associated deaths among US children, 1979-1997. *J. Infect. Dis. 183*, 16-22.

[4] Thompson,W.W. et al. (2003). Mortality associated with influenza and respiratory syncytial virus in the United States. *JAMA 289*, 179-186.

[5] Nair,H. et al. (2010). Global burden of acute lower respiratory infections due to respiratory syncytial virus in young children: a systematic review and meta-analysis. *Lancet 375*, 1545-1555.

[6] Wendt,C.H. & Hertz,M.I. (1995). Respiratory syncytial virus and parainfluenza virus infections in the immunocompromised host. *Semin. Respir. Infect. 10*, 224-231.

[7] Ison,M.G. & Hayden,F.G. (2002). Viral infections in immunocompromised patients: what's new with respiratory viruses? *Curr. Opin. Infect. Dis. 15*, 355-367.

[8] Han,L.L.; Alexander,J.P. & Anderson,L.J. (1999). Respiratory syncytial virus pneumonia among the elderly: an assessment of disease burden. *J Infect. Dis 179*, 25-30.

[9] Falsey,A.R. et al. (2005). Respiratory syncytial virus infection in elderly and high-risk adults. *N. Engl. J. Med. 352*, 1749-1759.

[10] Mufson,M.A. et al. (1985). Two distinct subtypes of human respiratory syncytial virus. *J Gen Virol 66 (Pt 10)*, 2111-2124.

[11] Anderson,L.J. et al. (1985). Antigenic characterization of respiratory syncytial virus strains with monoclonal antibodies. *J Infect. Dis 151*, 626-633.

[12] Johnson,P.R. et al. (1987). The G glycoprotein of human respiratory syncytial viruses of subgroups A and B: extensive sequence divergence between antigenically related proteins. *Proc. Natl Acad. Sci U. S. A 84*, 5625-5629.

[13] Becker,S.; Quay,J. & Soukup,J. (1991). Cytokine (tumor necrosis factor, IL-6, and IL-8) production by respiratory syncytial virus-infected human alveolar macrophages. *J Immunol. 147*, 4307-4312.

[14] Franke-Ullmann,G. et al. (1995). Alteration of pulmonary macrophage function by respiratory syncytial virus infection in vitro. *J Immunol. 154*, 268-280.

[15] Midulla,F. et al. (1989). Respiratory syncytial virus infection of human cord and adult blood monocytes and alveolar macrophages. *Am Rev Respir. Dis 140*, 771-777.

[16] Panuska,J.R. et al. (1990). Productive infection of isolated human alveolar macrophages by respiratory syncytial virus. *J Clin Invest 86*, 113-119.

[17] Hornung,V. et al. (2004). Replication-dependent potent IFN-alpha induction in human plasmacytoid dendritic cells by a single-stranded RNA virus. *J. Immunol. 173*, 5935-5943.

[18] Rico,M.A. et al. (2009). Human respiratory syncytial virus infects and induces activation markers in mouse B lymphocytes. *Immunol. Cell Biol. 87*, 344-350.

[19] Rico,M.A. et al. (2010). TLR4-independent upregulation of activation markers in mouse B lymphocytes infected by HRSV. *Mol. Immunol. 47*, 1802-1807.
[20] Everard,M.L. et al. (1994). Analysis of cells obtained by bronchial lavage of infants with respiratory syncytial virus infection. *Arch. Dis Child 71*, 428-432.
[21] Becker,S.; Quay,J. & Soukup,J. (1991). Cytokine (tumor necrosis factor, IL-6, and IL-8) production by respiratory syncytial virus-infected human alveolar macrophages. *J Immunol. 147*, 4307-4312.
[22] Pribul,P.K. et al. (2008). Alveolar macrophages are a major determinant of early responses to viral lung infection but do not influence subsequent disease development. *J Virol 82*, 4441-4448.
[23] Graham,B.S. et al. (1991). Respiratory syncytial virus infection in anti-mu-treated mice. *J Virol 65*, 4936-4942.
[24] Mills,J. et al. (1971). Experimental respiratory syncytial virus infection of adults. Possible mechanisms of resistance to infection and illness. *J Immunol. 107*, 123-130.
[25] Holberg,C.J. et al. (1991). Risk factors for respiratory syncytial virus-associated lower respiratory illnesses in the first year of life. *Am J Epidemiol 133*, 1135-1151.
[26] The IMpact-RSV Study Group (1998). Palivizumab, a humanized respiratory syncytial virus monoclonal antibody, reduces hospitalization from respiratory syncytial virus infection in high-risk infants. *Pediatrics 102*, 531-537.
[27] Connors,M. et al. (1991). Respiratory syncytial virus (RSV) F, G, M2 (22K), and N proteins each induce resistance to RSV challenge, but resistance induced by M2 and N proteins is relatively short-lived. *J Virol. 65*, 1634-1637.
[28] Lawless-Delmedico,M.K. et al. (2000). Heptad-repeat regions of respiratory syncytial virus F1 protein form a six-membered coiled-coil complex. *Biochemistry 39*, 11684-11695.
[29] López,J.A. et al. (1998). Antigenic structure of human respiratory syncytial virus fusion glycoprotein. *J. Virol. 72*, 6922-6928.
[30] Sakurai,H. et al. (1999). Human antibody responses to mature and immature forms of viral envelope in respiratory syncytial virus infection: significance for subunit vaccines. *J Virol 73*, 2956-2962.
[31] Singleton,R. et al. (2003). Inability to evoke a long-lasting protective immune response to respiratory syncytial virus infection in mice correlates with ineffective nasal antibody responses. J Virol *77*, 11303-11311.
[32] Walsh,E.E. & Falsey,A.R. (2004). Humoral and mucosal immunity in protection from natural respiratory syncytial virus infection in adults. *J Infect. Dis 190*, 373-378.
[33] Weltzin,R. et al. (1994). Intranasal monoclonal immunoglobulin A against respiratory syncytial virus protects against upper and lower respiratory tract infections in mice. *Antimicrob. Agents Chemother. 38*, 2785-2791.
[34] Fisher,R.G. et al. (1999). Passive IgA monoclonal antibody is no more effective than IgG at protecting mice from mucosal challenge with respiratory syncytial virus. *J Infect. Dis 180*, 1324-1327.
[35] Falsey,A.R. & Walsh,E.E. (1998). Relationship of serum antibody to risk of respiratory syncytial virus infection in elderly adults. *J Infect.* Dis *177*, 463-466.
[36] Juntti,H. et al. (2009). Cytokine responses in cord blood predict the severity of later respiratory syncytial virus infection. *J Allergy Clin Immunol. 124*, 52-58.

[37] Macaubas,C. et al. (2003). Association between antenatal cytokine production and the development of atopy and asthma at age 6 years. *Lancet 362*, 1192-1197.

[38] Gern,J.E. et al. (2006). Bidirectional interactions between viral respiratory illnesses and cytokine responses in the first year of life. *J Allergy Clin Immunol. 117*, 72-78.

[39] Murai,H. et al. (2007). IL-10 and RANTES are elevated in nasopharyngeal secretions of children with respiratory syncytial virus infection. *Allergol. Int 56*, 157-163.

[40] Larranaga,C.L. et al. (2009). Impaired immune response in severe human lower tract respiratory infection by respiratory syncytial virus. Pediatr Infect. *Dis J 28*, 867-873.

[41] Munir,S. et al. (2011). Respiratory syncytial virus interferon antagonist NS1 protein suppresses and skews the human T lymphocyte response. *PLoS. Pathog. 7*, e1001336.

[42] Schlender,J. et al. (2000). Bovine respiratory syncytial virus nonstructural proteins NS1 and NS2 cooperatively antagonize alpha/beta interferon-induced antiviral response. *J. Virol. 74*, 8234-8242.

[43] Anderson,L.J. & Heilman,C.A. (1995). Protective and disease-enhancing immune responses to respiratory syncytial virus. *J Infect. Dis. 171*, 1-7.

[44] Johnson,T.R. et al. (1998). Priming with secreted glycoprotein G of respiratory syncytial virus (RSV) augments interleukin-5 production and tissue eosinophilia after RSV challenge. *Journal of Virology 72*, 2871-2880.

[45] Alwan,W.H. & Openshaw,P.J. (1993). Distinct patterns of T- and B-cell immunity to respiratory syncytial virus induced by individual viral proteins. *Vaccine 11*, 431-437.

[46] De Graaff,P.M. et al. (2004). HLA-DP4 presents an immunodominant peptide from the RSV G protein to CD4 T cells. *Virology 326*, 220-230.

[47] Graham,B.S. et al. (1991). Role of T lymphocyte subsets in the pathogenesis of primary infection and rechallenge with respiratory syncytial virus in mice. *J. Clin. Invest. 88*, 1026-1033.

[48] Alwan,W.H.; Record,F.M. & Openshaw,P.J. (1992). CD4+ T cells clear virus but augment disease in mice infected with respiratory syncytial virus. Comparison with the effects of CD8+ T cells. *Clin Exp. Immunol. 88*, 527-536.

[49] Tang,Y.W. & Graham,B.S. (1997). T cell source of type 1 cytokines determines illness patterns in respiratory syncytial virus-infected mice. *J Clin Invest 99*, 2183-2191.

[50] Chiba,Y. et al. (1989). Development of cell-mediated cytotoxic immunity to respiratory syncytial virus in human infants following naturally acquired infection. *J Med Virol. 28*, 133-139.

[51] Isaacs,D.; Bangham,C.R. & McMichael,A.J. (1987). Cell-mediated cytotoxic response to respiratory syncytial virus in infants with bronchiolitis. *Lancet 2*, 769-771.

[52] Heidema,J. et al. (2007). CD8+ T cell responses in bronchoalveolar lavage fluid and peripheral blood mononuclear cells of infants with severe primary respiratory syncytial virus infections. *J Immunol. 179*, 8410-8417.

[53] Chang,J. & Braciale,T.J. (2002). Respiratory syncytial virus infection suppresses lung $CD8^+$ T-cell effector activity and peripheral $CD8^+$ T-cell memory in the respiratory tract. *Nat. Med. 8*, 54-60.

[54] Lee,Y.M. et al. (2008). IFN-gamma production during initial infection determines the outcome of reinfection with respiratory syncytial virus. *Am J Respir. Crit Care Med 177*, 208-218.

[55] Tregoning,J.S. et al. (2010). Genetic susceptibility to the delayed sequelae of neonatal respiratory syncytial virus infection is MHC dependent. *J Immunol. 185*, 5384-5391.

[56] Cherrie,A.H. et al. (1992). Human cytotoxic T cells stimulated by antigen on dendritic cells recognize the N, SH, F, M, 22K, and 1b proteins of respiratory syncytial virus. *J Virol. 66*, 2102-2110.

[57] Kulkarni,A.B. et al. (1993). Immunization of mice with vaccinia virus-M2 recombinant induces epitope-specific and cross-reactive K^d-restricted $CD8^+$ cytotoxic T cells. *J. Virol. 67*, 4086-4092.

[58] Openshaw,P.J. et al. (1990). The 22,000-kilodalton protein of respiratory syncytial virus is a major target for Kd-restricted cytotoxic T lymphocytes from mice primed by infection. *J Virol. 64*, 1683-1689.

[59] Pemberton,R.M. et al. (1987). Cytotoxic T cell specificity for respiratory syncytial virus proteins: fusion protein is an important target antigen. *J. Gen. Virol. 68*, 2177-2182.

[60] Olson,M.R.; Hartwig,S.M. & Varga,S.M. (2008). The number of respiratory syncytial virus (RSV)-specific memory CD8 T cells in the lung is critical for their ability to inhibit RSV vaccine-enhanced pulmonary eosinophilia. *J Immunol. 181*, 7958-7968.

[61] Shastri,N.; Schwab,S. & Serwold,T. (2002). Producing nature's gene-chips: the generation of peptides for display by MHC class I molecules. *Annu. Rev. Immunol. 20*, 463-493.

[62] Rock,K.L.; York,I.A. & Goldberg,A.L. (2004). Post-proteasomal antigen processing for major histocompatibility complex class I presentation. *Nat. Immunol. 5*, 670-677.

[63] Saveanu,L. et al. (2005). Concerted peptide trimming by human ERAP1 and ERAP2 aminopeptidase complexes in the endoplasmic reticulum. *Nat. Immunol. 6*, 689-697.

[64] Parker,K.C.; Bednarek,M.A. & Coligan,J.E. (1994). Scheme for ranking potential HLA-A2 binding peptides based on independent binding of individual peptide side-chains. *J. Immunol. 152*, 163-175.

[65] Rammensee,H.G. et al. (1999). SYFPEITHI: database for MHC ligands and peptide motifs. *Immunogenetics 50*, 213-219.

[66] Bjorkman,P.J. et al. (1987). Structure of the human class I histocompatibility antigen, HLA-A2. *Nature 329*, 506-512.

[67] Bjorkman,P.J. et al. (1987). The foreign antigen binding site and T cell recognition regions of class I histocompatibility antigens. *Nature 329*, 512-518.

[68] York,I.A. et al. (1999). Proteolysis and class I major histocompatibility complex antigen presentation. *Immunol. Rev. 172*, 49-66.

[69] Kulkarni,A.B. et al. (1993). The cytolytic activity of pulmonary CD8+ lymphocytes, induced by infection with a vaccinia virus recombinant expressing the M2 protein of respiratory syncytial virus (RSV), correlates with resistance to RSV infection in mice. *J. Virol. 67*, 1044-1049.

[70] Lee,S. et al. (2007). Tissue-specific regulation of CD8+ T-lymphocyte immunodominance in respiratory syncytial virus infection. *J. Virol. 81*, 2349-2358.

[71] Chang,J.; Srikiatkhachorn,A. & Braciale,T.J. (2001). Visualization and characterization of respiratory syncytial virus F-specific $CD8^+$ T cells during experimental virus infection. *J. Immunol. 167*, 4254-4260.

[72] Jiang,S. et al. (2002). Virus-specific CTL responses induced by an H-2K^d-restricted, motif-negative 15-mer peptide from the fusion protein of respiratory syncytial virus. *J. Gen. Virol. 83*, 429-438.

[73] Johnstone,C. et al. (2004). Shifting immunodominance pattern of two cytotoxic T-lymphocyte epitopes in the F glycoprotein of the Long strain of respiratory syncytial virus. *J. Gen. Virol. 85*, 3229-3238.

[74] Prince,G.A. et al. (1979). Respiratory syncytial virus infection in inbred mice. *Infect. Immun. 26*, 764-766.

[75] Rutigliano,J.A. et al. (2005). Identification of an H-2D(b)-restricted CD8+ cytotoxic T lymphocyte epitope in the matrix protein of respiratory syncytial virus. *Virology 337*, 335-343.

[76] Goulder,P.J. et al. (2000). Characterization of a novel respiratory syncytial virus-specific human cytotoxic T-lymphocyte epitope. *J Virol 74*, 7694-7697.

[77] Terrosi,C. et al. (2007). Immunological characterization of respiratory syncytial virus N protein epitopes recognized by human cytotoxic T lymphocytes. *Viral Immunol. 20*, 399-406.

[78] Venter,M. et al. (2003). Respiratory syncytial virus nucleoprotein-specific cytotoxic T-cell epitopes in a South African population of diverse HLA types are conserved in circulating field strains. *J. Virol. 77*, 7319-7329.

[79] Brandenburg,A.H. et al. (2000). HLA class I-restricted cytotoxic T-cell epitopes of the respiratory syncytial virus fusion protein. *J Virol 74*, 10240-10244.

[80] Rock,M.T. & Crowe,J.E. (2003). Identification of a novel human leucocyte antigen-A*01-restricted cytotoxic T-lymphocyte epitope in the respiratory syncytial virus fusion protein. *Immunology 108*, 474-480.

[81] Heidema,J. et al. (2004). Human CD8(+) T cell responses against five newly identified respiratory syncytial virus-derived epitopes. *J. Gen. Virol. 85*, 2365-2374.

[82] Samino,Y. et al. (2004). An endogenous HIV envelope-derived peptide without the terminal NH_3+ group is physiologically presented by major histocompatibility class I molecules. *J. Biol. Chem. 279*, 1151-1160.

[83] Samino,Y. et al. (2006). A long N-terminal-extended nested set of abundant and antigenic major histocompatibility complex class I natural ligands from HIV envelope protein. J. Biol. Chem. *281*, 6358-6365.

[84] Infantes,S. et al. (2011). Unusual viral ligand with alternative interactions is presented by HLA-Cw4 in human respiratory syncytial virus-infected cells. Immunol. *Cell Biol. 89*, 558-565.

[85] Falk,K. et al. (1991). Allele-specific motifs revealed by sequencing of self-peptides eluted from MHC molecules. Nature 351, 290-296.

[86] Meiring,H.D. et al. (2006). Stable isotope tagging of epitopes: a highly selective strategy for the identification of major histocompatibility complex class I-associated peptides induced upon viral infection. Mol. Cell Proteomics. 5, 902-913.

[87] Infantes,S. et al. (2010). Multiple, non-conserved, internal viral ligands naturally presented by HLA-B27 in human respiratory syncytial virus-infected cells. Mol. Cell. Proteomics 9, 1533-1539.

[88] Hall,C.B. (1994). Prospects for a respiratory syncytial virus vaccine. Science 265, 1393-1394.

[89] Murata,Y. (2009). Respiratory syncytial virus vaccine development. Clin Lab Med 29, 725-739.

[90] Suhrbier,A. (2002). Polytope vaccines for the codelivery of multiple CD8 T-cell epitopes. Expert. Rev Vaccines. 1, 207-213.

[91] Ovsyannikova,I.G. et al. (2007). Mass spectrometry and peptide-based vaccine development. Clin Pharmacol. Ther. 82, 644-652.

In: Respiratory Syncytial Virus
Editors: Haneul Nam and Gippeum Kun, pp. 165-178
ISBN 978-1-62100-835-4

Chapter 5

RESPIRATORY SYNCYTIAL VIRUS DISEASE AND SEVERITY OF ILLNESS

Parthak Prodhan, M.D.[1] ***and Natan Noviski, M.D.***[2*]

[1]Department of Pediatrics, Sections of Pediatric Critical Care, Pediatric Cardiology, College of Medicine, University of Arkansas Medical Sciences, Arkansas Children's Hospital, Little Rock, Arkansas, U. S.

[2]Pediatric Critical Care Medicine, Massachusetts General Hospital *for* Children, Harvard Medical School, 175 Cambridge Street (#524), Boston, Massachusetts, U. S.

ABSTRACT

RSV is an important respiratory pathogen of infants and young children and is the most common cause of lower respiratory tract infection-related hospitalization of children under one year of age.

RSV infects over 2/3 of the birth cohort within the first year of life. It has been estimated that more than 120,000 infants in the United States are hospitalized annually with RSV infection. Clinical symptoms are the result of increased mucous production, edema and significant air-trapping. Depending on the types and sizes of airways infected, RSV causes bronchiolitis and/or bronchopneumonia.

Severe RSV disease may also lead to hospitalization and/or PICU admission, requiring, occasionally, mechanical ventilation and even ECMO. Due to the magnitude of the RSV disease impact, and the large variation of the clinical picture, the ability to predict severe RSV illnesses has become important in order to provide appropriate resources for the management of severe RSV disease. Many investigators have described the risks factors that increase the likelihood of hospitalization and of severe RSV disease. This review describes the clinical variables associated with severe RSV illness. In addition, there are predictive models, as in the case of the Michigan and the Rotterdam models, which are based on clinical and epidemiological parameters, which address the ability to predict severe RSV disease in previously healthy infants.

* Author for Correspondence:
Tel: (617)-724-4380
Fax: 617-724-4391
E-mail: nnoviski@partners.org

The role of co- infection, viral and bacterial, and nosocomial RSV infection is reviewed as well. Additionally, the current status of genetic polymorphism in RSV disease is briefly highlighted.

Keywords: children; RSV; severity.

I. Introduction

A. Epidemiology

RSV is the most common cause of childhood acute lower respiratory tract infection (ALRI) and an important cause of death. Approximately 66,000–199,000 children <5 years of age die annually from RSV-associated ALRI, with 99% of deaths occurring in developing countries (1). In the United States, RSV accounts for 20% of hospitalizations, 18% of emergency department visits, and 15% of office visits for acute respiratory infections during the winter season (2, 3). Among RSV-infected children, those who were previously healthy infants represent the largest cohort to require hospitalization though mortality rates are low (<1% of all hospitalized, infected children) in these patients (2).

B. Pathogenesis

The virus, a labile paramyxovirus, enters the host via the nasal or conjunctival mucosa and replicates within the mucosal cells followed by ongoing peribronchial inflammation, respiratory epithelial necrosis/sloughing, increased tissue edema, and excessive mucus production. The airways may become partially or completely occluded causing air trapping, hyperinflation, and atelectasis which manifests clinically as impaired oxygenation and respiratory distress (4).

Both viral (viral inoculums load, RSV subtypes) and host factors (socio-epidemiologic factors, presence of comorbidities, concentration of neutralizing antibodies, non use of prophylaxis, etc.) may explain the clinical spectrum of RSV infection so as to identify why only a small sub-set of RSV-infected children progress and have more complicated and protracted clinical courses (5).

C. Clinical Presentations

The clinical presentation of RSV ranges from that of a mild self-limiting upper respiratory tract infection and progresses to include cough, wheeze, shortness of breath, increased respiratory rate, and retractions of the respiratory muscles, indicating lower respiratory tract involvement which may require hospitalization. Lower respiratory tract involvement can manifest either as acute bronchiolitis, involving nasal mucosa to bronchioles up to 75 to 300-mm in diameter, or bronchopneumonia if the airways beyond the bronchioles are involved (6). Bronchiolitis is the more commonly observed clinical pattern and is predominantly associated with small airway obstruction with a moderate degree of parenchymal disease. The radiographic changes of hyperinflation and atelectasis are consistent with this obstructive pathophysiology. In contrast, bronchopneumonia is indicative of a more severe parenchymal lung disease with small increases in airways resistance and shows features consistent with severe restrictive pulmonary function. This pattern affects about 25%–30% of infants with RSV-associated acute respiratory failure. Patients with this pattern typically show alveolar consolidation as the main radiographic feature and may progress to acute respiratory distress syndrome and the clinical course is usually more severe compared to those presenting with bronchiolitis (7,8,9).

RSV may also present with severe disease manifesting prominent extra-pulmonary involvement (cardiac, hepatic, neurologic, sepsis-like syndrome, neuroendocrine) (10). It is plausible that the involvement of the extra-pulmonary systems are due to the presence of a higher viral load (11), or a heightened host immune response to the virus (12) causing excessive tissue injury.

Cardiovascular failure, with hypotension and inotrope requirement, myocardial injury, cardiac arrhythmias (sinoatrial blocks, supraventricular tachycardia, complex atrial tachycardia, and complete heart block, ventricular tachycardia), and pericardial effusion with tamponade, can occur in RSV-infected children particularly in those cared for in the ICUs (13-16). Myocardial injury, measured by using troponin I levels, in previously healthy children with RSV infection admitted to the ICU, is more frequently seen in younger children (75% in <3 months old), and is associated with a greater need for mechanical ventilation and required inotrope support especially in those with the highest troponin I levels (15). A positive cardiac troponin I (>0.3 ng/mL) correctly identified RSV-infected children who require mechanical ventilation (16).

Elevated blood transaminase levels are seen in about 46% of ventilated patients for RSV infection (17,18). Those with elevated transaminases have a significantly longer duration of mechanical ventilation (mean 10.6 days versus 3.5 days) and more inotrope use. All deaths occurred in the group with elevated transaminase levels and the elevation was more often seen in those with congenital heart disease (86% in patients with congenital heart disease compared to 27% in those without congenital heart disease). This elevation in transaminases may be due to hepatitis in the patients; however in those with underlying congenital heart disease, ischemic hepatitis due to hepatic venous congestion from right ventricular failure may also be a contributing factor.

Acute neurological manifestations which include central apneas, seizures, lethargy, feeding or swallowing difficulties, abnormalities of tone or strabismus, cerebrospinal fluid abnormalities, abnormal diaphragmatic flutter, and electroencephalogram findings are found in up to 39% of RSV-positive patients admitted to ICUs (19-24). In those with milder RSV disease admitted to the general pediatric ward, neurological complications, excluding patients with simple febrile convulsions, were found in 1.2% of patients (19). Central apnea, one of the more common manifestations, may be the first sign of RSV disease in children. Apneas, defined as respiratory arrest >20 seconds and/or bradycardia with accompanying cyanosis or oxygen desaturation below 90% have been found in 16%– 21% of children admitted to hospitals with RSV infection (21). Patients with apnea tend to be younger, have significantly lower temperature, higher $pCO2$, lower pH at presentation, more atelectasis on chest radiographs, and a significantly increased probability of requiring ICU admission and mechanical ventilation. The relative risk for mechanical ventilation increases with the number of apneic episodes. Apnea at admission was also a strong predictor for recurrent apnea.

Seizures were also reported more commonly in those admitted to the ICU (6.6% versus 0.7% for pediatric ward admissions) and included both generalized tonic–clonic and partial/complex partial seizures with/without secondary generalization (24) with rare cases of status epilepticus.

D. Defining Disease Severity

Critical review of the literature related to RSV-related illness severity, and its prediction, requires the reader to be cognizant of the following issues: (a) severe RSV disease has been defined as the need for supplemental oxygen, hospitalization, transfer to a higher level of care once hospitalized and prolonged hospital length of stay. While for those requiring intensive care unit (ICU) admission, end-points may suggest a more complicated clinical course which includes mortality, length of mechanical ventilation and prolonged ICU stay; (b) whether studies included at-risk sub-groups or only previously healthy children as part of their study cohort; (c) variation in physician practice and indications for higher level of care among different countries across the world, and (d) whether the study was done in the pre-prophylaxis or the post-prophylaxis era as risk factors may have been modified with the use of prophylaxis.

II. Predictors of Severe Disease

Several epidemiologic, clinical, biochemical and genetic factors have been investigated to identify various sub-groups among those infected with RSV who are at risk for increased morbidity and mortality. This identification of risk factors has several important clinical and research implications, i.e., selection of patients for efficacy and effectiveness studies, validation of similar treatment groups, assessment of severity of illness status, length of stay adjustment from diverse hospital settings, and assessment of resource utilization so as to help select patient sub-groups who should receive expensive or limited available therapies.

A. Clinical Predictors

1. Socio-Economic Factors

Several environmental and demographic factors reported to be associated with severe RSV lower respiratory tract disease include male gender, age <6 months, birth during the first half of the RSV season, crowding/siblings, and daycare exposure are significant risk factors for severe RSV LRI (25). In contrast, many studies suggest that passively acquired maternal antibody and breast-feeding are protective against severe RSV disease (25).

2. Co-morbidities

Co-morbid conditions in RSV- infected children add substantially to the risk of having worse outcomes. Thorburn *et al* (26) reviewed their institutional ICU cohort of 406 RSV-positive children and noted that 98.5% required mechanical ventilation and 8.6 % of the children died (n=35). All children who died had pre-existing medical conditions. 54% (n=19) of children had pre-existing disease in 2 or more organ systems. The presence of multiple comorbidities has an additive adverse impact on outcomes (27). For instance, whereas prematurity itself, without chronic lung disease, adversely affects the outcome of RSV infection, the accompanying presence of chronic lung disease of prematurity has a much greater negative effect.

Comorbid conditions well described to date include the presence of underlying prematurity (28-30); underlying pulmonary disease (31-33) such as cystic fibrosis, recurrent aspiration pneumonia, pulmonary malformations, neurogenic disorders interfering with pulmonary toilet, congenital diaphragmatic hernia, and tracheoesophageal fistula; congenital/acquired immunodeficiency states (34-38) such as malignancy, organ transplants, congenital immunodeficiency, and human immunodeficiency virus infection; and heart disease (39-41).

Additional studies have recently identified additional comorbid conditions associated with worse outcomes in RSV-infected children. These include the presence of obesity (42), central nervous system anomalies (43), neuromuscular disorders (44), congenital malformations and chromosomal abnormalities, including Down syndrome (45,46). Neuromuscular impairment (NMI) was noted in 4.7% (n=73 children out of 1541 patients) of a large RSV-infected multi-center study cohort (44). Even though approximately half of these NMI patients had at least 1 additional risk factor to explain a severe clinical course, multivariate logistic regression confirmed NMI to be independently associated with pediatric ICU admission and need for mechanical ventilation. (44). Similarly, certain congenital malformations such as congenital hydrocephalus without spina bifida, choanal atresia, agenesis, hypoplasia, dysgenesis of the lung, and cleft lip/palate in RSV-infected children were associated with a prolonged hospital stay and a higher rate of mechanical ventilation in the first 2 years of life (43). A more severe clinical course may be due to impaired ability to clear airway secretions as a result of ineffective cough, respiratory muscle weakness, recurrent microaspiration, history of frequent exposure to antibiotics and hospitalizations, colonization with resistant pathogens, and impaired immunologic defense mechanisms due to severe malnutrition and cachexia. Any acute viral infection, in particular if associated with airway obstruction, could aggravate respiratory muscle fatigue and predispose children to severe hypoxemia and hypercapnia.

3. Nosocomial RSV Infection

During seasonal outbreaks, up to 6% of all RSV infection in hospitalized children may be attributed to nosocomial spread (47,48,49) of particle droplets shed and carried via hands or fomites with subsequent transfer to an uninfected person by patients or health care workers. Up to 45% of contacts can acquire RSV infection during such spreads (47). Within the ICUs, persistent shedders of RSV are an important potential source of nosocomial RSV infection. Nosocomial RSV infection causes increased morbidity and mortality particularly (26,47,48) in children with comorbidities who demonstrate a doubling in hospital stay attributable to RSV and a 10-fold increase in mortality risk (47). Up to 60% of mechanically ventilated cohorts with nosocomial RSV infection had at least 1 additional comorbid condition (48). The fact that half of the cases occurred in premature infants, particularly in those with severe chronic lung disease, highlights the importance of enforcing strict droplet precautions measures, deferring elective cardio-respiratory surgery to non-epidemic seasons, or to avoid if possible, admission of high-risk children to hospitals during the RSV outbreak season.

4. Co-infection

Co-infection with bacteria and other viruses in RSV-infected children is not uncommon. The incidence of serious bacterial infection (1.2%), bacteremia (0.6%) or urinary tract infection (2%) is low in young children with acute bronchiolitis, or more specifically, with RSV infection. (50-52). However, pulmonary bacterial co-infection among those requiring ICU care range from 17.5% to 44%, (53-56). Patients with bacterial co-infection require significantly longer ventilatory support and have a higher risk of mortality. Clinical features, routine laboratory tests, and radiologic finding do not reliably differentiate infants with RSV from those with co-infections. Among bacterial infection, co-infection with *Bordetella* requires special mention as pertussis (culture/ PCR positive) co-infection was noted in 16%–74% of infants hospitalized with RSV (57).

Recent molecular techniques for viral detection have further enhanced the ability to identify viral co-infection with RSV. Up to 60% of children co-infected with RSV and human metapneumovirus (hMPV) (58,59), which is closely related to RSV, may require ICU care (60). hMPV-RSV co-infection has been noted in up to 70% (61) of mechanically ventilated infants with severe bronchiolitis and is associated with a 10-fold increase in relative risk of admission to the ICU for mechanical ventilation (62).

5. Genetic Variations

More than 20 independent studies to date have assessed the impact of at least 40 genetic variations—mostly single nucleotide polymorphisms— in association studies to identify high-risk patients with RSV infection (63). Despite the amount of information available, we are still far from evolving a practical and cost-effective screening tool based on whether knowledge derived from case control studies can be applied to disease management practices. Flaws in many of these studies include inconsistently-defined phenotypes, small sample sizes, studies conducted with different ethnic groups, and false-positive and false-negative associations, have not been re-evaluated prospectively or their results have not been reproducible. Furthermore, many studies have failed to adequately assess the contribution of particular candidate gene locus as they have screened single nucleotide polymorphisms independently instead of screening haplotypes defined on the basis of linkage disequilibrium.

B. Prediction Models

Current investigations in developing prediction models, in contrast to earlier studies, have tended to include more homogenous patient sub-sets to identify high-risk groups among children with RSV infection. However, most scores or prediction models used in RSV-infected children have been criticized for their lack of reproducibility and inter-observer variability and are subject to era effect. Further, many of the prediction models have either not been rigorously developed or have not been tested in subsequent validation studies in diverse clinical settings.

The FLIP (**F**actors that most **L**ikely may lead to development of RSV related respiratory **I**nfection and subsequent hospital admission among **P**remature infants born 33–35 weeks) study (64) (n= 186 hospitalized infants with 371 age-matched controls from 50 Spanish hospitals during the 2002–2003 RSV season) identified 7 risk factors (birth within 10 weeks of the beginning of the RSV season, birth weight, breast fed <2 months, number of siblings >2 years, number of family members with atopy, number of family members with wheezing, and gender) with the highest probability of differentiating hospitalized and non-hospitalized infants with RSV. The model had a predictive accuracy of 71% and the area under the receiver-operator curve (AUC) of 0.79. This initial FLIP study model has subsequently been validated in multiple studies from Canada and Europe (65-67). However, a recent follow-up study by the FLIP investigators (FLIP 2) (68) to validate the findings from the original FLIP study found only 3 independent risk factors (absolute chronologic age of <10 weeks at the onset of RSV season, presence of school-age siblings or daycare attendance, and maternal smoking during pregnancy) that significantly increase the risk of RSV-related respiratory infection and hospitalization. Further validations of these results are required in future studies.

A practical, easy-to-use instrument, RSV risk scoring tool to guide judicious RSV prophylaxis for moderate- to high-risk, 33-35-wGA infants was similarly developed and validated in Canada (69). This scoring tool includes 7 risk factors: cosine transformation of birth month; subject or siblings attending daycare; more than 5 individuals in the home including the subject; small for gestational age (SGA); absence of eczema in the family history; gender; and more than 1 smoker in the household. Cutoff scores of 0–48, 49–64, and 65–100 for low-, moderate-, and high-risk subjects, respectively, were created. The tool had a sensitivity of 68.2% and a specificity of 71.9% in identifying those requiring hospitalization and was cost-effective in reducing hospitalization in infants who are most at-risk while avoiding prophylaxis in a large segment (81.9%) of their low-risk GA cohort. However, the risk scoring tool did not perform well when applied to term infants (70).

Ritveild, *et al*, (71) utilizing a retrospective Dutch cohort (2469 hospitalized children with RSV with 140,661 children who were 1,181,790 months at risk in the community) developed a clinical prediction rule to reliably estimate individual monthly risks of hospitalization for RSV infection and discriminate between high- and low-risk children. They found that age and the seasonal monthly RSV pattern were the strongest predictors, while gestational age, presence of bronchopulmonary dysplasia, birth weight, and gender were less important for identifying a high-risk group (AUC of the prediction rule for all children at risk= 0.80, premature children with gestational age <33 or 37 weeks, the AUCs were 0.75 and 0.80, respectively).

In term infants, Houben, *et al*, (72) using a prospective Dutch birth cohort study (n= 298), recently proposed a simple clinical prediction rule to identify those at risk of RSV LRTI in the first year of life. Significant predictors included daycare attendance and/or the presence of siblings, high parental education levels, birth weight of >4 kg, and month of birth between April and September [AUC 0.72 (95% confidence interval: 0.64–0.80)], and a scoring system (score ranged from 0 to 5 points) devised based on these predictors showed that the absolute risk of RSV LRTI was 3% for children with scores of ≤ 2 (20% of all children) and 32% for children with all 4 factors (i.e., a score of 5).

Moler, *et al* (73) developed a prediction model (Michigan model) using a retrospective cohort obtained from 9 RSV epidemics from 1983-1992 and reported that 9 predictor variables measured at admission/during first 24 hours of hospitalization (log weight, congenital heart disease, failure to thrive, premature birth, bronchopulmonary dysplasia, other pulmonary diseases, miscellaneous conditions, early mechanical ventilation, and early ribavirin treatment) better identified those more likely to require prolonged hospitalization (AUC= 0.89). Validation of the Michigan model was of particular interest for investigators in the Netherlands where the mean duration of hospitalization was approximately twice that in the United States. Kneyber *et al*, (74) studied an RSV cohort obtained from 1992-1995 (n=177 children <12 months of age) for validating the Michigan model using a Dutch study cohort. The Michigan model performed poorly when applied to the Dutch cohort (AUC=0.65). Using the same cohort, the Rotterdam model identified only weight and oxygen supplementation as independent predictors for a prolonged hospital stay (> 9 days, median for their database). The AUC for the developmental model was 0.65 and the validation model using another RSV patent cohort (from the 1995–1996 season) was poor (AUC= 0.52). Additional limitations of the Michigan model were that it did not include clinical variables like hypoxia or chest radiographic findings.

Few studies have investigated clinical variables to accurately identify among RSV infected infants seen in the emergency room or those on the general pediatric floor who would require ICU. Damore *et al,* (75) in a prospective multicenter ED-based (30 EDs in US) study cohort of 1,456 enrolled patients in 2004-2006 of children admitted for bronchiolitis identified four independent predictors of ICU admission (age <2 months, an ED visit the past week, moderate / severe retractions, and inadequate oral intake (AUC= 0.80). Surprisingly, the initial RR, initial oxygen saturation, and lowest oxygen saturation were not found to be independent predictors of ICU admission. However, this study was not specific to RSV infected infants only, and only created a derivational model and no validation, and issues concerning subjectivity in defining poor oral intake and degree of retractions were also noted.

Brook *et al,* (76) assessed variables obtained from the clinical history, physical examination, oximetry, and chest radiographic findings at the time of presentation to accurately identify among previously healthy infants with RSV infection hospitalized on a general pediatric floor clinical deterioration leading to ICU transfer. They found that a respiratory rate of >80/ minute and an oxygen saturation <85% at time of presentation in the ED each had a specificity >97% for predicting subsequent deterioration. Each parameter, however, had a sensitivity <30%. Other studies in infants bronchiolitis have found other cutoffs for respiratory rate (>45/breaths per minute), oxygen saturation (< 95% and < 90%) to be more predictive of ICU admission (77-81). The presence of lethargy, grunting, and an arterial partial pressure of CO2 of > 65 mmHg on initial presentation in the emergency department were also associated with the subsequent need for mechanical ventilation in the ICU (82).

Critically ill children with co-morbidities with RSV infection when hospitalized in the ICU have prolonged duration of mechanical ventilation, and ICU length of stay (83). In mechanically ventilated RSV infected infants without associated co-morbidities, the time course of intensive care may be predicted based on early respiratory and radiologic parameters during the first 48 hours of mechanical ventilation (8, 9). Tasker et al, initially, generated from a retrospective cohort of 45 infants, parameters which would identify infants with more severe lower airway disease, as demonstrated by four-quadrant consolidation on chest X-ray. During the first 24 hours of mechanical ventilator support, an alveolar arterial oxygen gradient of (AaDO2) > 400 and mean airway pressure (MAP) > 10 had a positive and negative predictive value of 100% and 97%, respectively; in the second 24 hours, AaDO2 >

300 and MAP > 10 had a positive and negative predictive value of 91% and 100%, respectively. Subsequently in a second study, a prospective, hypothesis-testing, analysis of length-of-stay in 44 infants stratified according to the above AaDO2 and MAP criteria demonstrated that it correlates with significantly longer ICU length of stay (median 17 versus 7 days).

CONCLUSION

Over the past 2 decades, many studies have attempted to identify "at-risk" groups to develop severe RSV disease. In the post-prophylaxis era many of the studies focus on identifying at-risk groups within sub-sets who should be candidates for passive immunization. In the current era of emphasis on personalized medicine, it is possible that severe RSV disease can be predicted through a combination of clinical and genetic factors.

ACKNOWLEDGEMENT

We acknowledge Ms Suzanne Speakers' contribution in editing the manuscript.

REFERENCES

[1] Nair H, Nokes DJ, Gessner BD, et al. Global burden of acute lower respiratory infections due to respiratory syncytial virus in young children: a systematic review and meta-analysis. *Lancet.* 2010;375:1545-55.

[2] Hall CB, Weinberg GA, Iwane MK, et al. The burden of respiratory syncytial virus infection in young children. *N Engl J Med.* 2009;360:588-98.

[3] Centers for Disease Control and Prevention (CDC). Respiratory syncytial virus activity - United States, July 2008-December 2009. *MMWR Morb Mortal Wkly Rep.* 2010;59:230-3.

[4] Spencer H. Pathology of the lung. Oxford, UK: Pergamon Press, 1985; 131–65.

[5] Welliver RC. Review of epidemiology and clinical risk factors for severe respiratory syncytial virus (RSV) infection. *J Pediatr.* 2003;143:S112-S117.

[6] Newth CJL. Time course of severe respiratory syncytial virus infection in mechanically ventilated infants. *Acta Paediatr.* 2000;89: 893-99.

[7] Hammer J, Numa A, CJL Newth. Acute respiratory distress syndrome caused by respiratory syncytial virus. *Pediatr. Pulmonol.* 1997;23:176–83.

[8] Tasker RC.Time course of severe respiratory syncytial virus infection in mechanically ventilated infants. *Acta Pædiatr.* 2000; 89:938–41.

[9] Prodhan P, Westra SJ, Lin J, Karni-Sharoor S, Regan S, Noviski N.Chest radiological patterns predict the duration of mechanical ventilation in children with RSV infection. *Pediatr Radiol.* 2009;39:117-23.

[10] Eisenhut M. Extrapulmonary manifestations of severe respiratory syncytial virus infection – a systematic review. *Crit Care.* 2006;10:R107-12.

[11] Fodha I, Vabret A, Ghedira L, et al. Respiratory syncytial virus infections in hospitalized infants: association between viral load, virus subgroup, and disease severity. *J Med Virol.* 2007;79:1951-58.

[12] Amanatidou V, Apostolakis S, Spandidos DA. Genetic diversity of the host and severe respiratory syncytial virus-induced lower respiratory tract infection. *Pediatr Infect Dis J.* 2009;28:135-40.

[13] Donnerstein RL, Berg RA, Shehab Z et al. Complex atrial tachycardias and respiratory syncytial virus infections in infants. *J Pediatr.*1994;125:23-8.

[14] Armstrong DS, Menahem S. Cardiac arrhythmias as a manifestation of acquired heart disease in association with paediatric respiratory syncitial virus infection. *J Paediatr Child Health.* 1993;29:309-11.

[15] Checchia PA, Appel HJ, Kahn S et al. Myocardial injury in children with respiratory syncytial virus infection. Pediatr Crit Care Med. 2000;1:146-50.

[16] Moynihan JA, Brown L, Sehra R et al. Cardiac troponin I as a predictor of respiratory failure in children hospitalized with respiratory syncytial virus (RSV) infections: a pilot study. *Am J Emerg Med.* 2003;21:479-82.

[17] Eisenhut M, Thorburn K: Hepatitis associated with severe respiratory syncytial virus positive lower respiratory tract infection. *Scand J Infect Dis.* 2002; 34:235-38.

[18] Eisenhut M, Thorburn K, Ahmed T. Transaminase levels in ventilated children with respiratory syncytial virus bronchiolitis. *Intensive Care Med.* 2004;30:931-34.

[19] Sweetman LL, Ng Y-T, Butler IJ, Bodensteiner JB: Neurologic complications associated with respiratory syncytial virus. *Pediatr Neurol.* 2005;32:307-10.

[20] Ng Y-T, Cox C, Atkins J, Butler IJ: Encephalopathy associated with respiratory syncytial virus bronchiolitis. *J Child Neurol.* 2001;16:105-08.

[21] Kneyber MC, Brandenburg AH, de Groot R, et al. Risk factors for respiratory syncytial virus associated apnoea. *Eur J Pediatr.* 1998 ;157:331-35.

[22] Zlateva KT, Van Ranst MV: Detection of subgroup B respiratory syncytial virus in the cerebrospinal fluid of a patient with respiratory syncytial virus pneumonia. *Pediatr Infect Dis J.* 2004;23:1065-66.

[23] Adams JA, Zabaleta IA, Sackner MA: Diaphragmatic flutter in three babies with bronchopulmonary dysplasia and respiratory syncytial virus bronchiolitis. *Pediatr Pulmono.l* 1995;19:312-16.

[24] Kho N, Kerrigan JF, Tong T, et al. Respiratory syncytial virus infection and neurologic abnormalities: retrospective cohort study. *J Child Neurol.* 2004;19:859-64.

[25] Simoes EAF. Environmental and demographic risk factors for respiratory syncytial virus lower respiratory tract disease. *J Pediatr.* 2003;143:S118-26.

[26] Thorburn K. Pre-existing disease is associated with a significantly higher risk of death in severe respiratory syncytial virus infection. *Arch Dis Child.*2009;94:99–103.

[27] Purcell K, Fergie J. Concurrent serious bacterial infections in 2396 infants and children hospitalized with respiratory syncytial virus lower respiratory tract infections. *Arch Pediatr Adolesc Med.* 2002;156:322–24.

[28] Simon A, Ammann RA, Wilkesmann A, et al. DSM RSV Paed Study Group. Respiratory syncytial virus infection in 406 hospitalized premature infants: results from a prospective German multicenter database. *Eur J Pediatr.* 2007;166:1273–83.

[29] Broughton S, Bhat R, Roberts A, et al. Diminished lung function, RSV infection, and respiratory morbidity in prematurely born infants. *Arch Dis Child.* 2006;91:26–30.

[30] Liese JG, Grill E, Fischer B, et al. Incidence and risk factors of respiratory syncytial virus-related hospitalizations in premature infants in Germany. *Eur J Pediatr.* 2003;162:230–36.
[31] Arnold SR, Wang EE, Law BJ, et al. Variable morbidity of respiratory syncytial virus infection in patients with underlying lung disease: a review of the PICNIC RSV database. Pediatric investigators collaborative network on infections in Canada. *Pediatr Infect Dis J.* 1999;18:866–69.
[32] Robinson KA, Odelola OA, Saldanha I, McKoy N. Palivizumab for prophylaxis against respiratory syncytial virus infection in children with cystic fibrosis. *Cochrane Database Syst Rev.* 2010;2:CD007743.
[33] Speer ME, Fernandes CJ, Boron M, Groothuis JR. Use of Palivizumab for prevention of hospitalization as a result of respiratory syncytial virus in infants with cystic fibrosis. *Pediatr Infect Dis J.*2008;27:559–61.
[34] Hall CB, Powell KR, MacDonald NE, et al. Respiratory syncytial viral infection in children with compromised immune function. *N Engl J Med.*1986;315:77–81.
[35] Madhi SA, Venter M, Madhi A, et al. Differing manifestations of respiratory syncytial virus-associated severe lower respiratory tract infections in human immunodeficiency virus type 1-infected and uninfected children. *Pediatr Infect Dis J.* 2001;20:164–70.
[36] Sung L, Alonzo TA, Gerbing RB, Aplenc R, et al. Children's Oncology Group. Respiratory syncytial virus infections in children with acute myeloid leukemia: a report from the Children's Oncology Group. *Pediatr Blood Cancer.* 2008;51:784-86.
[37] Khanna N, Widmer AF, Decker M, et al.. Respiratory syncytial virus infection in patients with hematological diseases: single-center study and review of the literature. Clin Infect Dis. 2008;46:402-12.
[38] El Saleeby CM, Somes GW, DeVincenzo JP, Gaur AH. Risk factors for severe respiratory syncytial virus disease in children with cancer: the importance of lymphopenia and young age. *Pediatrics.* 2008;121:235–43.
[39] Altman CA, Englund JA, Demmler G et al. Respiratory syncytial virus in patients with congenital heart disease: a contemporary look at epidemiology and success of preoperative screening. *Pediatr Cardiol.* 2000; 21:433-38.
[40] Kristensen K, Stensballe LG, Bjerre J, et al. Risk factors for respiratory syncytial virus hospitalisation in children with heart disease. *Arch Dis Child.* 2009;94:785–89.
[41] Feltes TF, Cabalka AK, Meissner HC, et al. Palivizumab prophylaxis reduces hospitalization due to respiratory syncytial virus in young children with hemodynamically significant congenital heart disease. *J Pediatr.* 2003;143:532–40.
[42] Akiyama N, Segawa T, Ida H, et al. Bimodal effects of obesity ratio on disease duration of respiratory syncytial virus infection in children. *Allergol Int.* 2011 Mar 25. [Epub ahead of print]
[43] Zachariah P, Ruttenber M, Simões EA. Hospitalizations due to respiratory syncytial virus in children with congenital malformations. *Pediatr Infect Dis J.* 2011;30:442-45.
[44] Wilkesmann A, Ammann RA, Schildgen O, et al. DSM RSV Ped Study Group. Hospitalized children with respiratory syncytial virus infection and neuromuscular impairment face an increased risk of a complicated course. *Pediatr Infect Dis J.* 2007;26:485–91.
[45] Megged O, Schlesinger Y. Down syndrome and respiratory syncytial virus infection. *Pediatr Infect Dis J.* 2010;29:672–73.

[46] Bloemers BL, van Furth AM, Weijerman ME, et al. Down syndrome: a novel risk factor for respiratory syncytial virus bronchiolitis—a prospective birth-cohort study. *Pediatrics*. 2007;120:e1076–81.

[47] Langley JM, LeBlanc JC, Wang EE, et al. Nosocomial respiratory syncytial virus infection in Canadian pediatric hospitals: a Pediatric Investigators Collaborative Network on Infections in Canada Study. *Pediatrics*. 1997;100:943-46.

[48] Simon A, Müller A, Khurana K, et al. DSM RSV Paed Study Group. Nosocomial infection: a risk factor for a complicated course in children with respiratory syncytial virus infection--results from a prospective multicenter German surveillance study. *Int J Hyg Environ Health*. 2008;211:241-50.

[49] Thorburn K, Kerr S, Taylor N, van Saene HK. RSV outbreak in a paediatric intensive care unit. *J Hosp Infect*. 2004;57:194-201.

[50] Melendez E, Harper MB. Utility of sepsis evaluation in infants 90 days of age or younger with fever and clinical bronchiolitis. *Pediatr Infect Dis J*. 2003;22:1053–56.

[51] Levine DA, Platt SL, Dayan PS, et al. Risk of serious bacterial infection in young febrile infants with respiratory syncytial virus infections. *Pediatrics*. 2004;113:1728 – 34.

[52] Titus MO, Wright SW. Prevalence of serious bacterial infections in febrile infants with respiratory syncytial virus infection. *Pediatrics*. 2003;112:282–84.

[53] Randolph AG, Reder L, Englund JA. Risk of bacterial infection in previously healthy respiratory syncytial virus-infected young children admitted to the intensive care unit. *Pediatr Infect Dis J*. 2004;23:990-94.

[54] Kneyber MC, Blussé van Oud-Alblas H, van Vliet M, et al. Concurrent bacterial infection and prolonged mechanical ventilation in infants with respiratory syncytial virus lower respiratory tract disease. *Intensive Care Med*. 2005;31:680-85.

[55] Duttweiler L, Nadal D, Frey B. Pulmonary and systemic bacterial co-infections in severe RSV bronchiolitis. *Arch Dis Child*. 2004;89:1155–57.

[56] Thorburn K, Harigopal S, Reddy V, et al. High incidence of pulmonary bacterial co-infection in children with severe respiratory syncytial virus (RSV) bronchiolitic. *Thorax*. 2006;61;611-61.

[57] Cosnes-Lambe C, Raymond J, Chalumeau M, Pons-Catalano C, et al. Pertussis and respiratory syncytial virus infections. *Eur J Pediatr*. 2008;167:1017–19.

[58] Aberle JH, Aberle SW, Pracher E, et al. Single versus dual respiratory virus infections in hospitalized infants. *Pediatr Infect Dis J*. 2005; 24:605–10.

[59] Wilkesmann A, Schildgen O, Eis-Hübinger AM, et al.Human metapneumovirus infections cause similar symptoms and clinical severity as respiratory syncytial virus infections. *Eur J Pediatr*. 2006;165: 467–75.

[60] Semple MG, Cowell A, Dove W, Greensill J, McNamara PS, Halfhide C, Shears P, Smyth RL, Hart CA. Dual infection of infants by human metapneumovirus and human respiratory syncytial virus is strongly associated with severe bronchiolitis. *J Infect Dis*. 2005; 191:382–86.

[61] Greensill J, McNamara PS, Dove W, et al. Human metapneumovirus in severe respiratory syncytial virus bronchiolitis. *Emerg Infect Dis*. 2003; 9: 372–75.

[62] Stempel HE, Martin ET, Kuypers J, et al. Multiple viral respiratory pathogens in children with bronchiolitis. *Acta Paediatr*. 2009;98:123-26.

[63] Amanatidou V, Apostolakis S, Sapndidos DA. Genetic diversity of the host and severe respiratory syncytial virus-induced lower respiratory tract infection. *Pediatr Infect Dis J.* 2009;28:135–40.

[64] Figueras-Aloy J, Carbonell-Estrany X, Quero J. IRIS Study Group. Case-control study of the risk factors linked to respiratory syncytial virus infection requiring hospitalization in premature infants born at a gestational age of 33–35 weeks in Spain. *Pediatr Infect Dis J.* 2004;23:815–20.

[65] Lanari M, Adorni F, Silvestri M, Coscia A, Musicco M and Italian Study Group on Risk Factors for RSV-related Hospitalization. The multicenter Italian birth cohort study on incidence and determinants of lower respiratory tract infection hospitalization in infants at 33 weeks GA or more: Preliminary results. *Early Hum Dev.* 2011;87S:S43–S46.

[66] Simoes EA, Carbonell-Estrany X, Fullarton JR, et al. A predictive model for respiratory syncytial virus (RSV) hospitalization of premature infants born at 33–35 weeks of gestational age, based on data from the Spanish FLIP study. *Respir Res.* 2008;9:78-83.

[67] Simões EA, Carbonell-Estrany X, Fullarton JR, et al. European risk factors' model to predict hospitalization of premature infants born 33–35 weeks gestational age with respiratory syncytial virus: validation with Italian data. J Matern Fetal Neonatal Med.2010 May 21 [Epub ahead of print].

[68] Figueras-Aloy J, Carbonell-Estrany X, Quero-Jiménez J, et al. FLIP-2 Study: risk factors linked to respiratory syncytial virus infection requiring hospitalization in premature infants born in Spain at a gestational age of 32 to 35 weeks. *Pediatr Infect Dis J.* 2008;27:788–93.

[69] Sampalis JS, Langley J, Carbonell-Estrany X, et al. Hospitalization in premature Infants born at 33 through 35 completed weeks of gestation development and validation of a Risk Scoring Tool to predict respiratory syncytial virus. *Med Decis Making.* 2008;28: 471-75.

[70] Paes B, Cole M, Latchman A, Pinelli J. Predictive value of the respiratory syncytial virus risk-scoring tool in the term infant in Canada. *Curr Med Res Opin.* 2009;25:2191-6.

[71] Rietveld E, Vergouwe Y, Steyerberg EW, et al. Hospitalization for respiratory syncytial virus infection in young children: development of a clinical prediction rule. *Pediatr Infect Dis J.* 2006;25:201–7.

[72] Houben ML, Bont L, Wilbrink B et al. Clinical prediction rule for RSV bronchiolitis in healthy newborns: *Prognostic Birth Cohort Study Pediatrics.* 2011;127;35-41.

[73] Moler FW, Ohmit SE. Severity of illness models for respiratory syncytial virus-associated hospitalisation. *Am J Respir Crit Care Med.* 1999;159:1234–40.

[74] Kneyber MCJ, Moons KGM, de Groot R, Moll HA. Prediction of duration of hospitalization in respiratory syncytial virus infection. *Pediatr Pulmonol.* 2002;33:453–57.

[75] Damore D, Mansbach JM, Clark S, Ramundo M, Camargo Jr CA. Prospective multicenter bronchiolitis study: Predicting intensive care unit admissions. *Acad Emer Med.* 2008; 15:887–94.

[76] Brooks AM, McBride JT, McConnochie KM, et al. Predicting deterioration in previously healthy infants hospitalized with respiratory syncytial virus infection. *Pediatrics*. 1999;104:463– 67.

[77] Wang EE, Law BJ, Stephens D and Pediatric Investigators Collaborative Network on Infections in Canada (PICNIC) prospective study of risk factors and outcomes in patients hospitalized with respiratory syncytial viral lower respiratory tract infection. J Pediatr. 1995;126:212–19.

[78] Opavsky MA, Stephens D, Wang EE. Testing models predicting severity of respiratory syncytial virus infection on the PICNIC RSV database. Pediatric Investigators Collaborative Network on Infections in Canada. *Arch Pediatr Adolesc Med*. 1995; 149:1217–20.

[79] McConnochie KM, Hall CB, Walsh EE, Roghmann KJ. Variation in severity of respiratory syncytial virus infections with subtype. *J Pediatr*. 1990; 117:52–62.

[80] Voets S, van Berlaer G, Hachimi-Idrissi S. Clinical predictors of the severity of bronchiolitis. *Eur J Emer Med*. 2006, 13:134–38.

[81] Prodhan P, Sharoor-Karni S, Lin J, Noviski N. Predictors of respiratory failure among previously healthy children with respiratory syncytial virus infection. *Am J Emerg Med*. 2011;29:168-73.

[82] Buckingham SC, Quasney MW, Bush AJ, DeVincenzo JP. Respiratory syncytial virus infections in the pediatric intensive care unit: Clinical characteristics and risk factors for adverse outcomes. *Pediatr Crit Care Med*. 2001; 2:318 –23.

INDEX

A

access, 9, 22, 28, 131
acid, vii, 2, 9, 10, 13, 53, 70, 85, 135, 157
acquired immunity, 92
adaptive immunity, 112
adenosine, 25, 111
adenovirus, 3, 4, 15, 79, 119, 158
adhesion, 101, 103, 105
adjustment, 168
adolescents, 79
aerosols, 128
age, vii, viii, ix, 1, 3, 4, 5, 6, 7, 8, 11, 12, 16, 20, 24, 25, 26, 28, 32, 35, 36, 37, 40, 41, 43, 44, 45, 46, 47, 48, 50, 51, 55, 56, 62, 79, 81, 84, 91, 93, 97, 99, 100, 101, 107, 117, 118, 123, 125, 126, 127, 128, 129, 137, 138, 140, 141, 142, 144, 161, 165, 166, 168, 171, 172, 175, 176
agonist, 20
allele, 154, 155, 158
allergens, 7
allergic asthma, 7, 97
allergy, 7, 55, 56, 97, 117, 118, 127, 141, 142
alters, 129
alveolar macrophage, 150, 159, 160
alveoli, 35, 39
anaphylaxis, 131
anencephaly, 42
antisense, 132, 133
antiviral agents, 30, 110
antiviral drugs, ix, 124, 132
antiviral therapy, 30, 158
apnea, 24, 25, 26, 28, 32, 61, 62, 63, 64, 127, 137, 142, 167
arrhythmias, 174
aspirate, 8, 12
aspiration, 39, 40, 43, 70, 126, 134, 169
assessment, 18, 24, 31, 47, 103, 159, 168
asthma, 7, 18, 26, 42, 48, 49, 55, 56, 97, 98, 99, 100, 101, 103, 104, 105, 115, 117, 118, 119, 126, 127, 141, 152, 161
asymptomatic, 38
atelectasis, 31, 62, 84, 166, 167
atopy, 6, 97, 99, 103, 140, 161, 171
attachment, 8, 33, 77, 87, 88, 113, 114, 125, 126, 128, 132, 133, 139, 141, 142, 150
auscultation, 83
authorities, 17
avian, 3, 9, 18
avoidance, viii, 2, 43, 118
awareness, 31

B

bacteremia, 24, 41, 62, 170
barriers, 19
base, 35, 103, 135
base pair, 135
beneficial effect, 104, 106, 137
benefits, 16, 18, 45, 93, 94, 144
benzodiazepine, 30, 132
beta interferon, 112, 113, 139, 161
biliary atresia, 43
bioinformatics, 157
biotin, 117
birth weight, 6, 26, 35, 68, 127, 144, 171
births, 42
blood, 8, 9, 33, 57, 93, 94, 131, 151, 152, 159, 160, 167
blood cultures, 94
blood monocytes, 159
bloodstream, 9
bone, 42, 46, 74, 84, 104
bradycardia, 167
bradypnea, 24
breakdown, 22

breast feeding, viii, 2, 35, 42, 52
breathing, 18, 28, 40, 61, 97
bronchitis, 3, 110, 126
bronchoconstriction, 20
bronchodilator, 19, 20, 22, 104, 136
bronchopneumonia, x, 165, 166
bronchopulmonary dysplasia, viii, 2, 29, 66, 67, 77, 127, 144, 171, 172, 174
bronchospasm, 22

C

cachexia, 169
caffeine, 23, 24, 25, 32, 63
cancer, 41, 42, 175
candidates, 26, 28, 51, 130, 132, 133, 138, 158, 173
capillary, 39
cardiac arrhythmia, 167
cardiovascular system, 25
caregivers, 30
cartilage, 84
causal relationship, 99, 101
central nervous system, 84, 169
cerebrospinal fluid, 167, 174
challenges, 78, 111
chemical, 130
chemokines, 87, 88, 91, 101, 103, 116, 126, 127, 141, 151
chemotaxis, 116
chemotherapy, 41
chest radiography, 8, 21, 22, 26, 28
chicken, 56
childhood, viii, 7, 56, 79, 80, 81, 99, 100, 101, 110, 111, 115, 117, 118, 119, 125, 126, 140, 153, 166
chlamydia, 69
cholesterol, 105
chromosomal abnormalities, 6, 169
cigarette smoking, 42
circulation, 9, 94, 142
circumpolar region, 42
classes, 99
classification, 20
cleavage, 30, 132
cleft lip, 169
climate, 128
climates, 5, 11
clusters, 128
collagen, 84
colonisation, 69
colonization, 38, 39, 70, 169
combination therapy, viii, 2, 22, 24, 27, 31
combined effect, 23, 30
commercial, vii, 2, 10, 16, 17, 18
communities, 42, 47, 48
community, vii, 1, 5, 8, 17, 19, 22, 24, 28, 29, 42, 43, 56, 95, 96, 106, 107, 117, 139, 171
comorbidity, 80
complement, 10, 35, 92, 116
complementary DNA, 135
complex partial seizure, 168
complexity, 39, 156
compliance, 29, 47, 66, 74
complications, 7, 40, 52, 111, 167, 174
compounds, 132, 137
computed tomography, 84
conjunctiva, 128, 129, 138
consciousness, 28
consensus, 29, 105
consolidation, 83, 105, 106, 167, 172
consumption, vii, 1
contamination, 43
control group, 7, 19, 28, 130
control measures, 16, 48, 52, 75
controlled studies, viii, 2, 9, 52, 103
controlled trials, viii, 2, 18, 32, 43, 44, 45, 74
controversial, 88, 103, 104
coronavirus, 3, 4, 9, 15, 57
correlation, 6, 8, 9, 27, 96
correlations, 10
cortex, 105
corticosteroids, 8, 105, 110, 119, 136, 137
cost, 3, 17, 32, 36, 37, 44, 48, 49, 50, 59, 66, 74, 75, 76, 96, 103, 106, 109, 110, 115, 134, 136, 158, 170, 171
cotton, 33, 50, 110, 120, 141, 144, 146
cough, 30, 79, 83, 126, 128, 131, 136, 166, 169
coughing, 40
critical period, 35
croup, 26, 39
crowded households, 42
culture, viii, 2, 4, 10, 11, 13, 14, 15, 16, 30, 57, 58, 59, 88, 93, 94, 95, 96, 106, 117, 133, 144, 170
cyanosis, vii, 1, 83, 167
cyanotic, 32, 33, 34, 51
cycles, 8
cysteine, 112
cystic fibrosis, 21, 38, 44, 48, 69, 70, 74, 77, 169, 175
cytoplasm, 8, 124, 132
cytotoxicity, 105

D

database, 60, 71, 155, 162, 172, 174, 175, 178
deaths, viii, 3, 6, 40, 41, 42, 51, 55, 79, 81, 123, 125, 129, 139, 150, 159, 166, 167

decongestant, 21, 61
defense mechanisms, 169
deficiencies, 41
deficiency, 29, 81, 153
degradation, 132, 153
dehiscence, 43
demographic factors, 168
denaturation, 51
dendritic cell, 9, 91, 115, 116, 150, 152, 159, 162
deposition, 92
depth, 31
derivatives, 132
destruction, 29
detectable, 38, 89
detection, vii, ix, 2, 3, 9, 10, 11, 12, 13, 14, 15, 25, 53, 57, 58, 59, 60, 94, 95, 96, 117, 123, 134, 135, 138, 144, 146, 170
diaphragm, 43
diaphragmatic hernia, 43, 47, 73, 74, 169
diarrhea, 131
dimorphism, 126
directors, 44
discomfort, 136
discrimination, vii, 2, 10
disease progression, 20, 29, 97
diseases, 25, 142, 175
disequilibrium, 170
disorder, 46
displacement, 10
distress, vii, 1, 3, 19, 22, 27, 28, 43, 69, 79, 84, 103, 136, 166
distribution, 17, 110, 128, 140
diuretic, 131
divergence, 142, 159
diversity, 126, 142, 174, 177
donors, 108, 130, 155
drug delivery, 18
drugs, viii, 2, 16, 119, 132, 133, 136, 138
dysphagia, 40
dysplasia, 32, 43
dyspnea, 83

E

economic evaluation, 50, 75
economic status, 6, 42
economics, 76
eczema, 35, 171
edema, vii, ix, 1, 20, 21, 165, 166
editors, 138
education, 6, 43, 171
effusion, 83
egg, 56
elderly population, viii, 123, 125, 129
electroencephalogram, 167
electron, 134
electron microscopy, 134
electrophoresis, 13
elongation, 8
emergency, vii, 1, 4, 5, 18, 19, 21, 22, 23, 24, 26, 27, 47, 53, 61, 166, 172
employment, 4
encephalopathy, 84, 111
encoding, 7, 149, 158
endocrine, 40
endotracheal intubation, 28
enterovirus, 3
environment, viii, 2, 5, 52, 87, 91, 98, 143
eosinophilia, 51, 77, 89, 114, 161, 162
eosinophils, 89, 102
epinephrine, vii, 2, 19, 20, 21, 22, 23, 25, 27, 31, 61, 119, 136
epithelial cells, 9, 38, 70, 87, 92, 93, 101, 113, 120, 151
epithelium, 9, 18, 84, 88, 101, 125, 151
epitopes, ix, 132, 149, 151, 153, 154, 155, 156, 158, 163
equipment, 95
ethnic groups, 170
ethnicity, 6
etiology, 2, 53, 82
evidence, viii, 2, 6, 18, 19, 22, 24, 25, 27, 28, 29, 31, 32, 38, 39, 44, 48, 52, 60, 74, 75, 92, 93, 101, 103, 104, 105, 127, 137, 143
evolution, 10, 141, 150
excitotoxicity, 84
exclusion, 49
excretion, 41
exposure, viii, 33, 38, 43, 52, 79, 101, 126, 127, 168, 169
external validation, 69
extraction, 12, 15, 17

F

failure to thrive, 172
fear, 104
fever, 8, 65, 83, 94, 126, 128, 131, 136, 176
fibroblasts, 84
fibrosis, 44
financial, 7, 45, 94
financial support, 45
fixation, 10
fluid, 21, 38, 60, 103, 161
formation, 8, 33, 35, 125, 132
fragments, 132

funding, 44
fungal infection, 92
fusion, viii, 2, 8, 13, 14, 33, 50, 51, 76, 77, 87, 108, 113, 124, 125, 128, 132, 133, 138, 143, 146, 155, 156, 157, 160, 162, 163

G

gastroenteritis, 131
gastroesophageal reflux, 39, 40, 71
gel, 13, 95, 135
genes, 7, 86, 88, 102, 124, 127, 128, 143
genome, 7, 8, 124, 125, 128, 138, 143, 149, 152, 158
genomic regions, 16
genotype, 142
genus, 7
glycoproteins, 33, 88, 108, 114, 125, 151, 152
grants, 138, 158
growth, 68
guidance, 18, 31
guidelines, 18, 31, 38, 46, 48, 109

H

haplotypes, 153, 170
health, ix, 6, 17, 18, 60, 133, 149, 150, 169
heart block, 167
heart disease, 26, 33, 34, 40, 47, 49, 50, 52, 71, 167, 169, 172, 174, 175
height, 96
helium, 26, 147
hematology, 43
hemisphere, 128
hemolytic anemia, 103
hemorrhage, 42
hepatitis, 65, 167
hepatitis d, 167
heredity, 98
hernia, 43, 47
heterogeneity, viii, 2, 18
high risk patients, 29, 48
histamine, 141
histocompatibility antigens, 162
history, 17, 24, 29, 35, 36, 52, 108, 169, 172
home oxygen therapy, 39
hormones, 105
hospitalization, vii, viii, ix, x, 1, 2, 3, 5, 6, 7, 8, 20, 23, 25, 31, 32, 33, 34, 35, 36, 37, 38, 39, 40, 43, 44, 45, 46, 47, 48, 49, 50, 51, 52, 53, 54, 66, 67, 68, 69, 72, 73, 74, 82, 91, 97, 101, 107, 114, 125, 127, 130, 133, 136, 137, 143, 144, 149, 151, 160, 165, 166, 168, 171, 175, 177
host, 8, 9, 42, 84, 85, 87, 89, 92, 93, 106, 112, 116, 124, 125, 127, 128, 129, 131, 132, 150, 152, 158, 159, 166, 167, 174, 177
human, ix, 3, 9, 17, 22, 25, 32, 33, 41, 53, 57, 59, 60, 62, 68, 71, 79, 101, 112, 113, 116, 117, 118, 120, 124, 126, 130, 134, 138, 139, 141, 142, 144, 146, 149, 150, 151, 153, 155, 156, 157, 159, 160, 161, 162, 163, 169, 170, 175, 176
humidity, 5, 128
humoral immunity, 115
hyaline, 84
hybridization, 13, 15, 59, 60, 95, 146
hydrocephalus, 169
hygiene, 52, 137
hyperinflation, 29, 134, 166, 167
hypersensitivity, 77, 131
hypertonic saline, viii, 2, 19, 20, 21, 22, 31, 60, 61, 137, 147
hypertrophy, 39
hypoplasia, 39, 43, 70, 169
hypotension, 167
hypothesis, 39, 173
hypoxemia, 169
hypoxia, 28, 107, 172

I

ideal, 129
identification, 30, 58, 60, 94, 96, 111, 134, 138, 140, 155, 156, 158, 163, 168
identity, 151
impairments, 26, 40, 44
improvements, 26, 33
in vitro, 18, 38, 50, 66, 90, 103, 113, 131, 133, 139, 144, 145, 146, 159
in vivo, 38, 66, 88, 92, 113, 115, 116, 131, 139, 144, 145, 150, 155
incidence, viii, 3, 5, 6, 22, 24, 28, 29, 31, 32, 35, 38, 39, 41, 43, 47, 50, 53, 62, 79, 81, 115, 120, 123, 125, 127, 129, 131, 151, 170, 176, 177
incubation period, 126, 128
index case, 48
induction, 41, 77, 88, 91, 92, 106, 112, 113, 153, 159
industrialized countries, 80
inferences, 106
inferiority, 51
inhibition, 10, 50, 90, 103, 106, 131, 132, 139, 150
inhibitor, 119, 132, 145
initiation, 25, 124
injections, 33, 47, 152
injury, 84, 103, 167, 174
innate immunity, 88
inoculation, 7, 10, 66, 120, 128, 129, 133, 138, 140

insertion, 89
institutions, vii, 1, 18, 26, 40
intensive care unit, 6, 22, 43, 48, 60, 63, 64, 65, 73, 75, 143, 168, 176, 177, 178
interference, 17, 90, 130, 132, 133, 146
interferon, 7, 53, 112, 113, 115, 118, 125, 139, 150, 161
intervention, vii, 2, 18, 23, 25, 28, 30, 32, 121, 132
intramuscular injection, 130
intravenous fluids, 103, 137
isolation, 9, 10, 11, 32, 43, 48, 66, 95, 134, 138, 143, 156
isotope, 157, 163
issues, 19, 44, 168, 172

K

kidney, 138
kinetics, 114, 121, 155

L

laboratory studies, 33
laboratory tests, 135, 170
laminar, 26
laryngitis, 3
lasers, 15
later life, 99, 101, 126
lead, ix, x, 3, 20, 21, 24, 30, 37, 38, 43, 86, 93, 100, 110, 118, 124, 136, 165, 171
lesions, 6, 33
lethargy, 136, 167, 172
leucocyte, 8, 163
leukemia, 41
leukocytes, 151
leukotrienes, vii, 2, 105, 121, 140, 141
life cycle, 132
lifetime, 48
ligand, 85, 86, 87, 155, 156, 157, 158, 163
light, 29
liquid chromatography, 156
liver, 41, 72
liver transplant, 41, 72
liver transplantation, 41, 72
locus, 170
longitudinal study, 5, 54, 141
low risk, 37, 44
low temperatures, 5
lower respiratory tract infection, vii, ix, 1, 3, 4, 5, 6, 39, 54, 56, 62, 65, 68, 69, 71, 72, 79, 114, 160, 165, 166, 174, 175, 177, 178
lumen, 84, 153

M

macrophages, 9, 29, 35, 88, 102, 113, 115, 150, 160
magnetic particles, 12
magnetic resonance, 39
magnitude, x, 101, 165
major histocompatibility complex, ix, 114, 115, 149, 153, 162, 163
majority, 5, 11, 26, 28, 38, 40, 42, 46, 48, 80, 130, 136, 137, 151
malaria, 158
malignancy, 72, 169
malnutrition, 6, 169
management, viii, ix, x, 1, 2, 10, 18, 24, 29, 31, 52, 60, 61, 62, 64, 96, 97, 117, 119, 120, 123, 124, 137, 140, 165, 170
marital status, 6
marketing, 44
marrow, 46
maternal smoking, 171
matrix, 8, 89, 125, 149, 155, 157, 163
measles, 131
measurement, 28
measurements, 27
median, 8, 9, 12, 26, 40, 41, 43, 44, 48, 172, 173
medical, vii, viii, 1, 2, 5, 6, 26, 34, 40, 42, 44, 46, 47, 52, 82, 131, 136, 169
medicine, 26, 146, 173
melanoma, 85
membranes, 84, 128
memory, 71, 77, 89, 93, 114, 129, 153, 154, 155, 161, 162
messenger RNA, 30
meta-analysis, 27, 29, 55, 61, 65, 105, 111, 119, 137, 147, 159, 173
metabolic disorder, 42
metabolism, 103
mice, 38, 56, 57, 70, 76, 77, 88, 89, 110, 113, 114, 115, 118, 127, 132, 133, 144, 146, 150, 151, 152, 153, 154, 155, 156, 157, 160, 161, 162, 163
microspheres, 15
migration, 92, 106
modelling, 75
models, ix, x, 7, 36, 37, 38, 48, 93, 101, 149, 151, 153, 165, 170, 177, 178
molecules, ix, 22, 30, 65, 103, 133, 149, 153, 155, 157, 158, 162, 163
monoclonal antibody, 9, 25, 33, 57, 63, 66, 67, 109, 110, 130, 131, 133, 138, 144, 145, 160
monolayer, 10, 134
montelukast, 25, 121

morbidity, vii, viii, 1, 6, 7, 31, 35, 43, 46, 56, 70, 71, 72, 74, 96, 100, 104, 110, 119, 123, 125, 129, 137, 168, 169, 174, 175
mortality, vii, viii, 1, 6, 25, 30, 31, 34, 41, 43, 46, 48, 55, 67, 72, 74, 80, 81, 84, 96, 104, 106, 107, 108, 110, 123, 125, 129, 137, 139, 140, 150, 159, 166, 168, 169, 170
mosaic, 84
motif, 154, 155, 156, 162
mucolysis, 22
mucosa, 21, 22, 32, 129, 133, 138, 166
mucus, vii, 1, 87, 91, 92, 116, 128, 166
multiplication, 131, 133
multivariate analysis, 40
mumps, 131
muscles, 64, 166
mutagenesis, 130
mutant, 51
mutations, 158

N

nanoparticles, 13, 16
nasopharynx, 125
necrosis, 84, 87, 126, 166
neonates, 9, 43, 57, 63, 74, 92, 108
nerve, 40
nervous system, 70
nested PCR, 13
neurological disease, 40
neutropenia, 42
neutrophils, 35, 38, 88, 150
next generation, 30
nitric oxide, 38
normal children, 39, 96
nucleic acid, vii, 2, 3, 4, 10, 15, 17, 53, 93, 95, 96, 133, 134, 135
nucleoprotein, 155, 163
nucleotides, 124
nursing, 32, 43, 134
nursing home, 134
nutrition, 137
nutritional status, 103

O

obesity, 169, 175
obstacles, 51
obstruction, 9, 20, 22, 26, 28, 29, 56, 84, 87, 104, 105, 115, 136, 166, 169
occlusion, 116, 126
old age, 127
oligomers, 132, 133, 146
opportunities, 78
organ, 41, 46, 74, 84, 169
oscillation, 106
otitis media, 3, 126, 129, 131, 141
outpatient, viii, 2, 5, 22, 34, 50, 81, 82, 110, 131, 136
oxygen, 8, 20, 22, 26, 27, 31, 32, 33, 34, 39, 51, 62, 64, 82, 84, 103, 106, 119, 136, 137, 147, 167, 168, 172

P

paediatric patients, 58, 65
palate, 169
palivizumab, viii, ix, 2, 25, 26, 29, 33, 34, 37, 39, 44, 45, 46, 47, 48, 49, 50, 51, 52, 63, 67, 69, 71, 73, 74, 75, 76, 106, 107, 109, 110, 120, 121, 123, 130, 131, 133, 138, 140, 144
paradigm shift, 31
parallel, 17
parenchyma, 18, 126
pathogenesis, 17, 38, 51, 65, 77, 84, 99, 104, 105, 110, 113, 115, 125, 140, 152, 161
pathogens, 3, 33, 53, 56, 57, 59, 97, 152, 158, 169, 176
pathology, 8, 33, 88, 89, 91, 92, 113, 120, 152
pathophysiology, 18, 20, 22, 28, 29, 131, 167
patient care, ix, 19, 123
pattern recognition, 85
pediatrician, 26
peptide, ix, 132, 149, 153, 154, 155, 156, 157, 161, 162, 163, 164
percentile, 35
perfusion, 21, 84
pericardial effusion, 167
perinatal, 84
peripheral blood, 57, 120, 152, 155, 161
peripheral blood mononuclear cell, 120, 152, 155, 161
permeability, 101
persistent asthma, 99, 118
pertussis, 170
phagocytosis, 106, 113
pharmacokinetics, 33, 67, 144, 145, 146
pharyngitis, 3, 83
phenotype, 89, 91, 152
phenotypes, 97, 170
phosphorylation, 87
physicians, 3, 10
physics, 26
physiology, viii, 2, 18, 20, 29, 31, 85
pigs, 127, 143
pilot study, 174

pipeline, viii, ix, 2, 123
placebo, 7, 25, 32, 33, 46, 50, 65, 66, 103, 104, 106, 119, 120, 132, 137, 145
placenta, 143
plaque, 14, 84
plasma membrane, 124
plasticity, 156
platform, 97
playing, 127
pneumococcus, 83
pneumonia, vii, viii, ix, 1, 3, 5, 9, 28, 39, 40, 41, 42, 43, 48, 56, 57, 67, 70, 79, 81, 83, 84, 106, 112, 115, 118, 125, 126, 128, 129, 137, 140, 142, 149, 150, 159, 174
pneumonitis, 18
polar, 124
polarization, 152
policy, 17, 43
pollutants, 42
polymerase, 8, 13, 14, 57, 58, 59, 75, 124, 125, 131, 132, 134, 135, 146, 149
polymerase chain reaction, 8, 57, 58, 59, 75, 134, 146
polymorphism, x, 166
polymorphisms, vii, 2, 10, 127, 170
polyp, 84
pools, ix, 149, 156
population, 5, 9, 23, 24, 25, 30, 31, 34, 42, 46, 47, 51, 58, 68, 76, 82, 83, 100, 106, 108, 125, 133, 153, 163
potential benefits, 95
prediction models, 170
predictive accuracy, 171
predictor variables, 171
pregnancy, 6, 36, 38, 171
premature infant, viii, 2, 6, 25, 33, 34, 35, 46, 47, 48, 51, 52, 66, 67, 68, 69, 71, 73, 75, 100, 109, 126, 127, 144, 169, 174, 175, 177
prematurity, 6, 24, 26, 35, 40, 41, 42, 67, 81, 82, 106, 169
preoperative screening, 175
preparation, iv, 30, 107
preschool, 35, 97
preschool children, 97
preterm infants, 24, 34, 35, 50, 63, 64, 68, 69, 75, 100, 110, 115, 118, 144
prevention, vii, viii, ix, 2, 4, 31, 32, 33, 46, 55, 63, 67, 69, 73, 74, 75, 77, 81, 99, 105, 107, 108, 109, 117, 119, 124, 126, 131, 133, 145, 146, 175
priming, 89
principles, 48
probability, 10, 24, 37, 43, 128, 167, 171
probe, 10
producers, 116
professionals, 44, 45, 103
prognosis, 9
pro-inflammatory, 105
proliferation, 84
promoter, 86, 124, 143
prophylactic, 48, 91
prophylaxis, viii, ix, 2, 7, 25, 26, 29, 31, 34, 36, 37, 41, 42, 44, 45, 46, 47, 48, 50, 52, 56, 63, 65, 66, 67, 69, 72, 73, 74, 75, 76, 106, 107, 110, 121, 123, 129, 138, 140, 142, 166, 168, 171, 173, 175
prostaglandins, 105
protection, ix, 33, 51, 52, 88, 92, 107, 120, 130, 142, 149, 150, 151, 152, 153, 160
protein blocks, 112
protein sequence, 154
protein structure, 155
protein synthesis, 10
proteins, 7, 10, 12, 29, 30, 33, 88, 89, 92, 112, 113, 114, 124, 125, 128, 132, 133, 138, 139, 142, 149, 151, 152, 153, 155, 156, 158, 159, 160, 161, 162
proteome, 158
prototype, 135
public health, 17
pulmonary diseases, 172
pulmonary hypertension, 39

Q

quality assurance, 17
quality control, 17
quantification, 97
questionnaire, 8

R

race, 6, 144
radiation, 5
radiography, 22
rales, 83
randomized controlled clinical trials, 44, 52
rash, 131
reactions, 25, 51
reactive airway disease, 25, 63, 119, 137
reactivity, 38, 76, 100, 143
reading, 7, 16, 124, 149
reagents, 13, 15, 96, 134
real time, 8, 15, 16
receptors, 85, 92, 93, 104, 113
recognition, 12, 33, 43, 85, 88, 93, 112, 113, 153, 162
recombinant DNA, 33, 109, 131, 158

recommendations, iv, 43, 67, 105, 140
recovery, 142
recurrence, 43
reflexes, 28
regions of the world, 5
Registry, 45, 47, 73
regression, 36, 169
regression model, 36
regulations, 22
rehydration, 21
relatives, 35
relaxation, 20
reliability, 96
repair, 43, 47
replication, viii, 2, 8, 9, 33, 50, 88, 105, 124, 125, 131, 132, 133, 139, 145, 150, 152
repressor, 86, 112
reproduction, 103
requirements, 84, 94, 137, 138
residues, 153, 154, 155, 157
resistance, vii, 2, 10, 21, 63, 106, 126, 154, 160, 162, 167
resolution, ix, 20, 149, 158
resource utilization, 7, 34, 168
resources, vii, x, 1, 17, 31, 165
restriction fragment length polymorphis, 13
restrictions, 109
reticulum, 153, 162
reverse transcriptase, 59, 135
rhinitis, 3, 129, 131
rhinorrhea, 83, 126, 128
rhonchi, 83
robotics, 17
rodents, 92
root, 35
routes, 23, 66, 140
rubber, 128
rubella, 131

S

safety, viii, 2, 25, 33, 46, 50, 51, 52, 61, 74, 77, 110, 132, 146
saliva, 32
saturation, 20, 84, 172
savings, 17
school, 35, 36, 38, 99, 100, 101, 171
scope, 26, 29
scripts, 60
seasonality, 17, 54, 142
secretion, 28, 102, 114, 134, 143, 151, 152
senescence, 71
sensitivity, 3, 10, 11, 12, 13, 14, 15, 16, 17, 25, 46, 48, 58, 94, 95, 96, 134, 135, 156, 171, 172
sensitization, 7, 89, 99, 100, 118, 119
sensors, 112
sepsis, 167, 176
sequencing, 13, 14, 163
serology, 4, 10, 93, 134, 135
serum, 9, 33, 57, 90, 91, 92, 107, 108, 114, 126, 127, 130, 150, 151, 160
severe acute respiratory syndrome, 3, 57
severe asthma, 101
sex, 6, 97, 144
shortage, 109
shortness of breath, 166
showing, 8, 85, 87, 91, 134
sibling, 35, 38, 39, 42
siblings, 6, 35, 36, 38, 50, 127, 168, 171
side effects, 106
signal transduction, 88
signaling pathway, 86, 87
signals, 93, 101, 124
signs, ix, 39, 83, 84, 106, 123, 126, 128, 131, 134
simulation, 75
single test, vii, 2, 10, 17, 18
skeleton, 39
skin, 32, 50, 128
smoke exposure, 6, 35
smoking, viii, 2, 6, 36, 38, 127
smooth muscle, 20, 104
societal cost, 18
software, 155, 157
solution, 61, 147
specialists, 46
species, 103, 157
speculation, 97
spina bifida, 42, 169
spleen, 150, 154
sputum, 17
stability, 128
stabilization, 28
standardization, 96
state, 43, 151
states, 169
status epilepticus, 168
steroids, vii, 2, 23, 41
stimulation, 21, 77, 90, 152
stoves, 42
strabismus, 167
stratification, 20
stridor, 26
structural protein, 150
structure, 19, 39, 68, 85, 127, 138, 160

subgroups, 33, 45, 46, 54, 81, 126, 132, 133, 142, 150, 151, 159
subjectivity, 172
submucosa, 21
supervision, 131
supplementation, 119, 137, 172
suppression, 107, 152
supraventricular tachycardia, 167
surface area, 35, 39
surfactant, 26, 29, 65, 88, 106, 113, 137
surveillance, 5, 40, 43, 54, 66, 140, 176
survival, 35, 46, 87, 128
survivors, 43, 73, 74
susceptibility, 35, 127, 153, 161
swelling, 105
symptoms, ix, 7, 12, 38, 83, 84, 105, 118, 123, 126, 127, 128, 134, 136, 165, 176
syndrome, 39, 64, 70, 167
synergistic effect, 22, 25
synthesis, 29, 124, 132, 133, 138, 140, 150

T

tachycardia, 25, 167
tachypnea, 83, 136
target, viii, 2, 16, 36, 50, 86, 87, 88, 102, 105, 108, 114, 124, 131, 132, 135, 137, 138, 162
teams, 22
technician, 96
techniques, vii, 1, 59, 60, 94, 96, 117, 134, 135, 146, 170
technologies, 158
technology, vii, 2, 33, 46, 60, 74, 95, 109, 131, 132, 156, 158
temperature, 51, 128, 144, 167
test data, 54
testing, 4, 9, 10, 11, 12, 13, 14, 16, 17, 58, 93, 130, 173
therapy, ix, 9, 18, 19, 20, 22, 23, 25, 26, 27, 29, 30, 31, 34, 41, 51, 64, 65, 66, 103, 104, 105, 106, 107, 119, 120, 123, 131, 137, 138, 147
threshold level, 114
time frame, 4
tissue, viii, 2, 35, 38, 39, 58, 84, 93, 94, 95, 133, 161, 166, 167
tobacco, 52, 127
tobacco smoke, 52
toddlers, 79
tonic, 168
toxicity, 133
tracheoesophageal fistula, 43, 169
transaminases, 167
transcription, 8, 10, 59, 60, 87, 88, 117, 124, 133, 146, 149
transcription factors, 87
transcripts, 146
transformation, 171
transmembrane glycoprotein, 128, 150
transmission, ix, 6, 32, 33, 50, 66, 73, 109, 124, 126, 128, 142, 143
transplant, 41, 46, 48, 74
transplantation, 9, 41, 57, 72, 75, 84
transport, 19, 96
transportation, 135
treatment, vii, ix, 2, 4, 7, 8, 9, 10, 18, 19, 20, 21, 22, 23, 25, 27, 30, 31, 33, 45, 46, 51, 52, 57, 60, 61, 62, 63, 64, 65, 91, 95, 97, 99, 103, 104, 107, 109, 110, 117, 119, 120, 123, 124, 130, 131, 132, 133, 136, 137, 138, 145, 146, 151, 168, 172
tremor, 25
trial, viii, 2, 7, 15, 18, 19, 20, 21, 24, 27, 28, 32, 33, 39, 44, 45, 46, 50, 61, 62, 63, 64, 65, 76, 77, 104, 106, 119, 120, 121, 137, 145
triggers, 88
tumor, 41, 143, 159, 160
turbinates, 50

U

umbilical cord, 152
underlying mechanisms, 92
upper airways, 21, 151
upper respiratory infection, 96
upper respiratory tract, vii, 1, 5, 9, 50, 79, 83, 96, 126, 141, 166
urban, 42, 49, 50
urinary tract, 24, 170
urinary tract infection, 24, 170

V

vaccine, viii, ix, 2, 51, 65, 76, 77, 78, 89, 91, 107, 108, 110, 120, 123, 126, 129, 130, 133, 138, 139, 143, 144, 149, 158, 162, 163, 164
valence, 12, 121
validation, 17, 68, 69, 168, 170, 172, 177
variables, vii, x, 35, 37, 100, 165, 172
variations, 170
vasculature, 21
vasoconstriction, 21
vector, 158
ventilation, 7, 19, 21, 24, 26, 27, 28, 29, 32, 38, 62, 64, 65, 68, 106, 120, 137, 167, 169, 172
ventricular tachycardia, 167

viral gene, 88, 124
viral infection, 17, 18, 38, 41, 55, 57, 60, 69, 71, 75, 84, 92, 93, 94, 96, 99, 111, 112, 115, 117, 118, 126, 134, 135, 139, 141, 145, 150, 163, 169, 175
viral pathogens, ix, 29, 30, 74, 79, 88, 90, 123
virology, 9, 58, 139
virus infection, 3, 4, 8, 10, 17, 18, 53, 54, 60, 67, 69, 76, 85, 89, 91, 94, 117, 135, 141, 143, 146, 154, 159, 160, 162, 174, 176
virus replication, 9, 113, 139
viruses, vii, viii, 2, 3, 4, 8, 9, 10, 11, 13, 14, 15, 16, 17, 32, 42, 53, 55, 56, 57, 59, 60, 66, 72, 79, 80, 88, 94, 95, 96, 111, 112, 117, 126, 130, 137, 140, 146, 152, 158, 159, 170
viscosity, 22, 33
vomiting, 30, 131

W

war, 43, 107
water, 21, 32
weakness, 40, 169
wealth, 17
web, 155
weight gain, 35
wheeze, 7, 20, 55, 56, 83, 97, 98, 99, 100, 117, 142, 166
wheezing, viii, 7, 8, 35, 36, 56, 57, 62, 79, 80, 83, 97, 99, 100, 101, 104, 105, 110, 111, 117, 118, 119, 126, 127, 128, 131, 136, 140, 141, 142, 171
wild type, 153
wood, 42
workers, 169
worldwide, vii, viii, 1, 38, 80, 84, 110, 123, 125, 129, 150

X

x-rays, 83

Y

yield, 68
young adults, 140
young people, 96